Meningococcal Vaccines

METHODS IN MOLECULAR MEDICINE™

John M. Walker, Series Editor

Meningococcal Vaccines

Methods and Protocols

Edited by

Andrew J. Pollard, MD, PhD

BC Research Institute for Children's and Women's Health, Vancouver, BC, Canada

and

Martin C. J. Maiden, PhD

Wellcome Trust Centre for the Epidemiology of Infectious Disease, Oxford, UK

Foreword by

E. Richard Moxon, MB, BChir

Department of Pediatrics, Oxford University, Oxford, UK

Humana Press ✳ Totowa, New Jersey

Cover design by Patricia F. Cleary.

Production Editor: Mark J. Breaugh.

For additional copies, pricing for bulk purchases, and/or information about other Humana titles, contact Humana at the above address or at any of the following numbers: Tel.: 973-256-1699; Fax: 973-256-8341; E-mail: humana@humanapr.com; Website: http://humanapress.com

Printed in the United States of America. 10 9 8 7 6 5 4 3 2 1

Library of Congress Cataloging in Publication Data

Main entry under title: Methods in molecular medicine™.

Meningococcal vaccines: methods and protocols / edited by Andrew J. Pollard and
Martin C.J. Maiden.
        p. ; cm. -- (Methods in molecular medicine ; 66)
    Companion volume to: Meningococcal disease.
    Includes bibliographical references and index.
    ISBN 0-89603-801-7 (alk. paper)
    1. Bacterial vaccines--Laboratory manuals. 2. Neisseria meningitidis--Laboratory
manuals. 3. Meningitis--Laboratory manuals. I. Pollard, Andrew J. II. Maiden, Martin C.
J. III. Meningococcal disease. IV. Series.
    [DNLM: 1. Meningitis, Meningococcal--drug therapy. 2. Meningococcal
Vaccines--therapeutic use. WC 245 M5457 2001]
    QR189.5.B33 M46 2001
    616.8'2--dc21

Foreword

Since the first recognition of outbreaks of cerebrospinal or spotted fever at the end of the nineteenth and the beginning of the twentieth centuries, the menace of the meningococcus has been high on the list of public health priorities. Few if any pathogens surpass the meningococcus in the rapidity and severity with which it devastates previously healthy individuals. The challenge of understanding the biology of this fascinating microbe is immense, but few will doubt that successful control of meningococcal meningitis and septicemia will only transpire through the application of a body of extraordinary detailed information, including key minutiae of its molecular biology.

In the first of two companion volumes, *Meningococcal Vaccines*, the team of experts gathered by Andy Pollard and Martin Maiden converge to provide an impressive accumulation of molecular tools with which to lay bare the secrets of the meningococcus. The results of this ambitious and welcome volume represent an exciting and much needed resource for all of us in the field. Time and again, on reading through the carefully prepared texts, I found the contents not only enlightening and relevant to my own research program, but also a source of new ideas and approaches—with the wherewithal to move forward all there in front of me!

Despite the pernicious behavior of the meningococcus in causing devastating disease, the new developments and tools afforded by molecular microbiology and epidemiology can surely be used to turn the tide on this pathogen. No scholar or investigator of *Neisseria meningitidis* will want to be without the riches contained within this work whose pages, I predict, will rapidly show evidence of repeated use in the many laboratories and offices of those who pursue the challenges of the meningococcus.

E. Richard Moxon, MB, BChir

Preface

Meningococcal disease, which occurs chiefly as either septicemia or meningitis, represents a major health problem worldwide. In Europe, the Americas, and Australasia these syndromes, which can occur by themselves or in combination, are principally diseases of early childhood and adolescence, whereas in Africa and Asia, especially China, large-scale epidemic or pandemic outbreaks can involve the whole community. In many industrialized countries there are few childhood diseases that parents fear more than "meningitis," the term commonly used to refer to meningococcal disease.

There are a number of good reasons for this fear. Meningococcal disease is sporadic, unpredictable, and difficult to diagnose. The disease progresses in a matter of hours from apparently trivial symptoms to a life-threatening medical emergency. Even in the presence of treatment, a positive outcome is uncertain and, frequently, victims are left with severe disabling sequelae ranging from brain damage to limb loss. Finally, the apparently most rational approach to controlling meningococcal disease, childhood vaccination, is hindered by the lack of a suitable comprehensive vaccine, a fact that can leave public health officials feeling helpless in the face of meningococcal disease outbreaks.

Many of these factors are a consequence of the natural history of *Neisseria meningitidis*, the causative agent in meningococcal disease. Perhaps the most important consideration in this regard is paradoxical for one of the most feared pathogens: the meningococcus is a normally harmless member of the commensal flora of adult humans. Asymptomatic colonization of the nasopharynx is very common, averaging at about 10% of the population in many countries, peaking at higher levels, 30–40%, in some age groups. Probably as a consequence of this ubiquity, meningococcal populations contain bewildering antigenic and genetic diversity. There are thousands of distinct meningococcal variants described to date and each of these has a sophisticated mechanism for varying its surface coat in response to immune attack. In summary, this bacterium is very well adapted indeed to living with the human immune system. This adaptation is the principal reason for the difficulties in vaccine development.

Safe, effective vaccines against meningococcal disease have been available since the late 1960s. These target the polysaccharide coat of the meningococcus, which is essential for the organism's survival in the bloodstream. From the dozen or so such coats available to the meningococcus, only five, those which define serogroups A, B, C, Y, and W-135, are associated with disease. Unfortu-

nately, vaccines that include unmodified polysaccharides are poorly immunogenic, eliciting only a temporary immune response in adults and none at all in
infants. Serogroup B polysaccharide is problematic because its especially poor
immunogenicity may result from immunological identity to human polysaccharides, raising concern about the safety of any vaccine based on this molecule. In
addition to these polysaccharides, many research and development programs
have targeted the protein components of the meningococcal coat but, as yet,
despite some promising reports, none of these has resulted in a wholly satisfactory vaccine.

However, at the beginning of the 21st century, nearly 120 years after the
first isolation of the meningococcus and its association with human disease in
1887, there is optimism that solutions to meningococcal disease may be on the
horizon, even if comprehensive solutions remain elusive in the short or even
medium term. Polysaccharide–protein conjugate vaccines, which will provide
infants with life time immunity against meningococci that express the serogroup
A, C, Y, and W-135 antigens, are likely to be available soon. The completion of
the whole genome sequences of two meningococci and the start of the postgenomic age will provide a host of novel data and approaches to research on the
development of new meningococcal vaccines. Molecular methods, combined
with phylogenetic and theoretical approaches, promise accurate molecular and
epidemiological descriptions of those meningococci responsible for disease,
adding further knowledge to the arsenal that can be brought to bear on this difficult problem.

Meningococcal Vaccines is designed to provide a comprehensive discussion of current molecular and cellular methods relevant to meningococcal
vaccine development and evaluation. The first two chapters provide the context
for the book, by reviewing vaccination strategies and describing the mechanisms
of immunity that are relevant to natural and vaccine-induced protection against
disease. The succeeding chapters deal in detail with the many approaches available for vaccine design and the assessment of immune responses to vaccine candidates and novel vaccine formulations. The book concludes with a discussion
of the implementation of a new meningococcal vaccine, based on recent experience in the United Kingdom. A companion text, *Meningococcal Disease,* is available from Humana Press; this includes overview chapters and detailed methods
in the areas of diagnostic microbiology, bacterial characterization, epidemiology, host–pathogen interactions, and clinical studies.

Finally, some words of thanks to the many people who have made this
book possible: the series editor, John Walker, and the staff of Humana Press for
commissioning this book and seeing it through to press; the chapter authors for

their hard and always enthusiastic work in response to (frequently unreasonable) goading by the editors; our immediate colleagues who, over the years, have generously shared their knowledge, ideas, and expertise with us; and last, but by no means least, the legion of physicians and scientists who have labored in the fight against meningococcal disease since its first definitive description in 1805.

Andrew J. Pollard, md, phd
Martin C. J. Maiden, phd

Contents

Contributors

AUDUN AASE • *Department of Vaccinology, National Institute of Public Health, Oslo, Norway*

LOEK VAN ALPHEN • *Laboratory of Vaccine Research, National Institute of Public Health and the Environment, Bilthoven, The Netherlands*

CARMEN ARIGITA • *Department of Pharmaceutics, Utrecht Institute of Pharmaceutical Sciences, Utrecht, The Netherlands*

RAY BORROW • *Manchester Public Health Laboratory, Withington Hospital, Manchester, UK*

PAUL J. BRETT • *Division of Bacteriology, National Institute for Biological Standards and Control, Hertfordshire, UK*

GEORGE M. CARLONE • *Respiratory Diseases Immunology Section, National Center for Infectious Diseases, Atlanta, GA*

BAMBOS M. CHARALAMBOUS • *Department of Medical Microbiology, Royal Free & University College Medical School, London, UK*

MYRON CHRISTODOULIDES • *Molecular Microbiology and Infection Group, School of Medicine, University of Southampton, Southampton, UK*

RICHARD F. COLLINS • *Department of Biomolecular Sciences, University of Manchester Institute of Science and Technology, Manchester, UK*

ALEXEI A. DELVIG • *Department of Microbiology and Immunology, Newcastle University, Newcastle, UK*

JEREMY P. DERRICK • *Department of Biomolecular Sciences, University of Manchester Institute of Science and Technology, Manchester, UK*

LEANNE M. DEWINTER • *Department of Microbiology & Infectious Diseases, University of Calgary, Calgary, AB, Canada*

JOHN J. DONNELLY • *Vaccines Research and Development, Chiron Corporation, Emeryville, CA*

PADDY FARRINGTON • *Department of Statistics, The Open University, Milton Keynes, UK*

IAN M. FEAVERS • *Division of Bacteriology, National Institute of Biological Standards & Control, Hertfordshire, UK*

CARL E. FRASCH • *Division of Bacterial Products, Center for Biologics Evaluation and Research, Rockville, MD*

DAVID GOLDBLATT • *Immunobiology Unit, Institute of Child Health, London, UK*

ANDREW R. GORRINGE • *Center for Applied Microbiology and Research, Salisbury, UK*

MATHIJS R. GRAAF • *Department of Pharmaceutics, Utrecht Institute of Pharmaceutical Sciences, Utrecht, The Netherlands*

DAN M. GRANOFF • *Children's Hospital Oakland Research Institute, Oakland, CA*

ZHONGWU GUO • *Institute for Biological Science, National Research Council of Canada, Ottawa, ON, Canada*

BJØRN HANEBERG • *Department of Vaccinology, National Institute of Public Health, Oslo, Norway*

JOHN E. HECKELS • *Molecular Microbiology and Infection Group, School of Medicine, University of Southampton, Southampton, UK*

JOHAN HOLST • *Department of Vaccinology, National Institute of Public Health, Oslo, Norway*

CATHERINE A. ISON • *Department of Infectious Diseases & Microbiology, Imperial College School of Medicine, London, UK*

HAROLD JENNINGS • *Institute for Biological Science, National Research Council of Canada, Ottawa, ON, Canada*

WIM JISKOOT • *Department of Pharmaceutics, Utrecht Institute of Pharmaceutical Sciences, Utrecht, The Netherlands*

KEITH A. JOLLEY • *Department of Zoology, University of Oxford, Oxford, UK*

HELENA KÄYHTY • *Department of Vaccines, National Public Health Institute, Helsinki, Finland*

GIDEON F. A. KERSTEN • *Department of Product and Process Development, National Institute of Public Health and the Environment, Bilthoven, The Netherlands*

PETER VAN DER LEY • *Laboratory of Vaccine Research, National Institute of Public Health and the Environment, Bilthoven, The Netherlands*

MARTIN C.J. MAIDEN • *Department of Zoology, University of Oxford, Oxford, UK*

TERJE E. MICHAELSEN • *Department of Vaccinology, National Institute of Public Health, Oslo, Norway*

ELIZABETH MILLER • *Immunization Division, PHLS Communicable Disease Surveillance Center, London, UK*

LISBETH MEYER NÆSS • *Department of Vaccinology, National Institute of Public Health, Oslo, Norway*

E. RICHARD MOXON • *Molecular Infectious Diseases Group, Oxford University Department of Pediatrics, Oxford, UK*

FREDRIK OFTUNG • *Department of Vaccinology, National Institute of Public Health, Oslo, Norway*

ANDREW J. POLLARD • *BC Research Institute for Children's & Women's Health, Vancouver, BC, Canada*

JAN T. POOLMAN • *Bacterial Vaccine R&D Program, SmithKline Beecham Biologicals, Rixensart, Belgium*

KAREN M. REDDIN • *Center for Applied Microbiology and Research, Salisbury, UK*

JOHN H. ROBINSON • *Department of Microbiology and Immunology, Newcastle University, Newcastle, UK*

EINAR ROSENQVIST • *Department of Vaccinology, National Institute of Public Health, Oslo, Norway*

DAVID M. SALISBURY • *Department of Health, London, UK*

ANTHONY B. SCHRYVERS • *Department of Microbiology & Infectious Diseases, University of Calgary, Calgary, AB, Canada*

LIANA STEEGHS • *Laboratory of Vaccine Research, National Institute of Public Health and the Environment, Bilthoven, The Netherlands*

JANET SUKER • *Division of Bacteriology, National Institute for Biological Standards & Control, Hertfordshire, UK*

PIERRE VOET • *Bacterial Immunology, SmithKline Beecham Biologicals, Rixensart, Belgium*

ELISABETH WEDEGE • *Department of Vaccinology, National Institute of Public Health, Oslo, Norway*

LEE WETZLER • *Evans Biomedical Research Center, Boston University School of Medicine, Boston, MA*

QINGLING YANG • *Institute for Biological Science, National Research Council of Canada, Ottawa, ON, Canada*

1

Meningococcal Vaccines and Vaccine Developments

Ian M. Feavers

1. Introduction

Despite rapid advances in the diagnosis of bacterial infections and the availability of effective antibiotics, meningococcal disease continues to represent a substantial public health problem for most countries (1–4). Disease usually develops rapidly, is notoriously difficult to distinguish from other febrile illnesses, and generally has a high case-fatality rate. The death of an otherwise fit and healthy individual can occur within a very short time from the first appearance of symptoms, those who survive frequently suffer from permanent tissue damage and neurological problems (4,5). Consequently, the development and implementation of effective immunoprophylaxis is a *sine qua non* for the comprehensive control of meningococcal disease. From an historical perspective, many meningococcal vaccines have been developed and evaluated in clinical trials; unfortunately, no vaccine so far offers comprehensive protection. This overview traces the development of the existing licensed vaccines and examines the prospects of vaccine candidates that are currently under development or subject to clinical evaluation.

The challenges faced by the vaccine developer in designing meningococcal vaccines that are safe, comprehensive, and efficacious in the age groups most at risk of disease are a consequence of the complex biology of *Neisseria meningitidis*. It is a Gram-negative, encapsulated organism that is naturally competent for transformation with DNA. It only thrives in the human host and is not known to colonize any other animal or environmental niches. Meningococcal carriage is very much more common than disease (6) and, notwithstanding the devastating impact of meningococcal disease, it may be more

From: *Methods in Molecular Medicine, vol. 66: Meningococcal Vaccines: Methods and Protocols*
Edited by: A. J. Pollard and M. C. J. Maiden © Humana Press Inc., Totowa, NJ

appropriate to consider this bacterium as a commensal that rarely causes disease rather than as a strict pathogen. The meningococcus is, therefore, specifically adapted to the colonization of humans and has evolved a battery of mechanisms that enable it to evade the human immune response.

Meningococcal meningitis and septicaemia are ostensibly childhood diseases, with highest attack rates in infants *(7)*. Carbohydrate antigens, such as capsular polysaccharide or lipopolysaccharide (LPS), are poorly immunogenic in the very young and frequently mimic host cell structures *(8–10)* posing a dilemma for the vaccine developer: can immunity to a carbohydrate be enhanced in infants and, if so, would such a vaccine elicit an autoimmune response? Protein vaccine candidates present a different problem; they are generally better immunogens than carbohydrates, but the more immunogenic meningococcal surface-protein antigens suffer from the disadvantage that they are also antigenically highly variable *(11,12)*. In this case, the vaccine developer is faced with producing a vaccine that offers adequate cross-protection against the majority of virulent meningococci circulating in the population.

Besides hiding behind a camouflage of poorly immunogenic and highly variable cell-surface structures, meningococci utilize a variety of genetical mechanisms to facilitate their persistent colonization of humans. These simultaneously provide them with the potential to circumvent anything less than comprehensive immune protection. The mosaic structure of the genes and operons that encode major cell surface structures provides evidence of the importance of horizontal genetical exchange, mediated by transformation and recombination, in the generation of meningococcal antigenic diversity *(13,14; see* also Chapter 24). It has profound implications for both the development and evaluation of vaccine candidates, as well as for the implementation of vaccination programs *(15)*, as it provides a mechanism for the reassortment of antigen-encoding genes among meningococcal clones and increases the prospect of meningococci evading host immunity *(16,17)*. In addition, the expression of many antigen genes is tightly regulated so that critical antigens are not continuously expressed in vivo *(18–22)*.

Like many other medically important bacteria, the meningococcus has historically been characterized serologically on the basis of its surface antigens *(23–26)*. It can synthesize one of a number of polysaccharide capsules that define the serogroup; pathogenic isolates invariably belong to one of five serogroups, A, B, C, W135, or Y. Serogroups are further subdivided into serotypes and serosubtypes on the basis the serological reactivity of major outer membrane proteins (OMPs) and into immunotypes on the basis of differences in LPS structure. Perhaps not surprisingly, the capsular antigens have been critical in the development of the licensed vaccines. Arguably, if it had been possible to produce a pentavalent vaccine based on the capsular polysaccharide of the pathogenic serogroups that was safe and effective in infants, comprehensive control of meningococcal disease through routine immunization would already be possible. However, the use of serogroup B capsule presents particular problems, and as a result many of the other surface antigens are under consideration as potential components of future vaccines (for review, *see* **ref. 27**).

1.1. Historical Perspective

Historically, attempts to prevent meningococcal disease by immuno-prophylaxis seem to have been inspired by successes in the prevention of other important diseases through vaccination. Following the use of killed whole-cell vaccines for the prevention of typhoid at the turn of the last century *(28)*, numerous studies explored the potential of immunization with heat-killed meningococcal cells to prevent disease *(29)*. Many of the clinical trials that were conducted with whole cell formulations were poorly controlled and the efficacy of these preparations was at best questionable. This, together with the unacceptable reactogenicity caused by their high endotoxin content, ultimately resulted in the abandonment of the killed whole-cell vaccine approach.

In the 1930s, the successful prevention of diphtheria and tetanus by immunization with toxoids prompted the search for a meningococcal toxin in cell-free culture supernatants. Kuhns et al. evaluated the vaccine potential of culture filtrates in studies that provided limited evidence for the efficacy of this approach *(30,31)*. Because the culture supernatants would have been contaminated with capsular polysaccharide, endotoxin, and OMPs, it is impossible to attribute the protection observed to a particular antigen. These preliminary observations do not appear to have been pursued further. In common with research on vaccines against other infectious diseases at that time, perhaps the optimism surrounding the introduction of antibiotics suppressed interest in meningococcal vaccine development.

During the early 1940s, the association of meningococcal disease with the increase in the recruitment of Allied Forces rekindled interest in vaccination to control disease outbreaks. Once again it was a vaccine against another pathogen that was to provide the inspiration for subsequent developments. Promising results with a multivalent pneumococcal polysaccharide vaccine indicated that capsular polysaccharides may be able to elicit protective immune responses *(32)*. The clinical evaluations of early preparations of meningococcal serogroup A and C polysaccharides were far from encouraging, probably because the capsular material was degraded to low molecular-weight oligosaccharides by the purification methods employed at the time. However, during the 1960s the development of an innovative purification procedure permitted the production of highly purified, high molecular-weight meningococcal capsular polysaccharides *(33)*. Polysaccharides produced in this way have proved to be safe and immunogenic in adults and older children *(34–36)*. They form the basis of the currently licensed meningococcal polysaccharide vaccine formulations.

Unfortunately, polysaccharides are usually T-cell independent antigens. Consequently, they are poorly immunogenic in the very young, they fail to stimulate a good anamnestic response, and they often elicit low-avidity antibody responses. Meningococcal capsular polysaccharides are no exception *(37)*; the currently licensed polysaccharide vaccines are not indicated for children under 2 yr of age and the vaccines are not used in long-term immunization programs. Recently, the successful introduction of the *Hib* vaccine into a number of national immunization programs *(38)* has been followed by the rapid development of meningococcal glycoconjugate vaccines *(39–41)*. These consist of partially hydrolyzed, size-fractionated oligosaccharides chemically conjugated to either tetanus or diphtheria toxoids as carrier proteins. In clinical studies they have proved to be safe, immunogenic, and to give a good anamnestic response regardless of the age of the vaccinee *(42–49)*. The first such vaccine was licensed in the UK at the end of 1999 and has since been licensed for use in a number of other European countries.

Assuming that such glycoconjugate vaccines prove to be effective in infant immunization schedules, the development of safe and effective vaccines that offer protection against serogroup B disease remains a major challenge. Today serogroup B organisms are responsible for most meningococcal disease in developed countries *(7)*. However, attempts to develop vaccines based upon serogroup B polysaccharide have proved unsuccessful *(9)*. Purified B polysaccharide, a polymer of α 2-8 linked sialic acid, has failed to elicit a significant increase in antibody responses in clinical trials. The lack of response in man may be explained by immunological tolerance to similar sialic-acid structures on human cells and raises the question of whether a serogroup B polysaccharide vaccine that overcame tolerance would be acceptable in terms of its safety.

2. Vaccines

2.1. Polysaccharide Vaccines

The currently licensed polysaccharide vaccines include two formulations— a bivalent A and C vaccine and a tetravalent formulation containing A, C, W135, and Y polysaccharides—that are produced by a number of European and North American companies. The high molecular size polysaccharides used in these vaccines are produced by essentially the same method as first described by Gotschlich et al. *(33)*. All four polysaccharide components have been shown to be immunogenic in adults and older children *(34,50,51)*, although it has only been possible to demonstrate protective efficacy against infection with serogroup A and C organisms because of the low incidence of W135 and Y disease. In early protective efficacy trials in US military recruits, monovalent serogroup C vaccines were demonstrated to have an efficacy in the region of 90% *(35)*. Similar levels of protection were observed when serogroup A vaccines were studied in Africa and Finland *(36)*.

Serum bactericidal antibodies play a crucial role in the protection of the host against meningococcal disease. The evidence for this includes an association between the lack of serogroup specific bactericidal antibodies and occurrence of disease among military recruits *(52)* and the susceptibility of individuals, who congenitally lack complement components in the membrane-attack complex, to repeated meningococcal infections *(53)*. Although there has been considerable debate over the way in which the assay should be performed, the serum bactericidal-antibody titer provides an important immunological surrogate for protection, without which the subsequent development of glycoconjugate vaccines would have been severely hampered.

The size and duration of the immune response is age-dependent, reflecting the fact that meningococcal polysaccharides, like other carbohydrate antigens, are T-independent antigens, and suggests that B-cell maturation is critical for an effective immune response *(37,54,55)*. The serogroup C response was not effective in children under 2 yr of age and the licensed vaccines are consequently not indicated for use below this age. Serogroup A polysaccharide appears to be more immunogenic than C polysaccharide in young children but neither is capable of inducing long-term immunological memory. The polysaccharide vaccines are therefore generally not used in routine immunization programs due to the lack of protection that they offer in infancy and the relatively short-lived immune response that they elicit. Nevertheless, they are frequently offered to individuals who are at particular risk of infection including: military recruits, undergraduate students, patients with immunodeficiencies, and travelers to the so-called "meningitis belt" countries and the Haj pilgrimage *(27,56)*. They are also used together with chemotherapy to control localized outbreaks of serogroup C disease in schools and colleges in industrialized countries *(57)*. In the meningitis belt, polysaccharide vaccine has proved effective at controlling the spread of serogroup A epidemics *(58,59)* and recently the World Health Organization (WHO) has established a stock of vaccine that can be dispatched to sub-Saharan Africa at short notice whenever a sudden increase in disease rate indicates the potential onset of an epidemic.

2.2. Glycoconjugate Vaccines

The success of the *Hib* glycoconjugate vaccine has highlighted the advantages of converting polysaccharides into T-dependent antigens by chemical conjugation to protein-carrier molecules *(38,60,61)* and has led to the clinical development of similar vaccines based on the meningococcal serogroup A and C capsular polysaccharides *(41,62)*. Size-fractionated oligosaccharides derived from purified capsular polysaccharides conjugated to either the nontoxic, cross-reacting mutant of diphtheria toxin, CRM197, or tetanus toxoid have been evaluated for their safety and immunogenicity in clinical trials. The depolymerization, activation, and conjugation of meningococcal serogroup C polysaccharide to tetanus toxoid is detailed in Chapter 4.

Miller and Farrington, in Chapter 6 of this volume, review the rationale behind the conduct of clinical trials and the particular problems encountered in the evaluation of meningococcal vaccines. Generally, meningococcal-conjugate vaccines have been well-tolerated; both local and systemic reactions have been relatively mild and similar to those expected for unconjugated polysaccharide vaccines. They have proved to be highly immunogenic over a wide age range, including very young infants *(42–45,47–49)*. Studies in which infants have received three doses of vaccine at 2, 3, and 4 mo have shown that serogroup C- CRM197 conjugates induce high levels of high-avidity, anti-C polysaccharide antibodies that are bactericidal. Richmond et al. also demonstrated that the immune response of infants primed with the conjugate vaccine was boosted by the administration of serogroup C polysaccharide, confirming that the vaccine induces immunological memory *(49)*. These data indicate the successful induction of a T-cell dependent antibody response by serogroup C-CRM197 conjugate vaccines. Other clinical studies have shown that serogroup C conjugates in which tetanus toxoid has been used as the carrier protein or the C polysaccharide is *O*-deacetylated to be similarly immunogenic and well-tolerated *(46)*.

Three serogroup C conjugate vaccines have been licensed in the UK to date. Given the low incidence of disease caused by serogroup C organisms, it was impractical to conduct controlled protective efficacy studies and the license was granted on the basis that: 1) the conjugate was more immunogenic than the existing licensed polysaccharide vaccine, particularly in the very young; 2) it induced a good anamnestic response; and 3) the success of glycoconjugate vaccine technology in reducing disease had been established with the *Hib* vaccine. Careful monitoring of serogroup C disease throughout the phased introduction of the vaccine into national immunization schedules should provide some assessment of the effectiveness of these vaccines.* Provided that there is sufficient vaccine coverage, the introduction of serogroup C conjugate vaccine

---

*Recent estimates based on surveillance during the first 9 mo following the introduction of the serogroup C conjugate in England indicate that the short-term efficacy of the vaccine was 97% (95% CI 77–99) for teenagers and 92% (65–98) for toddlers (Ramsay, Andrews, Kaczmarski and Miller, 2001, *Lancet* **357**, 195, 196).

can reasonably be expected to parallel the previous success of the *Hib* vaccine, eventually leading to the eradication of serogroup C disease. Although drawing such parallels has been expeditious in the development of the new vaccines this optimism is, however, tempered by the knowledge that certain aspects of meningococcal disease and invasive *Haemophilus influenzae* type b disease are quite different *(15)*.

Type b organisms account for almost all septicaemic isolates of *H. influenzae*, whereas several different meningococcal serogroups cause invasive infections. In addition, there is little evidence that virulent isolates of non-type b *H. influenzae* arise through the genetical exchange of capsular polysaccharide loci *(63)*, whereas there is extensive evidence that virulent meningococci frequently exchange antigen genes, including those encoding their capsular polysaccharides *(17,64,65)*. The licensed serogroup C conjugate vaccines offer no cross-protective immunity to the non-serogroup C meningococci that are responsible for most of the meningococcal disease in industrialized countries, and that may arise as consequence of capsular switching. With the widespread use of monovalent serogroup C conjugate vaccines, the associated increase in the level of serogroup C specific salivary antibody together with the induction of immunological memory in the vaccinated population is likely to serve to reduce nasopharyngeal carriage, thereby increasing herd immunity *(66)*. This would represent a important shift in the immunological selection acting on meningococci circulating in the vaccinated population and could ultimately result in an increase in disease caused by the other pathogenic serogroups. Further development of meningococcal glycoconjugate components will inevitably lead to the availability of more comprehensive formulations comprising combinations of serogroup A, C, W135, and Y conjugates, but the development of an effective vaccine offering protection against disease caused by serogroup B organisms clearly remains the decisive obstacle in the elimination of meningococcal disease.

The poor immunogenicity of vaccine candidates consisting of native serogroup B polysaccharide conjugated to carrier proteins has been attributed to immunological tolerance associated with the presence of sialylated glycopeptides in human and animal tissues *(10)*. During embryonic and neonatal development, the neural cell adhesion molecule (N-CAM), which is widely distributed in human tissue, has long polysialic acid chains that are recognized by anti-serogroup B antibodies *(67)*. A number of studies have shown that the sialylation of N-CAM modulates cell-cell interactions during organogenesis and has led to concern that pregnancy or fetal development may be adversely affected by high levels of high avidity cross-reacting antibodies produced in response to a serogroup B conjugate vaccine. Jennings et al. postulated that chemical modification of the polysaccharide might overcome immunological tolerance and induce a safe and protective immune response *(68)*. A modified B polysaccharide, in which the *N*-acetyl groups at position C-5 of the sialic acid residues are replaced with *N*-propionyl groups, conjugated to tetanus toxoid proved to be immunogenic in mice. More recently, *N*-propionylated serogroup B polysaccharide conjugated to a recombinant meningococcal outer-membrane protein (rPorB) has been shown to be highly immunogenic in non human primates *(69)*. Importantly, no adverse reactions to the trial vaccine were observed in these studies, providing grounds for optimism, although the absence of an autoimmune response and the overall safety of such a vaccine remain to be substantiated by clinical trials, and it will inevitably take many years to establish its long-term safety. The preparation and characteristics of *N*-propionylated serogroup B polysaccharide conjugated to tetanus toxoid are described in Chapter 5.

2.3. Protein Vaccines

Concern over the safety of vaccines based on the serogroup B capsular polysaccharide has focused attention on alternative cell-surface antigens as vaccine candidates (**Table 1**). The most advanced of these, in terms of their clinical development, consist of meningococcal outer-membrane vesicles (OMVs) *(70–72)* or purified outer-membrane proteins (OMPs) *(73)*. Grown in broth culture, *N. meningitidis* produces substantial quantity of outer-membrane blebs, containing the same complement of OMPs as the organism itself *(74)*. These vesicles can be readily purified from detergent treated meningococcal cultures to form the basis of vaccine formulations (Chapters 6 and 7). Unfortunately, such vaccines suffer from significant drawbacks: 1) the most immunogenic antigens they contain are also the most variable, suggesting that OMV vaccines may not offer comprehensive protection against all meningococci; 2) their protective efficacy in young infants, the group most at risk of meningococcal disease, has not been demonstrated; and 3) protection appears to be short-lived. It has been suggested that mucosally administered OMV formulations may overcome some of these shortcomings and to explore this possibility immunogenicity studies have been performed in human volunteers (*see* Chapter 16) *(75)*.

Efficacy trials have been conducted with both OMV and purified OMP formulations. In response to an outbreak of disease in Cuba in the late 1980s, the Finlay Institute produced an OMV vaccine, based on this B:4:P1.19,15 (ET-5 complex) isolate, that also contained serogroup C capsular polysaccharide. Case controlled studies using the Cuban vaccine in Brazil revealed that protective efficacy was age-dependent; an efficacy of greater than 70% was recorded for children older than four years, while in younger children no efficacy was demonstrated *(76)*. Similarly, an increase in meningococcal disease in Norway caused by a B:15:P1.7,16 isolate belonging to the ET5 complex prompted the

Table 1
Summary of Protein-Vaccine Candidates That Might Offer Protection Against Serogroup B Disease

Vaccine candidate	Stage of development	Reference
Outer membrane vesicle:		
Finlay Institute	Licensed in some Central and Southern American countries	*(70)*
NIPH	Completed efficacy (phase III) studies in teenagers	*(71)*
RIVM	Immunogenicity (phase II) studies in various age groups	*(72,85)*
Purified outer membrane proteins	Efficacy studies	*(73)*
Transferrin binding protein B (TbpB)	Preliminary clinical studies in adult volunteers	*(87)*
Neisseria surface protein (NspA)	Preclinical research	*(113)*
Transferrin binding protein A (TbpA)	Preclinical research	*(114)*
FrpB	Preclinical research	*(115)*
Recombinant PorA	Preclinical research	*(116)*
Peptides from PorA	Preclinical research	*(117)*
TspA	Preclinical research	*(118)*

development of an OMV vaccine, the protective efficacy of which proved to be 57% in a double-blind, placebo-controlled trial conducted in secondary-school pupils *(71)*. A serotype-specific outbreak of serogroup B meningococcal disease in Iquique, Chile during the 1980s lead to the evaluation of a vaccine consisting of purified meningococcal OMPs noncovalently complexed to serogroup C polysaccharide in a randomized, controlled trial. The vaccine efficacy was 70% in the volunteers aged from 5–21 yr, but was not protective in children aged between 1 and 4 yr *(73)*. In all three studies, which used two dose schedules, there was evidence of better protection early after immunization, indicating that protection is short-lived and leading to suggestions that a third dose of vaccine may improve protective efficacy *(27)*. Each of these vaccines was based on a specific meningococcal isolate. Given the antigenic diversity of *N. meningitidis* isolates, this raises concerns that they cannot be relied upon to offer cross-protection against all virulent meningococci; fears that have been substantiated by immunogenicity studies showing that the ability of OMV vaccines to elicit cross-protective bactericidal antibodies is limited *(77)*.

Meningococci express two major OMPs, the class 1 OMP (PorA) and either a class 2 or class 3 OMP (PorB2 or PorB3, respectively), which are the most abundant proteins in OMVs *(78)*. PorA is particularly immunogenic in humans and is often seen as the critical component of OMV vaccines. The increase in antibodies directed against PorA observed in the serum of patients convalescing from meningococcal disease *(79)*, the ability of PorA to elicit bactericidal-antibody responses *(80)*, and the sequence variability of PorA, a likely consequence of immunoselective pressure in humans *(81)*, together provide compelling evidence for the expression of PorA in vivo and the protective potential of PorA as an antigen.

In an attempt to overcome the variability of PorA yet capitalize on its immunogenicity, researchers at the RIVM in the Netherlands have developed a candidate OMV vaccine that is multivalent with respect to its PorA epitopes *(82)*. The vaccine consists of OMVs from two meningococcal isolates in which the *porB*, *rmpM*, and an *opa* gene have been inactivated, each genetically engineered so as to express three different *porA* genes (six different serosubtypes in total) *(83)*. The methodology used for the construction of strains bearing different *porA* alleles is described detailed in Chapter 11 by van der Ley and van Alphen. They also contain genetic lesions that prevent the expression of capsular polysaccharide and the lacto-N-neotetraose moeity of meningococcal lipopolysaccharide to reduce the risk of inducing a cross-reactive antibody responses with human antigens. Approximately 90% of the protein content of the vaccine consists of PorA and all the epitopes expressed are recognized by their corresponding serosubtype specific monoclonal antibody (MAb) *(84)*. Although clinical trials to determine the protective efficacy of this vaccine have yet to be completed, immunogenicity trials in Gloucestershire and Rotterdam indicate that, in groups of children encompassing a range of ages, it elicits bactericidal antibody responses to strains bearing homologous PorA epitopes *(72,85)*. However, during the course of these studies, the use of panels of isogenic strains expressing heterologous PorA epitopes demonstrated that even relatively minor changes in the amino acid sequence of a PorA epitope could alleviate complement-mediated killing of the organism (*see* Chapter 11 for information on the construction of isogenic strains) *(86)*.

Together the poor protective efficacy of OMVs in infants and concerns that they would not offer protection against antigenically diverse meningococci raise serious doubts about their suitability for pediatric immunization programs. Furthermore, there are fears that the immnoselective pressure, resulting from the widespread use of a vaccine that fails to offer comprehensive protection against all virulent meningococci, is likely to increase the rate of antigenic change and hence the frequency with which such a vaccine would have to be reformulated if it were to remain effective against disease (*see* Chapter 7). Nevertheless, appropriately formulated OMV vaccines have considerable potential for the disruption of outbreaks of meningococcal disease caused by a single strain in older children and teenagers.

Reservations over the safety and effectiveness of polysaccharide and OMV vaccines against serogroup B disease have stimulated the search for the "Holy Grail" vaccine candidate that is antigenically highly conserved and yet elicits a safe and protective immune response. Most alternative vaccine candidates have not so far progressed beyond preclinical research and development (*see* Table 1). Only the transferrin-binding protein, TbpB, which is important for the acquisition of iron from human transferrin by the meningococcus in vivo, has been evaluated in preliminary clinical studies *(87)*. The rationale for the use of Tbps in vaccines as well as methods for the purification of native TbpB from *N. meningitidis* and recombinant TbpB from *Escherichia coli* are reviewed in Chapter 8. Despite evidence that TbpB offers protection against meningococcal septicemia in animal models *(88)*, initial clinical studies have failed to demonstrate a satisfactory bactericidal-antibody response in man *(87)*. TbpB like other cell-surface expressed antigens is variable and the poor immune response may, in part, be explained by the choice of TbpB variant. The smallest naturally occurring TbpB protein, lacking most of the larger regions of antigenic variation, presumably the principal targets of the immune response in man, was used for these studies. A number of other protein-vaccine candidates known to be expressed on the surface of *N. meningitidis* have shown promise in preclinical studies but their potential to elicit broadly cross-protective immune responses in humans awaits clinical scrutiny.

Recent developments in bacterial genomics and proteomics provide powerful new approaches to the identification of candidate antigens for the development vaccines offering protection against bacterial infections. The nucleotide sequences of the genomes of two meningococcal isolates, the serogroup A (subgroup IV) isolate Z2491 *(89)* and a derivative of the serogroup B (ET5 complex) isolate MC58 *(22)*, have already been completed and a third, the serogroup C (ET37 complex) isolate FAM18, is currently being determined. Scientists at Chiron Vaccines have screened the entire genome of MC58 to identify open reading frames (ORFs) encoding novel vaccine candidates *(90)*. A total of 570 ORFs encoding potential novel surface-exposed or exported proteins was identified by screening the genome sequence with various computer algorithms. These were then amplified by the polymerase chain reaction (PCR) and cloned into an *E. coli* expression system. The products of 350 of the ORFs were successfully expressed including: 70 possible lipoproteins; 96 predicted periplasmic proteins; 87 cytoplasmic membrane proteins; and 45 potential OMPs. The purified proteins were used to raise antisera in mice which were analyzed by enzyme-linked immunosorbent assay (ELISA) and fluorescence-activated cell sorting (FACS) analysis, to determine whether the proteins were immunogenic and present on the surface of a range of meningococcal isolates, respectively. The sera were also tested for their bactericidal activity. Eighty-five proteins proved to be strongly positive in one or more of these assays and seven were chosen for further study on the basis that they gave a good response in all three assays but were not encoded by genes that appeared to be phase variable. The antigenic variability of the candidate vaccine antigens was assessed by sequencing the corresponding genes in a diverse collection of meningococcal isolates. The identification of highly conserved proteins, expressed at the surface of the meningococcus and capable of inducing bactericidal antibodies, provides novel vaccine candidates that can be taken forward into clinical development. Whether such proteins are expressed and exposed to the human immune response in vivo and whether they elicit a protective response in humans are the crucial questions that must now be addressed.

2.4. Other Antigens

Besides the capsular polysaccharide and cell-surface proteins, meningococcal LPS has received much attention as a possible vaccine candidate (91–93). N. menigitidis expresses a number of different glycoforms of LPS, defining the meningococcal immunotype, and many of the LPS structures have been determined (94–98). The production of immunotype L3,7,9 LPS is a characteristic particularly associated with isolates from invasive disease (99,100) and the serum from individuals recovering from infection contains antibodies that recognize LPS epitopes (101). Although OMV vaccines retain some LPS, no clinical studies with vaccine candidates based solely on meningococcal LPS or LPS conjugates have been reported to date. Preclinical immunogenicity studies with detoxified LPS and with L3,7,9-toxoid conjugates indicates that LPS vaccines may tend to induce opsonic rather than bactericidal antibody responses (93). As a result of recent advances in the structure and biosynthesis of meningococcal LPS and its role in the pathogenesis of meningococcal disease, the candidacy of LPS as a vaccine component is likely to be the subject of further research and development in the future.

Recent studies have shown that peptide immunogens that mimic the conformation of carbohydrates can elicit cross-reactive antibody responses to bacterial polysaccharides (102,103). The feasibility of this approach was first established with peptide immunogens whose sequences were identified from the antigen-binding sites of anti-idiotypic antibodies raised against a serogroup C specific MAb (104). Mice immunized with peptides based on the primary sequence of the CDR loops of anti-idiotypic meningococcal capsular polysaccharide antibodies were shown to protect against lethal challenge of meningococcal cells *(105)*. The panning of phage-display libraries expressing peptides with random sequences of amino acids by carbohydrate-specific MAbs provides an alternative approach to identifying peptides that are potential conformational mimotopes. Peptide antigen mimics of carbohydrates are isolated by "bio-panning" random linear peptides expressed on the surface of bacteriophage with an anti-carbohydrate MAb. From these peptides, a consensus amino acid sequence is determined and immune response induced by the corresponding peptide can then be evaluated. This approach has also been applied to identify peptide mimics of serogroup A *(106)* and serogroup B *(107)* capsular polysaccharides as well as meningococcal LPS (*see* Chapter 14). So far most of the antigen mimics studied have failed to stimulate strong bactericidal-antibody responses, suggesting that either the immune response to the existing peptides requires further optimization or better, structurally defined, peptides are required before clinical studies can be contemplated.

The development of protective immunity in infants to meningococcal disease occurs at an age when the rates of carriage of *N. meningitidis* are very low *(108)*, suggesting that colonization by nonpathogenic *Neisseria* species and other bacteria expressing cross-reactive antigens may contribute to protection early in life. This observation has lead to the suggestion by several researchers that studies of the cell-surface structures of commensal *Neisseria* provide new opportunities for the design and development of meningococcal vaccines *(109,110)*. Even the intentional colonization of individuals with *N. lactamica* has been proposed as a possible means of enhancing protective immunity. No prophylactic measures against meningococcal disease based on commensal organisms or their antigens have been evaluated in clinical trials to date.

As novel vaccine candidates emerge and perhaps, in due course, combinations of antigens are employed in an attempt to develop more comprehensive vaccine formulations, it will be essential that appropriate assay systems are developed and standardized to permit the immunological contribution of each antigen to be established. The serum bactericidal assay has been widely accepted as the "gold standard" for the determination of the potential potency of meningococcal vaccines *(111)*. However, while there is convincing evidence that the presence of bactericidal antibodies correlates with protection against meningococcal disease *(52,112)*, the absence of bactericidal antibodies does not necessarily imply a lack of protection. A dogmatic expectation that meningococcal vaccine components should elicit bactericidal antibodies may result in the rejection of antigens that offer protection against serogroup B disease mediated by an alternative immunological mechanism.

References

1. Cartwright, K. A. V. (1995) *Meningococcal Disease.* John Wiley and Sons, Chichester, UK.
2. Tzeng, Y. and Stephens, D. S. (2000) Epidemiology and pathogenesis of *Neisseria meningitidis. Microbes. Infect.* **2,** 687–700.
3. Schwartz, B., Moore, P. S., and Broome, C. V. (1989) Global epidemiology of meningococcal disease. *Clin. Microbiol. Rev.* **2,** s118–s124.
4. Peltola, H. (1983) Meningococcal disease: still with us. *Rev. Infect. Dis.* **5,** 71–91.
5. Steven, N. and Wood, M. (1995) The clinical spectrum of meningococcal disease, in *Meningococcal Disease* (Cartwright, K., ed.), John Wiley and Sons, Chichester, UK, pp. 177–205.
6. Cartwright, K. A. V. (1995) Meningococcal carriage and disease, in *Meningococcal Disease* (Cartwright, K. A. V., ed.), John Wiley and Sons, Chichester, UK, pp. 115–146.
7. Jones, D. M. (1995) Epidemiology of meningococcal disease in Europe and the USA, in *Meningococcal Disease* (Cartwright, K. A. V., ed.), John Wiley and Sons, Chichester, UK, pp. 147–157.
8. Reingold, A. L., Broome, C. V., Ajello, G. W., Hightower, A. W., Bolan, G. A., Adamsbaum, C., et al. (1985) Age-specific differences in duration of clinical protection after vaccination with meningococcal polysaccharide A vaccine. *Lancet* **ii,** 114–118.
9. Wyle, F. A., Artenstein, M. S., Brandt, B. L., Tramont, E. C., Kasper, D. L., Altieri, P. L., et al. (1972) Immunologic response of man to group B meningococcal polysaccharide vaccines. *J Infect. Dis.* **126,** 514–521.
10. Finne, J., Leinonen, M., and Makela, P. H. (1983) Antigenic similarities between brain components and bacteria causing meningitis: implications for vaccine development and pathogenesis. *Lancet* **ii,** 355–357.
11. Poolman, J. T. (1995) Development of a meningococcal vaccine. *Infect. Agents Dis.* **4,** 13–28.
12. Zollinger, W. D. (1997) New and Improved Vaccines Against Meningococcal Disease, in *New Generation Vaccines* (Levine, M. M., Woodrow, G. C., Kaper, J. B., and Cobon, G. S., eds.), Marcel Dekker, New York, pp. 469.
13. Maiden, M. C. J. and Feavers, I. M. (1995) Population genetics and global epidemiology of the human pathogen *Neisseria meningitidis*, in *Population Genetics of Bacteria* (Baumberg, S., Young, J. P. W., Saunders, J. R., and Wellington, E. M. H., eds.), Cambridge University Press, Cambridge, UK, pp. 269–293.
14. Stephens, D. S. (1999) Uncloaking the meningococcus: dynamics of carriage and disease. *Lancet* **353,** 941–942.
15. Maiden, M. C. and Spratt, B. G. (1999) Meningococcal conjugate vaccines: new opportunities and new challenges. *Lancet* **354,** 615–616.
16. Frosch, M. and Meyer, T. F. (1992) Transformation-mediated exchange of virulence determinants by co-cultivation of pathogenic Neisseriae. *FEMS Microbiol. Lett.* **100,** 345–349.

17. Wang, J.-F., Caugant, D. A., Morelli, G., Koumaré, B., and Achtman, M. (1993) Antigenic and epidemiological properties of the ET-37 complex of *Neisseria meningitidis. J Infect. Dis.* **167**, 1320–1329.

18. Hammerschmidt, S., Hilse, R., van Putten, J. P., Gerardy Schahn, R., Unkmeir, A., and Frosch, M. (1996) Modulation of cell surface sialic acid expression in *Neisseria meningitidis* via a transposable genetic element. *EMBO J.* **15**, 192–198.

19. Hammerschmidt, S., Muller, A., Sillmann, H., Muhlenhoff, M., Borrow, R., Fox, A., et al. (1996) Capsule phase variation in *Neisseria meningitidis* serogroup B by slipped-strand mispairing in the polysialyltransferase gene (*siaD*): correlation with bacterial invasion and the outbreak of meningococcal disease. *Mol. Microbiol.* **20**, 1211–1220.

20. Jennings, M. P., Srikhanta, Y. N., Moxon, E. R., Kramer, M., Poolman, J. T., Kuipers, B., and van der Ley, P. (1999) The genetic basis of the phase variation repertoire of lipopolysaccharide immunotypes in *Neisseria meningitidis*. *Microbiology* **145**, 3013–3021.

21. van der Ende, A., Hopman, C. T., Zaat, S., Essink, B. B., Berkhout, B., and Dankert, J. (1995) Variable expression of class 1 outer membrane protein in *Neisseria meningitidis* is caused by variation in the spacing between the -10 and -35 regions of the promoter. *J. Bacteriol.* **177**, 2475–2480.

22. Tettelin, H., Saunders, N. J., Heidelberg, J., Jeffries, A. C., Nelson, K. E., Eisen, J. A., et al. (2000) Complete genome sequence of *Neisseria meningitidis* serogroup B strain MC58. *Science* **287**, 1809–1815.

23. Frasch, C. E., Zollinger, W. D., and Poolman, J. T. (1985) Serotype antigens of *Neisseria meningitidis* and a proposed scheme for designation of serotypes. *Rev. Infect. Dis.* **7**, 504–510.

24. Abdillahi, H. and Poolman, J. T. (1987) Whole-cell ELISA for typing *Neisseria meningitidis* with monoclonal antibodies. *FEMS Microbiol. Lett.* **48**, 367–371.

25. Vedros, N. A. (1987) Development of meningococcal serogroups, in *Evolution of Meningococcal Disease.* (Vedros, N. A., ed.), CRC Press, Boca Raton, FL, pp. 33–37.

26. Tsai, C. M., Mocca, L. F., and Frasch, C. E. (1987) Immunotype epitopes of *Neisseria meningitidis* lipooligosaccharide types 1 through 8. *Infect. Immun.* **55**, 1652–1656.

27. Frasch, C. E. (1995) Meningococcal vaccines: past, present and future, in *Meningococcal Disease* (Cartwright, K., ed.), John Wiley and Sons, Chichester, UK, pp. 245–284.

28. Wright, A. E. (1897) Remarks on vaccination against typhoid fever. *BMJ* **1**, 256–259.

29. Underwood, E. A. (1940) Recent knowledge of the incidence and control of cerebospinal fever. *BMJ* **i**, 757–763.

30. Kuhns, D. (1936) The control of meningococcic meningitis epidemics by active immunization with meningococcus soluble toxin: a preliminary report. *JAMA* **107**, 5–11.

31. Kuhns, D., Kisner, P., Williams, M. P., and Moorman, P. L. (1938) The control of meningococcic meningitis epidemics by active immunization with meningococcus soluble toxin: further studies. *JAMA* **110,** 484–487.

32. MacLeod, C. M., Hodges, R. G., Heidelberger, M., and Bernhard, W. G. (1945) Prevention of pneumococcal pneumonia by immunization with specific capsular polysaccharides. *J. Exp. Med.* **82,** 445–465.

33. Gotschlich, E. C., Liu, T. Y., and Artenstein, M. S. (1969) Human immunity to the meningococcus. III. Preparation and immunochemical properties of the group A, group B and group C meningococcal polysaccharides. *J. Exp. Med.* **129,** 1349–1365.

34. Gotschlich, E. C., Goldschneider, I., and Artenstein, M. S. (1969) Human immunity to the meningococcus IV. Immunogenicity of group A and group C meningococcal polysaccharides. *J. Exp. Med.* **129,** 1367–1384.

35. Artenstein, M. S., Gold, R., Zimmerly, J. G., Wyle, F. A., Schneider, H., and Harkins, C. (1970) Prevention of meningococcal disease by group C polysaccharide vaccine. *New England J. Med.* **282,** 417–420.

36. Peltola, H., Makela, H., Kayhty, H., Jousimies, H., Herva, E., Hallstrom, K., et al. (1977) Clinical efficacy of meningococcus group A capsular polysaccharide vaccine in children three months to five years of age. *New Engl. J. Med.* **297,** 686–691.

37. Gold, R., Lepow, M. L., Goldschneider, I., Draper, T. L., and Gotschlich, E. C. (1975) Clinical evaluation of group A and group C meningococcal polysaccharide vaccines in infants. *J. Clin. Invest.* **56,** 1536–1547.

38. Adams, W. G., Deaver, K. A., Cochi, S. L., Plikaytis, B. D., Zell, E. R., Broome, C. V., and Wenger, J. D. (1993) Decline of childhood *Haemophilus influenzae* type b (*Hib*) disease in the *Hib* vaccine era. *JAMA* **269,** 221–226.

39. Jennings, H. J. and Lugowski, C. (1982) Immunochemistry of groups A, B and C meningococcal polysaccharide-tetanus toxoid conjugates. *J. Immunol.* **127,** 1011–1018.

40. Beuvery, E. C., Miedema, F., van Delft, R. W., Haverkamp, J., Leussink, A. B., te Pas, B. J., et al. (1983) Preparation and physicochemical and immunological characterisation of polysaccharide-outer membrane protein complexes of *Neisseria meningitidis*. *Infect. Immun.* **40,** 369–380.

41. Costantino, P., Viti, S., Podda, A., Velmonte, M. A., Nencioni, L., and Rappuoli, R. (1992) Development and phase 1 clinical testing of a conjugate vaccine against meningococcus A and C. *Vaccine* **10,** 691–698.

42. Campagne, G., Garba, A., Fabre, P., Schuchat, A., Ryall, R., Boulanger, D., Bybel, M., et al. (2000) Safety and immunogenicity of three doses of a *Neisseria meningitidis* A + C diphtheria conjugate vaccine in infants from Niger. *Pediatr. Infect. Dis. J.* **19,** 144–150.

43. Leach, A., Twumasi, P. A., Kumah, S., Banya, W. S., Jaffar, S., Forrest, B. D., et al. (1997) Induction of immunologic memory in Gambian children by vaccination in infancy with a group A plus group C meningococcal polysaccharide-protein conjugate vaccine. *J. Infect. Dis.* **175,** 200–204.

44. Lieberman, J. M., Chiu, S. S., Wong, V. K., Partridge, S., Chang, S.-J., Chiu, C.-Y., et al. (1996) Safety and immunogenicity of a serogroups A/C *Neisseria*

meningitidis oligosaccharide-protein conjugate vaccine in young children. *JAMA* **275,** 1499–1503.

45. MacDonald, N. E., Halperin, S. A., Law, B. J., Forrest, B., Danzig, L. E., and Granoff, D. M. (1998) Induction of immunologic memory by conjugated vs plain meningococcal C polysaccharide vaccine in toddlers: a randomized controlled trial. *JAMA* **280,** 1685–1689.

46. Richmond, P., Goldblatt, D., Fusco, P. C., Fusco, J. D., Heron, I., Clark, S., et al. (1999) Safety and immunogenicity of a new *Neisseria meningitidis* serogroup C- tetanus toxoid conjugate vaccine in healthy adults. *Vaccine* **18,** 641–646.

47. Twumasi, P. A., Jr., Kumah, S., Leach, A., O'Dempsey, T. J., Ceesay, S. J., Todd, J., et al. (1995) A trial of a group A plus group C meningococcal polysaccharide-protein conjugate vaccine in African infants. *J. Infect. Dis.* **171,** 632–638.

48. Fairley, C. K., Begg, N., Borrow, R., Fox, A. J., Jones, D. M., and Cartwright, K. (1996) Conjugate meningococcal serogroup A and C vaccine: reactogenicity and immunogenicity in United Kingdom infants. *J. Infect. Dis.* **174,** 1360–1363.

49. Richmond, P., Borrow, R., Miller, E., Clark, S., Sadler, F., Fox, A., et al. (1999) Meningococcal serogroup C conjugate vaccine is immunogenic in infancy and primes for memory. *J. Infect. Dis.* **179,** 1569–1572.

50. Kayhty, H., Karanko, V., Peltola, H., Sarna, S., and Makela, P. H. (1980) Serum antibodies to capsular polysaccharide vaccine of group A *Neisseria meningitidis* followed for three years in infants and children. *J. Infect. Dis.* **142,** 861–868.

51. Lepow, M. L., Beeler, J., Randolph, M., Samuelson, J. S., and Hankins, W. A. (1986) Reactogenicity and immunogenicity of a quadravalent combined meningococcal polysaccharide vaccine in children. *J. Infect. Dis.* **154,** 1033–1036.

52. Goldschneider, I., Gotschlich, E. C., and Artenstein, M. S. (1969) Human immunity to the meningococcus. I. The role of humoral antibodies. *J. Exp. Med.* **129,** 1307–1326.

53. Figueroa, J., Andreoni, J., and Densen, P. (1993) Complement deficiency states and meningococcal disease. *Immunol. Res.* **12,** 295–311.

54. Lepow, M. L., Goldschneider, I., Gold, R., Randolph, M., and Gotschlich, E. C. (1977) Persistence of antibody following immunization of children with groups A and C meningococcal polysaccharide vaccines. *Pediatrics* **60,** 673–680.

55. Goldblatt, D. (1998) immunization and the maturation of infant immune responses. *Dev. Biol. Stand.* **95,** 125–132.

56. WHO (2000) Health conditions for travellers to Saudi Arabia. *Wkly. Epidemiol. Record* **75,** 7–8.

57. Begg, N. (1995) Outbreak Management, in *Meningococcal Disease* (Cartwright, K., ed.), John Wiley and Sons, Chichester, UK, pp. 285–305.

58. Greenwood, B. M. and Wali, S. S. (1980) Control of meningococcal infection in the African meningitis belt by selective vaccination. *Lancet* **1,** 729–732.

59. Mohammed, I., Obineche, E. N., Onyemelukwe, G. C., and Zaruba, K. (1984) Control of epidemic meningococcal meningitis by mass vaccination. I. Further epidemiological evaluation of groups A and C vaccines in northern Nigeria. *J. Infect.* **9,** 190–196.

60. Eskola, J., Takala, A. K., and Kayhty, H. (1993) *Haemophilus influenzae* type b polysaccharide-protein conjugate vaccines in children. *Curr. Opin. Pediatr.* **5,** 55–59.

61. Moxon, E. R., Heath, P. T., Booy, R., Azzopardi, H. J., Slack, M. P., and Ramsay, M. E. (1999) 4th European conference on vaccinology: societal value of vaccination. The impact of Hib conjugate vaccines in preventing invasive *H. influenzae* diseases in the UK. *Vaccine* **17,** S11–S13.

62. Goldblatt, D. (1998) Recent developments in bacterial conjugate vaccines. *J. Med. Microbiol.* **47,** 563–567.

63. Lipsitch, M. (1999) Bacterial vaccines and serotype replacement: lessons from Haemophilus influenzae and prospects for *Streptococcus pneumoniae. Emerg. Infect. Dis.* **5,** 336–345.

64. Caugant, D. A., Mocca, L. F., Frasch, C. E., Froholm, L. O., Zollinger, W. D., and Selander, R. K. (1987) Genetic structure of *Neisseria meningitidis* populations in relation to serogroup, serotype, and outer membrane protein pattern. *J. Bacteriol.* **169,** 2781–2792.

65. Swartley, J. S., Marfin, A. A., Edupuganti, S., Liu, L. J., Cieslak, P., Perkins, B., et al. (1997) Capsule switching of *Neisseria meningitidis. Proc. Natl. Acad. Sci. USA* **94,** 271–276.

66. Borrow, R., Fox, A. J., Cartwright, K., Begg, N. T., and Jones, D. M. (1999) Salivary antibodies following parenteral immunization of infants with a meningococcal serogroup A and C conjugated vaccine. *Epidemiol. Infect.* **123,** 201–208.

67. Finne, J. and Makela, P. H. (1985) Cleavage of the polysialosyl units of brain glycoproteins by a bacteriophage endosialidase. Involvement of a long oligosaccharide segment in molecular interactions of polysialic acid. *J. Biol. Chem.* **260,** 1265–1270.

68. Jennings, H. J., Roy, R., and Gamian, A. (1986) Induction of meningococcal group B polysaccharide-specific IgG antibodies in mice by using an N-propionylated B polysaccharide-tetanus toxoid conjugate vaccine. *J. Immunol.* **137,** 1708–1713.

69. Fusco, P. C., Michon, F., Tai, J. Y., and Blake, M. S. (1998) Preclinical evaluation of a novel group B meningococcal conjugate vaccine that elicits bactericidal activity in both mice and non-human primates. *J. Infect.* Dis. *175, 364–372.*

70. Sierra, G. V., Campa, H. C., Varcacel, N. M., Garcia, I. L., Izquierdo, P. L., Sotolongo, P. F., et al. (1991) Vaccine against group B *Neisseria meningitidis:* protection trial and mass vaccination results in Cuba. *NIPH. Ann.* **14,** 195–207.

71. Bjune, G., Hoiby, E. A., Gronnesby, J. K., Arnesen, O., Fredriksen, J. H., Halstensen, A., et al. (1991) Effect of outer membrane vesicle vaccine against group B meningococcal disease in Norway. *Lancet* **338,** 1093–1096.

72. de Kleijn, E. D., de Groot, R., Labadie, J., Lafeber, A. B., van den, D. G., van Alphen, L., et al. (2000) Immunogenicity and safety of a hexavalent meningococcal outer-membrane-vesicle vaccine in children of 2–3 and 7–8 years of age. *Vaccine* **18,** 1456–1466.

73. Boslego, J., Garcia, J., Cruz, C., Zollinger, W., Brandt, B., Ruiz, S., et al. (1995) Efficacy, safety, and immunogenicity of a meningococcal group B (15:P1.3) outer

membrane protein vaccine in Iquique, Chile. Chilean National Committee for Meningococcal Disease. *Vaccine* **13**, 821–829.

74. Frasch, C. E. and Peppler, M. S. (1982) Protection against group B *Neisseria meningitidis* disease: preparation of soluble protein and protein-polysaccharide immunogens. *Infect. Immun.* **37**, 271–280.

75. Haneberg, B., Dalseg, R., Wedege, E., Hoiby, E. A., Haugen, I. L., Oftung, F., et al. (1998) Intranasal administration of a meningococcal outer membrane vesicle vaccine induces persistent local mucosal antibodies and serum antibodies with strong bactericidal activity in humans. *Infect. Immun.* **66**, 1334–1341.

76. de Moraes, J. C., Perkins, B. A., Camargo, M. C., Hidalgo, N. T., Barbosa, H. A., Sacchi, C. T., et al. (1992) Protective efficacy of a serogroup B meningococcal vaccine in Sao Paulo, Brazil. *Lancet* **340**, 1074–1078.

77. Tappero, J. W., Lagos, R., Ballesteros, A. M., Plikaytis, B., Williams, D., Dykes, J., et al. (1999) Immunogenicity of 2 serogroup B outer-membrane protein meningococcal vaccines: a randomized controlled trial in Chile. *JAMA* **281**, 1520–1527.

78. Tsai, C.-M., Frasch, C. E., and Mocca, L. F. (1981) Five structural classes of major outer membrane proteins in *Neisseria meningitidis*. *J. Bacteriol.* **146**, 69–78.

79. Guttormsen, H.-K., Wetzler, L. M., and Solberg, C. O. (1994) Humoral immune response to class 1 outer membrane protein during the course of meningococcal disease. *Infect. Immuni.* **62**, 1437–1443.

80. Wedege, E. and Froholm, L. O. (1986) Human antibody response to a group B serotype 2a meningococcal vaccine determined by immunoblotting. *Infect. Immun.* **51**, 571–578.

81. Feavers, I. M., Fox, A. J., Gray, S., Jones, D. M., and Maiden, M. C. (1996) Antigenic diversity of meningococcal outer membrane protein PorA has implications for epidemiological analysis and vaccine design. *Clin. Diagn. Lab. Immunol.* **3**, 444–450.

82. van der Ley, P. and Poolman, J. T. (1992) Construction of a multivalent meningococcal vaccine strain based on the class 1 outer membrane protein. *Infect. Immun.* **60**, 3156–3161.

83. van der Ley, P., van der Biezen, J., and Poolman, J. T. (1995) Construction of *Neisseria meningitidis* strains carrying multiple chromosomal copies of the *porA* gene for use in the production of a multivalent outer membrane vesicle vaccine. *Vaccine* **13**, 401–407.

84. Claassen, I., Meylis, J., van der Ley, P., Peeters, C., Brons, H., Robert, J., et al. (1996) Production, characterization and control of a *Neisseria meningitidis* hexavalent class 1 outer membrane protein containing vesicle vaccine. *Vaccine* **14**, 1001–1008.

85. Cartwright, K., Morris, R., Rumke, H., Fox, A., Borrow, R., Begg, N., et al. (1999) Immunogenicity and reactogenicity in UK infants of a novel meningococcal vesicle vaccine containing multiple class 1 (PorA) outer membrane proteins. *Vaccine* **17**, 2612–2619.

86. van der Voort, E. R., van Dijken, H., Kuipers, B., van der Biezen, J., van der Ley, P., Meylis, J., et al. (1997) Human B- and T-cell responses after immunization

with a hexavalent PorA meningococcal outer membrane vesicle vaccine. _Infect. Immun._ **65,** 5184–5190.

87. Danve, B., Lissolo, L., Guinet, F., Boutry, E., Speck, D., Cadoz, M., et al. (1998) Safety and immunogenicity of a _Neisseria meningitidis_ group B transferrin binding protein vaccine in adults, in _Eleventh International Pathogenic Neisseria Conference_ (Nassif, X., Quentin-Millet, M. J., and Taha, M. K., eds.), EDK, Paris, pp. 53–53.

88. Danve, B., Lissolo, L., Mignon, M., Dumas, P., Colombani, S., Schryvers, A. B., and Quentin-Millet, M. J. (1993) Transferrin-binding proteins isolated from _Neisseria meningitidis_ elicit protective and bactericidal antibodies in laboratory animals. _Vaccine_ **11,** 1214–1220.

89. Parkhill, J., Achtman, M., James, K. D., Bentley, S. D., Churcher, C., Klee, S. R., et al. (2000) Complete DNA sequence of a serogroup A strain of _Neisseria meningitidis_ Z2491. _Nature_ **404,** 502–506.

90. Pizza, M., Scarlato, V., Masignani, V., Giuliani, M. M., Arico, B., Comanducci, M., et al. (2000) Identification of vaccine candidates against serogroup B meningococcus by whole-genome sequencing. _Science_ **287,** 1816–1820.

91. Gu, X. X. and Tsai, C.-M. (1993) Preparation, characterisation and immunogenicity of meningococcal lipooligosaccharide-derived oligosaccharide-protein conjugates. _Infect. Immun._ **61,** 1873–1880.

92. Jennings, H. J., Lugowski, C., and Ashton, F. E. (1984) Conjugation of meningococcal lipopolysaccharide R-type oligosaccharides to tetanus toxoid as route to a potential vaccine against group B _N. meningitidis. Infect. Immun._ **43,** 407–412.

93. Verheul, A. F. M., Snippe, H., and Poolman, J. T. (1993) Meningococcal lipopolysaccharides: virulence factor and potential vaccine component. _Microbiol. Rev._ **57,** 34–45.

94. DiFabio, J. L., Michon, F., Brisson, J.-R., and Jennings, H. J. (1990) Structure of the L1 and L6 core oligosaccharide epitopes of _Neisseria meningitidis. Can. J. Chemi._ **68,** 1029–1034.

95. Jennings, H. J., Beurret, M., Gamian, A., and Michon, F. (1987) Structure and immunochemistry of meningococcal lipopolysaccharides. _Antonie van Leeuwenhoek_ **53,** 519–522.

96. Kogan, G., Uhrin, D., Brisson, J. R., and Jennings, H. J. (1997) Structural basis of the _Neisseria meningitidis_ immunotypes including the L4 and L7 immunotypes. _Carbohydr. Res._ **298,** 191–199.

97. Verheul, A. F., Boons, G. J., van der Marel, G. A., van Boom, J. H., Jennings, H. J., Snippe, H., et al. (1991) Minimal oligosaccharide structures required for induction of immune responses against meningococcal immunotype L1, L2, and L3, 7,9 lipopolysaccharides determined by using synthetic oligosaccharide-protein conjugates. _Infect. Immun._ **59,** 3566–3573.

98. Scholten, R. J., Kuipers, B., Valkenburg, H. A., Dankert, J., Zollinger, W. D., and Poolman, J. T. (1994) Lipo-oligosaccharide immunotyping of _Neisseria_

meningitidis by a whole-cell ELISA with monoclonal antibodies. *J. Med. Microbiol.* **41,** 236–243.

99. Jones, D. M., Borrow, R., Fox, A. J., Gray, S., Cartwright, K. A., and Poolman, J. T. (1992) The lipooligosaccharide immunotype as a virulence determinant in *Neisseria meningitidis. Microb. Pathog.* **13,** 219–224.

100. Zollinger, W. D. and Moran, E. (1991) Meningococcal vaccines—present and future. *Trans. R. Soc. Trop. Med. Hyg.* **85(Suppl. 1),** 37–43.

101. Estabrook, M., Mandrell, R. E., Apicella, M. A., and Griffiss, J. M. (1990) Measurement of the human response to meningococcal lipooligosaccharide antigens by using serum to inhibit monoclonal antibody binding to purified lipooligosaccharide. *Infect. Immun.* **58,** 2204–2213.

102. Pincus, S. H., Smith, M. J., Jennings, H. J., Burritt, J. B., and Glee, P. M. (1998) Peptides that mimic the group B streptococcal type III capsular polysaccharide antigen. *J. Immunol.* **160,** 293–298.

103. De, B. X, Laurent, T., Tibor, A., Godfroid, F., Weynants, V., Letesson, J. J., and Mertens, P. (1999) Antigenic properties of peptidic mimics for epitopes of the lipopolysaccharide from Brucella. *J. Mol. Biol.* **294,** 181–191.

104. Westerink, M. A. J., Giardina, P. C., Apicella, M. A., and Kieber-Emmons, T. (1995) Peptide mimicry of the meningococcal group C capsular polysaccharide. *Proc. Natl. Acad Sci. USA* **92,** 4021–4025.

105. Westerink, M. A., Giardina, P. C., Apicella, M. A., and Kieber-Emmons, T. (1995) Peptide mimicry of the meningococcal group C capsular polysaccharide. *Proc. Natl. Acad. Sci. USA* **92,** 4021–4025.

106. Grothaus, M. C., Srivastava, N., Smithson, S. L., Kieber-Emmons, T., Williams, D. B., Carlone, G. M., and Westerink, M. A. (2000) Selection of an immunogenic peptide mimic of the capsular polysaccharide of *Neisseria meningitidis* serogroup A using a peptide display library. *Vaccine* **18,** 1253–1263.

107. Moe, G. R., Tan, S., and Granoff, D. M. (1999) Molecular mimetics of polysaccharide epitopes as vaccine candidates for prevention of *Neisseria meningitidis* serogroup B disease. *FEMS Immunol. Med. Microbiol.* **26,** 209–226.

108. Gold, R., Goldschneider, I., Lepow, M. L., Draper, T. F., and Randolph, M. (1978) Carriage of *Neisseria meningitidis* and *Neisseria lactamica* in infants and children. *J. Infect. Dis.* **137,** 112–121.

109. Troncoso, G., Sanchez, S., Moreda, M., Criado, M. T., and Ferreiros, C. M. (2000) Antigenic cross-reactivity between outer membrane proteins of *Neisseria meningitidis* and commensal *Neisseria* species. *FEMS Immunol. Med. Microbiol.* **27,** 103–109.

110. Griffiss, J. M., Yamasaki, R., Estabrook, M., and Kim, J. J. (1991) Meningococcal molecular mimicry and the search for an ideal vaccine. *Trans. R. Soc. Trop. Med. Hyg.* **85(Suppl. 1),** 32–36.

111. Maslanka, S. E., Gheesling, L. L., Libutti, D. E., Donaldson, K. B., Harakeh, H. S., Dykes, J. K., et al. (1997) Standardization and a multilaboratory compari-

son of *Neisseria meningitidis* serogroup A and C serum bactericidal assays. The Multilaboratory Study Group. *Clin. Diagn. Lab. Immunol.* **4,** 156–167.

112. Goldschneider, I., Gotschlich, E. C., and Artenstein, M. S. (1969) Human immunity to the meningococcus. II. Development of natural immunity. *J. Exp. Med.* **129,** 1327–1348.

113. Cadieux, N., Plante, M., Rioux, C. R., Hamel, J., Brodeur, B. R., and Martin, D. (1999) Bactericidal and cross-protective activities of a monoclonal antibody directed against *Neisseria meningitidis* NspA outer membrane protein. *Infect. Immun.* **67,** 4955–4959.

114. Pintor, M., Gomez, J. A., Ferron, L., Ferreiros, C. M., and Criado, M. T. (1998) Analysis of TbpA and TbpB functionality in defective mutants of *Neisseria meningitidis. J. Med. Microbiol.* **47,** 757–760.

115. Ala'Aldeen, D. A., Davies, H. A., and Borriello, S. P. (1994) Vaccine potential of meningococcal FrpB: studies on surface exposure and functional attributes of common epitopes. *Vaccine* **12,** 535–541.

116. Christodoulides, M., Brooks, J. L., Rattue, E., and Heckels, J. E. (1998) Immunization with recombinant class 1 outer-membrane protein from *Neisseria meningitidis*: influence of liposomes and adjuvants on antibody avidity, recognition of native protein and the induction of a bactericidal immune response against meningococci. *Microbiology* **144,** 3027–3037.

117. Christodoulides, M. and Heckels, J. E. (1994) Immunization with a multiple antigen peptide containing defined B- and T-cell epitopes: production of bactericidal antibodies against group B *Neisseria meningitidis. Microbiology* **140,** 2951–2960.

118. Kizil, G., Todd, I., Atta, M., Borriello, S. P., Ait-Tahar, K., and Ala'Aldeen, D. A. (1999) Identification and characterization of TspA, a major CD4(+) T-cell- and B-cell-stimulating Neisseria-specific antigen. *Infect. Immun.* **67,** 3533–3541.

2

Immune Response and Host–Pathogen Interactions

Andrew J. Pollard and David Goldblatt

1. Introduction

For the most part, the relationship between the pathogen, *Neisseria meningitidis*, and humans is uneventful. Colonization of the human nasopharynx at various times during life is an almost universal experience but clinically overt disease is unusual except during epidemics. This overview considers the relationship between the meningococcus and humans, reviewing current immunological and molecular understanding of this interaction of relevance to development of immunogenic vaccines.

2. Mucosal Infection
2.1. Adhesion and Invasion

In non-epidemic situations, 10–25% of the general population are colonized in the nasopharynx by meningococci (*1*). Carriage may be intermittent or prolonged. During close contact with a colonized individual transmission of *N. meningitidis* to a susceptible recipient may occur. It has been suggested, at least in the case of children, that transmission is often from outside of the immediate family (*2*). Following transmission, probably by aerosol, to the nasopharynx of the recipient, the organism must adhere in order to avoid ingestion and destruction in the intestine. Adherence occurs through interaction between human epithelial cells and bacterial surface structures including pili (*3*), Opa, and Opc (*4*). Initial adherence is probably mediated by pili (*5*), and antigenic and phase variation in pilin, the subunit that forms pili, both affects the adhesiveness of the bacteria and is probably an immune-evasion mechanism (*5*). CD46 on the epithelial cell is one probable receptor for host-pathogen pilin interactions (*4,6*). Adhesion is increased by cell contact-

From: *Methods in Molecular Medicine, vol. 66: Meningococcal Vaccines: Methods and Protocols*
Edited by: A. J. Pollard and M. C. J. Maiden © Humana Press Inc., Totowa, NJ

dependent transcriptional upregulation of the PilC1 protein that is required for pilin assembly *(7)*. However, tighter adherence between the organism and the epithelial cell is mediated by the bacterial Class 5 outer-membrane proteins (OMPs) including Opa, which binds to the epithelial-cell membrane surface receptor, CD66 *(8)*. Another class 5 meningococcal OMP, Opc, is involved with adhesion of meningococci but is also critical for successful invasion of acaspulate organisms *(9)* via interaction with heparan sulphate proteoglycans *(10)* or integrins *(11)* on the epithelial cell surface. The polysaccharide capsule of *N. meningtidis* may interfere with these host-pathogen interactions, and it is likely that phase variation in capsule expression (by slipped-strand mispairing in the polsialyltransferase gene) facilitates adherence and invasion in vivo *(12)*.

Methods used in the study of interactions of meningococci with epithelia and endothelial cells are considered in "Meningococcal Disease," edited by A. J. Pollard and M. C. J. Maiden, *(12a)*. It appears that there are several bacterial-surface structures critical for adhesion to and invasion through the human nasopharyngeal mucosa. Such structures may be important constituents of future vaccines and induce mucosal immune responses.

2.2. Mucosal Immune Mechanisms and Their Avoidance

Various host factors provide some resistance to infection of the mucosa by *N. meningitidis*. Continuous washing of the nasopharyngeal mucosal surface by saliva and mucosal secretions probably plays an important role in reducing the opportunity for bacteria to adhere. Other nonspecific immune mechanisms, including the action of salivary enzymes and pH, may be of importance too. Specific immunity via immunoglobulin (Ig) A and other immunoglobulin classes can be measured in nasopharyngeal secretions and may be an important means of host defense *(13,14)*. However, pathogenic meningococci produce IgA1 proteases, which cleave IgA1, generating (Fab) 2 IgA fragments that block binding of complement-fixing antibodies *(15,16)*, although the significance of this and the anti-protease antibody that blocks its activity remains uncertain in vivo.

2.3. Other Nasopharyngeal Flora

Of likely importance in meningococcal colonization of the human nasopharynx is the presence of competing, commensal flora, notably *Neisseria lactamica*. *N. lactamica* colonizes the nasopharynx in over 20% of children at 18 mo *(1)* and over 90% of 12–18-yr-olds have bactericidal antibody to this organism in the UK *(17)*. Conversely, colonization by pathogenic Neisseria at this age is uncommon with <0.71% of children under 4 yr of age carrying *N. meningitidis (1)*.

2.4. Host Genetic Susceptibility

Genetic variation in the host, particularly in the genes encoding receptors involved in bacterial adhesion and invasion, may play an important role in determining the success of this human-bacterial interaction. Few data are available concerning these host susceptibility factors. Meningococcal disease is more common in nonsecretors of the ABO blood-group antigens (*18*) and these individuals also produce lower levels of IgM in their nasopharyngeal secretions (*18*).

2.5. Integrity of the Mucosal Barrier and Disease

The observation of an association between recent influenza infection and invasive meningococcal disease and the increased risk of meningococcal disease and carriage associated with exposure to tobacco smoke (*19*) both suggest that the integrity of the mucosal surface is important in resisting colonization and invasion by meningococci. Recent data suggest that the charge and hydrophobicity of the mucosa are affected by exposure to tobacco smoke and that this in turn increases bacterial adhesion (*20*).

Following invasion into the epithelial cell, capsulate organisms appear to be enclosed in large vacuoles and acapsulate bacteria are found within membrane-bound vesicles (*21*). The bacteria translocate through the mucosa and some traverse the endothelium into the blood.

3. Bacteraemia

Both during invasion through the mucosa and when meningococci gain access to the blood, there are a number of host-immune mechanisms to be overcome. In the immunologically-naïve individual, innate immune mechanisms provide defense for the host. Various bacterial virulence factors resist these host immunologic mechanisms. Methods for measuring opsonophagocytosis (*see* **Chapter 23**) are considered and methods for measuring specific antibody (*see* **Chapters 18** and **19**) or measuring functional antibody levels (*see* **Chapters 20** and **21**) are described in this volume.

3.1. Phagocytosis

The relative contribution of phagocytes to natural immunity to meningococci in healthy individuals is unknown. The polysaccharide capsule of the meningococcus is antiphagocytic and resists this immune mechanism. Nonopsonic phagocytosis of bacteria probably occurs in the tissues or circulation through the interaction of bacteria with phagocyte pattern-recognition receptors such as macrophage mannose receptor, macrophage scavenger receptor, CD14 (which recognizes lipopolysaccharide; LPS), and complement receptor-3 (CR3). Non-opsonic phagocyte interactions may be directed at Opa and Opc on the bacterial surface, through receptors such as CD66, which is known to the host receptor for bacterial Opa *(8)*. However, such interactions may be inhibited by sialylation of surface polysaccharide *(22,23)*. Nonspecific serum opsonins, including complement- and mannan-binding lectin, are important in enhancing phagocytosis. Opsonophagocytosis by specific antibody is also likely to be an important immunologic mechanism for host defense, particularly for serogroup B meningococci *(24)*. For serogroup A and Y meningococci, anticapsular polysaccharide antibodies enhance phagocytosis in vitro *(25)* and opsonic antibody, which seems to be directed at conserved regions, is also generated against other surface structures after infection *(26)*.

Opsonized bacteria are probably removed from the circulation by splenic phagocytes, because asplenia and splenectomy are risk factors for disease *(27,28)*.

3.2. Complement-Mediated Bacteriolysis

The role of complement in protection against infection with *N. meningitidis* is reviewed in some detail in "Meningococcal Disease," edited by A. J. Pollard and M.C.J. Maiden *(12a)*. Presence of complement-fixing antibody in the blood correlates with immunity to serogroup A and C meningococci and induction of such antibodies is the goal of vaccination. In immunization studies, serum bactericidal antibody is measured as an in vitro correlate of immunity. Complement may be directly deposited on the bacterial surface or deposited following activation by Mannan Binding Lectin (MBL)-associated serine proteases, leading to the formation of the membrane-attack complex and lysis of the organism. However, antipolysaccharide-capsule specific complement-binding antibody is believed to be the primary acquired immune mechanism that protects against the non-B serogroups of meningococci. The presence of in vitro serum bactericidal activity against serogroups A, B, and C is inversely correlated with the age-related incidence of disease *(29)*. Moreover, presence of anti group A or C serum bactericidal antibody in blood protects against disease during an outbreak *(30–33)*, providing compelling evidence that anticapsular antibodies are important in host defense. Indeed, *complement* is essential for the protection afforded by specific antibody as witnessed by the increased risk of disease in individuals with complement deficiency *(34)*, who nevertheless may have adequate levels of specific antibody. Antibody is required, as shown by the increased risk of disease in individuals with hypogammaglobulinaemia *(35,36)*. It seems necessary that this antibody should bind the bacteria with high avidity to facilitate complement-mediated lysis of all serogroups of meningococci *(37,38)*.

For serogroup B meningococci, the polysaccharide covering of the organism does not seem to be an important target for antibody-mediated bacteriolysis because the capsule of this organism is both poorly immunogenic (so there are low antibody titers) *(39)* and resists complement deposition *(40,41)*. Although often assumed, it is not clear if bactericidal antibody directed against other outer-membrane structures contributes significantly to natural immunity to serogroup B meningococci, although in vitro most bactericidal activity seems to be directed at noncapsular antigens *(42)*. However, the presence of hypermutable regions in the genes encoding the surface exposed sequences of these antigens (*see* **Subheading 5.2.2.**) suggests that meningococci have evolved means of evading this host-immune mechanism, and further suggesting that these antibodies exert evolutionary pressure on the bacteria. Indeed, there are likely to be a number of genes expressed following entry into the blood that enable metabolic adaptation and may be targets for antibody.

In addition to complement deficiency and deficiency of MBL *(43)*, which enhances susceptibility to meningococcal infection, there are probably several more subtle polymorphisms in the genes encoding the effector mechanisms of the immune response to meningococci that increase susceptibility. For example, CD32 (FcγRIIa) polymorphisms are found more commonly in children with meningococcal disease *(44)* and a combination of FcγRIIa and FcγRIIIb polymorphisms are associated with an increased risk of meningococcal disease in individuals with a late complement component deficiency *(45)*.

3.3. The Endothelium and the Inflammatory Response

During growth in the blood, meningococci, in common with other Gram-negative bacteria, shed LPS-containing blebs of outer membrane. These blebs contain a full complement of meningococcal surface exposed structures and might act as a decoy for the host-immunologic defenses. Proliferation of meningococci in the blood lead to endothelial activation *(46,47)* and LPS activates the inflammatory cascade following binding to CD14 on macrophages. In turn, inflammatory mediators are released by the macrophage (including those resident in the spleen and liver), inducing a range of downstream effects that culminate in shock. However, because bacteraemia is possible in the absense of shock (indeed, this is the more usual situation), it seems likely that there is a dose-dependent relationship between the amount of LPS in the circulation and the inflammatory response. Support for this comes from the observation that the number of bacteria in the blood *(48,49)* and the concentration of LPS in the blood *(50,51)* correlates with the severity of disease. Thus, in individuals with mild disease, bacteria may be present at <1–240 cfu/mL *(52)* and in severe disease levels from 5×10^2–10^5 cfu/mL have been recorded *(51–53)*.

Methods for studying interactions of meningococci with endothelia are described in Chapter 38 in "Meningococcal Disease," edited by A. J. Pollard and M. C. J. Maiden *(12a)*.

4. Central Nervous System Infection

Invasion from the blood to the central nervous system (CNS), or to other sites following bacteraemia, is thought to follow pilus-mediated adhesion to the endothelium *(54,55)*. Expression of PilC may be an important factor in this interaction *(55,56)* and invasion of endothelial cells may be enhanced by Opc expression *(9,11)*. It is not certain how or where the meningococci cross the blood-brain barrier (BBB) and enter the CNS. This subject is discussed in more detail in "Meningococcal Disease," edited by A. J. Pollard and M. C. J. Maiden, drawing on data from in vivo and in vitro models *(12a)*. After invasion through the endothelium, meningococci gain access to the sub-arachnoid space, probably via the choroid plexus. In the CSF meningococci proliferate, shed LPS *(57)* and induce the release of pro- and anti-inflammatory cytokines *(58–60)*.

5. The Host-Immune Response

Previously we have considered the innate and acquired immune-effector mechanisms that must engage the meningococci during infection. It remains unclear how the different effector mechanisms relate to one another in importance for the host, although it seems certain that high-avidity, complement-binding antibody directed at the polysaccharide capsule is the most effective mechanism for non-serogroup B organisms. It is likely that opsonophagocytosis and innate immune mechansims also play a role.

5.1. Acquisition of Immunity

Antimeningococcal-specific immunity develops during childhood and there is thus likely to be variation in the importance of different effector mechanisms dependent on the age of the child. Immunity is almost certainly acquired through exposure to related Neisseria *(61,62)* and other bacteria in the gut and nasopharynx whose antigenic constituents cross-react with those of *N. meningitidis (26,63–65)*, inducing and boosting immune responses *(66)*. In the newborn, disease is rare as a result of placental transfer of maternal antibody, providing passive protection through opsonization or bacteriolysis *(29)*. The peak incidence in most industrialized countries of disease occurs between the ages of 6 mo to 2 yr. For children in this age group, susceptibility to disease is the consequence of a number of factors, including the loss of maternal antibody, the inability of young children to respond to pure polysaccharide antigens, and insufficient opportunity for immunity to develop through exposure to antigenic stimuli from related species. During this time, innate immune mechanisms may be central to protection including non-opsonic phagocytosis, opsonic phagocytosis with nonspecific opsonins (such as complement and MBL), and direct bacteriolysis following deposition of complement on the bacterial surface.

As a result of exposure to related bacteria during childhood, adult levels of antibody are reached in the second decade and are able to mediate opsonophagocytosis and antibody-directed, complement-mediated bacteriolysis. A comprehensive array of acquired and innate immune mechanisms is thus active from early adulthood, and the incidence of disease is lowered considerably.

5.2. Specificity of Antibody

5.2.1. Polysaccharide

As mentioned earlier, the specificity of antibody in vivo that it responsible for acquired immunity is unknown, although it is likely that the most effective protection for non-group B organisms following vaccination resides in anticapsular polysaccharide, complement-binding IgG. Antibody responses to the majority of pure polysaccharides (with *N. meningitidis* an important exception) are known to be age dependent and are designated T-independent, as T-lymphocytes are not required or ordinarily involved in induction of immune responses directed against them *(67)*. T-independent responses are age dependent (not usually seen in those under 18 mo) and do not result in the generation of memory. Conjugation of capsular polysaccharides can overcome the nonresponsiveness of young infants to polysaccharide antigens and can induce memory *(67)*.

The immune response to capsular polysaccharide when encountered on the surface of organisms in vivo is not as well-characterized as the response to pure polysaccharides when used as vaccine antigens. Recent data from studies on the naturally acquired immune response to the capsular polysaccharide of *Haemophilus influenzae* type b and pneumococcus would suggest that such antibodies are induced by a T-dependent mechanism *(68,69)*. Thus the observed rise in antibody titers in older children and adults following vaccination with plain meningococcal polysaccharide *(70)*, probably represent secondary immune responses following the induction of memory brought about by natural exposure to capsular polysaccharides cross-linked to other meningococcal surface structures.

The delay in the acquisition of naturally induced meningococcal anticapsular polysaccharide antibodies in those under 2 yr of age may thus be a general manifestation of the immaturity of the developing immune system.

Repeated dosing with meningococcal serogroup C vaccines induces hyporesponsiveness as measured by antibody titers *(70,71)*. Plain polysaccharide may induce terminal differentiation of polysaccharide-specific B cells, without generation of new memory B cells. Repeated dosing could deplete the polysaccharide-specific B-cell pool leading to a diminishing antibody response until a further conjugate stimulus generates new memory cells and boosts the immune response *(72)*. Conversely, A/C conjugate vaccines generate immunologic memory and boosting of antibody levels with subsequent doses *(70)* and can also overcome the hyporesponsiveness induced by prior administration of plain A/C polysaccharide *(73)*.

The quality of antibody induced following natural exposure or vaccination may vary depending on a number of factors, including the age of the individual being studied and the type of vaccine administered. The measurement of such qualitative aspects of antibody function is increasingly being recognized as an important component of such studies. The discrepancy between the level of antibody induced by plain meningococcal C polysaccharides vaccine (as measured by enzyme-linked immunosorbent assay ELISA) and antibody function as measured by a bactericidal activity has led to modifications of the ELISA as described in Chapter 21. The improvement in correlation between ELISA and bactericidal activity is most likely owing to restricting the ELISA to the measurement of higher avidity, and by implication more functional, antibody. Antibody responses to conjugate vaccines are, by virtue of the T-cell help induced, of higher avidity and thus modifications to the standard ELISA in the context of sera from conjugate vaccine recipients are probably not required. In addition to the correlation between avidity and function, antibody avidity has recently been used as a surrogate marker for the successful generation of memory following conjugate vaccination *(74)*. Owing to the T-cell help recruited by the glycoconjugate vaccines, antibody avidity increases in the naïve recipient in the weeks and months following vaccination and this can be measured by a modified ELISA. After a single dose of Men C Conjugate vaccine, avidity has been noted to increase, suggesting that a single dose is sufficient to induce immunological memory *(75)*.

The polysaccharide capsule of meningococci is highly conserved between strains, with only A, B, C, Y, and W135 polysaccharides being commonly associated with disease and providing the possibility of inclusion of a limited number of antigens in a broadly protective vaccine. Such a vaccine based on the plain polysaccharides of serogroup A, C, Y, and W135 is widely used for protection of travelers and in outbreak control *(76,77)*. Serogroup C conjugate vaccines have been recently introduced in the UK, and appear effective against this serogroup *(78)*. A combination conjugate A, C, Y, and W135 vaccine is likely to be available within the next few years. Unfortunately, serogroup B polysaccharide is poorly immunogenic, and no vaccines have yet been produced that have successfully provided protection against disease in humans using this bacterial product. Chemical modification of the serogroup B polysaccharide is being studied as a means of overcoming the immunogenicity problems described earlier *(79)* although the structural homology between B capsular polysaccharide and human neural-cell adhesion molecule (NCAM) *(80)* raises concerns about this approach. Development of a vaccine against serogroup B meningococci is mainly directed at noncapsular antigens and it is likely that these are also the targets of the natural immune response to this organism. Antibody directed against noncapsular antigens of other serogroups are also present in sera of adults or after infection, but their role in defense against disease caused by these organisms in contrast to that of polysaccharide is unknown.

5.2.2. Noncapsular Antigens

Noncapsular antigens are also targets of the antibody response following colonization, infection, or vaccination. It seems unlikely that natural acquired immunity to meningococci resides in opsonic or complement-binding antibody directed against a single antigen or epitope. Specific immunity in older children and adults probably results from the combined effect of antibody directed against a variety of antigens on the meningococcal surface. Indeed, antibody directed at PorA *(81)*, PorB *(82)*, Class 5 proteins *(83)*, lipopolysaccharide *(84)*, IgA1 protease *(85)*, neisserial surface protein A *(86)*, transferrin-binding proteins *(87)*, H.8 *(88)*, ferric-binding proteins *(89)*, and lactoferrin-binding protein A *(90)* have all been documented following infection. Methods for analysis of B-cell epitopes on these proteins are considered in Chapter 26. Unfortunately, the relative importance of each of these outer-membrane components in directing immune responses via opsonization or complement-mediated bacteriolysis is unclear. The availability of the meningococcal genome will introduce many more candidates to be considered as targets for natural immunity and vaccine development in the future.

5.3. T-Cell Immune Responses

T cells are important in providing help for antibody production in the generation of specific immunity against meningococci. In vitro T-cell proliferative responses (*see* Chapter 24) to PorA, Opa, Opc, and outer-membrane vesicles (OMVs) have been documented in normal adults *(91)* and after vaccination *(92,93)* or infection *(94)*. T-cell epitopes for PorA and Por B proteins appear to be in highly conserved regions of these porin proteins *(95–97)*. T-cell epitope mapping is described in Chapter 25. The pattern of cytokines produced by T cells following meningococcal infection or colonization *(94)* may be important in directing maturation of the antibody response and age-dependent differences in T-cell responses or their interactions with B cells could be responsible for the low-avidity antibody observed in young children *(37)*.

6. Conclusion

The nature of the human immune response to *N. meningitidis* has been evaluated in vitro and through epidemiologic observation, but the relative contribution of various immunologic factors to natural immunity to this organism remains incompletely understood. The chapters in this book provide the tools for the further investigation of these fundamental issues relevant to a better understanding of meningococcal pathophysiology. A better understanding of these will allow more rational development of not only better therapeutic strategies but also better vaccine design. Antibodies to the non-B serogroup meningococci have been proven be critical for protection and polysaccharide vaccines are able to induce this in the short term. With protein-polysaccharide conjugate vaccines for serogroup C meningococci available, and others on the horizon, the potential to provide life-long protection is tantalizingly in our grasp. For serogroup B meningococci, further evaluation of the nature of natural immunity and the immunogencity of noncapsular surface antibodies may hold the key to developing a protective vaccine directed against all disease-associated serogroups of meningococci. It is here that postgenomic science is likely to make a major contribution.

References

1. Gold, R., Goldschneider, I., Lepow, M. L., Draper, T. F., and Randolph, M. (1978) Carriage of Neisseria meningitidis and Neisseria lactamica in infants and children. *J. Infect. Dis.* **137,** 112–121.
2. Cartwright, K. A., Stuart, J. M., and Robinson, P. M. (1991) Meningococcal carriage in close contacts of cases. *Epidemiol. Infect.* **106,** 133–141.
3. Virji, M., Alexandrescu, C., Ferguson, D. J., Saunders, J. R., and Moxon, E. R. (1992) Variations in the expression of pili: the effect on adherence of Neisseria meningitidis to human epithelial and endothelial cells. *Mol. Microbiol.* **6,** 1271–1279.
4. Dehio, C., Gray-Owen, S. D., and Meyer, T. F. (2000) Host cell invasion by pathogenic Neisseriae. *Subcell. Biochem.* **33,** 61–96.
5. Nassif, X., Lowy, J., Stenberg, P., O'Gaora, P., Ganji, A., and So, M. (1993) Antigenic variation of pilin regulates adhesion of Neisseria meningitidis to human epithelial cells. *Mol. Microbiol.* **8,** 719–725.

6. Kallstrom, H., Islam, M. S., Berggren, P. O., and Jonsson, A. B. (1998) Cell signaling by the type IV pili of pathogenic Neisseria. *J. Biol. Chem.* **273,** 21,777–21,782.
7. Taha, M. K., Morand, P. C., Pereira, Y., Eugene, E., Giorgini, D., Larribe, M., and Nassif, X. (1998) Pilus-mediated adhesion of Neisseria meningitidis: the essential role of cell contact-dependent transcriptional upregulation of the PilC1 protein. *Mol. Microbiol.* **28,** 1153–1163.
8. Virji, M., Makepeace, K., Ferguson, D. J., and Watt, S. M. (1996) Carcinoembryonic antigens (CD66) on epithelial cells and neutrophils are receptors for Opa proteins of pathogenic neisseriae. *Mol. Microbiol.* **22,** 941–950.
9. Virji, M., Makepeace, K., Ferguson, D. J., Achtman, M., Sarkari, J., and Moxon, E. R. (1992) Expression of the Opc protein correlates with invasion of epithelial and endothelial cells by Neisseria meningitidis. *Mol. Microbiol.* **6,** 2785–2795.
10. de Vries, F. P., Cole, R., Dankert, J., Frosch, M., and van Putten, J. P. (1998) Neisseria meningitidis producing the Opc adhesin binds epithelial cell proteoglycan receptors. *Mol. Microbiol.* **27,** 1203–1212.
11. Virji, M., Makepeace, K., and Moxon, E. R. (1994) Distinct mechanisms of interactions of Opc-expressing meningococci at apical and basolateral surfaces of human endothelial cells; the role of integrins in apical interactions. *Mol. Microbiol.* **14,** 173–184.
12. Hammerschmidt, S., Muller, A., Sillmann, H., Muhlenhoff, M., Borrow, R., Fox, A., et al. (1996) Capsule phase variation in Neisseria meningitidis serogroup B by slipped-strand mispairing in the polysialyltransferase gene (siaD): correlation with bacterial invasion and the outbreak of meningococcal disease. *Mol. Microbiol.* **20,** 1211–1220.
12a. Pollard, A. J. and Maiher, M. C. J., eds. (2001) *Meningococcal Disease*, Humana Press, Totowa, NJ.
13. Brandtzæg, P. (1992) Humoral immune response patterns of human mucosae: induction and relation to bacterial respiratory tract infections. *J. Infect. Dis.* **165(Suppl. 1),** S167–S176.
14. Hamadeh, R. M., Galili, U., Zhou, P., and Griffiss, J. M. (1995) Anti-alpha-galactosyl immunoglobulin A (IgA), IgG, and IgM in human secretions. *Clin. Diagn. Lab. Immunol.* **2,** 125–131.
15. Jarvis, G. A. and Griffiss, J. M. (1991) Human IgA1 blockade of IgG-initiated lysis of Neisseria meningitidis is a function of antigen-binding fragment binding to the polysaccharide capsule. *J. Immunol.* **147,** 1962–1967.
16. Kobayashi, K., Fujiyama, Y., Hagiwara, K., and Kondoh, H. (1987) Resistance of normal serum IgA and secretory IgA to bacterial IgA proteases: evidence for the presence of enzyme-neutralizing antibodies in both serum and secretory IgA, and also in serum IgG. *Microbiol. Immunol.* **31,** 1097–1106.
17. Zorgani, A. A., James, V. S., Stewart, J., Blackwell, C. C., Elton, R. A., and Weir, D. M. (1996) Serum bactericidal activity in a secondary school population fol-

lowing an outbreak of meningococcal disease: effects of carriage and secretor status. *FEMS Immunol. Med. Microbiol.* **14,** 73–81.

18. Zorgani, A. A., Stewart, J., Blackwell, C. C., Elton, R. A., and Weir, D. M. (1992) Secretor status and humoral immune responses to Neisseria lactamica and Neisseria meningitidis. *Epidemiol. Infect.* **109,** 445–452.

19. Stuart, J. M., Cartwright, K. A., Robinson, P. M., and Noah, N. D. (1989) Effect of smoking on meningococcal carriage. *Lancet* **2,** 723–725.

20. El Ahmer, O. R., Essery, S. D., Saadi, A. T., Raza, M. W., Ogilvie, M. M., Weir, D. M., and Blackwell, C. C. (1999) The effect of cigarette smoke on adherence of respiratory pathogens to buccal epithelial cells. *FEMS Immunol. Med. Microbiol.* **23,** 27–36.

21. Stephens, D. S., Hoffman, L. H., and McGee, Z. A. (1983) Interaction of Neisseria meningitidis with human nasopharyngeal mucosa: attachment and entry into columnar epithelial cells. *J. Infect. Dis.* **148,** 369–376.

22. Estabrook, M. M., Zhou, D., and Apicella, M. A. (1998) Nonopsonic phagocytosis of group C Neisseria meningitidis by human neutrophils. *Infect. Immun.* **66,** 1028–1036.

23. McNeil, G. and Virji, M. (1997) Phenotypic variants of meningococci and their potential in phagocytic interactions: the influence of opacity proteins, pili, PilC and surface sialic acids. *Microb. Pathol.* **22,** 295–304.

24. Ross, S. C., Rosenthal, P. J., Berberich, H. M., and Densen, P. (1987) Killing of Neisseria meningitidis by human neutrophils: implications for normal and complement-deficient individuals. *J. Infect. Dis.* **155,** 1266–1275.

25. Roberts, R. B. (1967) The interaction in vitro between group B meningococci and rabbit polymorphonuclear leukocytes. Demonstration of type specific opsonins and bactericidins. *J. Exp. Med.* **126,** 795–818.

26. Guttormsen, H. K., Bjerknes, R., Næss, A., Lehmann, V., Halstensen, A., Sørnes, S., and Solberg, C. O. (1992) Cross-reacting serum opsonins in patients with meningococcal disease. *Infect. Immun.* **60,** 2777–2783.

27. Styrt, B. (1990) Infection associated with asplenia: risks, mechanisms, and prevention. *Am. J. Med.* **88,** 33N–42N.

28. Ellison, E. C. and Fabri, P. J. (1983) Complications of splenectomy. Etiology, prevention and management. *Surg. Clin. North Am.* **63,** 1313–1330.

29. Goldschneider, I., Gotschlich, E. C., and Artenstein, M.S. (1969) Human immunity to the meningococcus. I. The role of humoral antibodies. *J. Exp. Med.* **129,** 1307–1326.

30. Wahdan, M. H., Sallam, S. A., Hassan, M. N., Abdel Gawad, A., Rakha, A. S., Sippel, J. E., et al. (1977) A second controlled field trial of a serogroup A meningococcal polysaccharide vaccine in Alexandria. *Bull. WHO* **55,** 645–651.

31. Peltola, H., Mäkelä, H., Käyhty, H., Jousimies, H., Herva, E., Hallstrom, K., et al. (1977) Clinical efficacy of meningococcus group A capsular polysaccharide vaccine in children three months to five years of age. *N. Engl. J. Med.* **297,** 686–691.

32. Amato Neto, V., Finger, H., Gotschlich, E. C., Feldman, R. A., de Avila, C. A., Konichi, S. R., and Laus, W. C. (1974) Serologic response to serogroup C menin-

gococcal vaccine in Brazilian preschool children. *Rev. Inst. Med. Trop. Sao Paulo* **16,** 149–153.

33. Goldschneider, I., Gotschlich, E. C., and Artenstein, M. S. (1969) Human immunity to the meningococcus. II. Development of natural immunity. *J. Exp. Med.* **129,** 1327–1348.

34. Nicholson, A. and Lepow, I. H. (1979) Host defense against Neisseria meningitidis requires a complement-dependent bactericidal activity. *Science* **205,** 298–289.

35. Salit, I. E. (1981) Meningococcemia caused by serogroup W135. Association with hypogammaglobulinemia. *Arch. Intern. Med.* **141,** 664–665.

36. Hobbs, J. R., Milner, R. D., and Watt, P. J. (1967) Gamma-M deficiency predisposing to meningococcal septicaemia. *BMJ* **4,** 583–586.

37. Pollard, A. J. and Levin, M. (2000) Production of low-avidity antibody by infants after infection with serogroup B meningococci. *Lancet* **356,** 2065–2066.

38. Granoff, D. M., Maslanka, S. E., Carlone, G. M., Plikaytis, B. D., Santos, G. F., Mokatrin, A., and Raff, H. V. (1998) A modified enzyme-linked immunosorbent assay for measurement of antibody responses to meningococcal C polysaccharide that correlate with bactericidal responses. *Clin. Diagn. Lab. Immunol.* **5,** 479–485.

39. Finne, J., Bitter-Suermann, D., Goridis, C., and Finne, U. (1987) An IgG monoclonal antibody to group B meningococci cross-reacts with developmentally regulated polysialic acid units of glycoproteins in neural and extraneural tissues. *J. Immunol.* **138,** 4402–4407.

40. Jarvis, G. A. and Vedros, N. A. (1987) Sialic acid of group B Neisseria meningitidis regulates alternative complement pathway activation. *Infect. Immun.* **55,** 174–180.

41. Hammerschmidt, S., Birkholz, C., Zahringer, U., Robertson, B. D., van Putten, J., Ebeling, O., and Frosch, M. (1994) Contribution of genes from the capsule gene complex (cps) to lipooligosaccharide biosynthesis and serum resistance in Neisseria meningitidis. *Mol. Microbiol.* **11,** 885–896.

42. Zollinger, W. D. and Mandrell, R. E. (1983) Importance of complement source in bactericidal activity of human antibody and murine monoclonal antibody to meningococcal group B polysaccharide. *Infect. Immun.* **40,** 257–264.

43. Bax, W. A., Cluysenaer, O. J. J., Bartelink, A. K. M., Aerts, P., Ezekowitz, R. A. B., and Van Dyk, H. (1999) *Familiar Deficiency of Mannose-Binding Lectin Predisposing to Meningococcal Disease.* American Society for Microbiology, San Francisco, pp. 401.

44. Bredius, R. G., Derkx, B. H., Fijen, C. A., de Wit, T. P., de Haas, M., Weening, R. S., et al. (1994) Fc gamma receptor IIa (CD32) polymorphism in fulminant meningococcal septic shock in children. *J. Infect. Dis.* **170,** 848–853.

45. Fijen, C. A., Bredius, R. G., Kuijper, E. J., Out, T. A., De Haas, M., De Wit, A. P., et al. (2000) The role of Fcgamma receptor polymorphisms and C3 in the immune defence against Neisseria meningitidis in complement-deficient individuals. *Clin. Exp. Immunol.* **120,** 338–345.

46. Baines, P. B., Marzouk, O., Thomson, A. P., Sills, J. A., Riordan, F. A., and Hart, C. A. (1999) Endothelial cell adhesion molecules in meningococcal disease. *Arch. Dis. Child.* **80,** 74–76.

47. Heyderman, R. S., Klein, N. J., Daramola, O. A., Hammerschmidt, S., Frosch, M., Robertson, B. D., et al. (1997) Induction of human endothelial tissue factor expression by Neisseria meningitidis: the influence of bacterial killing and adherence to the endothelium. *Microb. Pathol.* **22,** 265–274.

48. La Scolea, L. J., Jr., Dryja, D., Sullivan, T. D., Mosovich, L., Ellerstein, N., and Neter, E. (1981) Diagnosis of bacteremia in children by quantitative direct plating and a radiometric procedure. *J. Clin. Microbiol.* **13,** 478–482.

49. La Scolea, L. J., Jr. and Dryja, D. (1984) Quantitation of bacteria in cerebrospinal fluid and blood of children with meningitis and its diagnostic significance. *J. Clin. Microbiol.* **19,** 187–190.

50. Brandtzæg, P., Sandset, P. M., Joo, G. B., Øvstebø, R., Abildgaard, U., and Kierulf, P. (1989) The quantitative association of plasma endotoxin, antithrombin, protein C, extrinsic pathway inhibitor and fibrinopeptide A in systemic meningococcal disease. *Thromb. Res.* **55,** 459–470.

51. Zwahlen, A. and Waldvogel, F. A. (1984) Magnitude of bacteremia and complement activation during Neisseria meningitidis infection: study of two co-primary cases with different clinical presentations. *Eur. J. Clin. Microbiol.* **3,** 439–441.

52. Brandtzæg, P., Kierulf, P., Gaustad, P., Skulberg, A., Bruun, J. N., Halvorsen, S., and Sørensen, E. (1989) Plasma endotoxin as a predictor of multiple organ failure and death in systemic meningococcal disease. *J. Infect. Dis.* **159,** 195–204.

53. Sullivan, T. D. and LaScolea, L. J., Jr. (1987) Neisseria meningitidis bacteremia in children: quantitation of bacteremia and spontaneous clinical recovery without antibiotic therapy. *Pediatrics* **80,** 63–67.

54. Virji, M., Käyhty, H., Ferguson, D. J., Alexandrescu, C., Heckels, J. E., and Moxon, E. R. (1991) The role of pili in the interactions of pathogenic Neisseria with cultured human endothelial cells. *Mol. Microbiol.* **5,** 1831–1841.

55. Pron, B., Taha, M. K., Rambaud, C., Fournet, J. C., Pattey, N., Monnet, J. P., et al. (1997) Interaction of Neisseria maningitidis with the components of the blood-brain barrier correlates with an increased expression of PilC. *J. Infect. Dis.* **176,** 1285–1292.

56. Virji, M., Makepeace, K., Peak, I., Payne, G., Saunders, J. R., Ferguson, D. J., and Moxon, E. R. (1995) Functional implications of the expression of PilC proteins in meningococci. *Mol. Microbiol.* **16,** 1087–1097.

57. Brandtzæg, P., Ovsteboo, R., and Kierulf, P. (1992) Compartmentalization of lipopolysaccharide production correlates with clinical presentation in meningococcal disease. *J. Infect. Dis.* **166,** 650–652.

58. van Furth, A. M., Seijmonsbergen, E. M., Langermans, J. A., Groeneveld, P. H., de Bel, C. E., and van Furth, R. (1995) High levels of interleukin 10 and tumor necrosis factor alpha in cerebrospinal fluid during the onset of bacterial meningitis. *Clin. Infect. Dis.* **21,** 220–222.

59. Rusconi, F., Parizzi, F., Garlaschi, L., Assael, B. M., Sironi, M., Ghezzi, P., and Mantovani, A. (1991) Interleukin 6 activity in infants and children with bacterial

meningitis. The Collaborative Study on Meningitis. *Pediatr. Infect. Dis. J.* **10,** 117–121.

60. van Deuren, M., van der Ven-Jongekrijg, J., Bartelink, A. K., van Dalen, R., Sauerwein, R. W., and van der Meer, J. W. (1995) Correlation between proinflammatory cytokines and antiinflammatory mediators and the severity of disease in meningococcal infections. *J. Infect. Dis.* **172,** 433–439.

61. Mitchell, M. S., Rhoden, D. L., and King, E. O. (1965) Lactose fermenting organisms resembling Neisseria meningitidis. *J. Bacteriol.* **90,** 560.

62. Hollis, D. G., Wiggins, G. L., Weaver, R. E., and Schubert, J. H. (1970) Current status of lactose-fermenting Neisseria. *Ann. NY Acad. Sci.* **174,** 444–449.

63. Hoff, G. E. and Høiby, N. (1978) Cross-reactions between Neisseria meningitidis and twenty-seven other bacterial species. *Acta. Pathol. Microbiol. Scand.* **86,** 87–92.

64. Glode, M. P., Robbins, J. B., Liu, T. Y., Gotschlich, E. C., Orskov, I., and Orskov, F. (1977) Cross-antigenicity and immunogenicity between capsular polysaccharides of group C Neisseria meningitidis and of Escherichia coli K92. *J. Infect. Dis.* **135,** 94–104.

65. Grados, O. and Ewing, W. H. (1970) Antigenic relationship between Escherichia coli and Neisseria meningitidis. *J. Infect. Dis.* **122,** 100–103.

66. Reller, L. B., MacGregor, R. R., and Beaty, H. N. (1973) Bactericidal antibody after colonization with Neisseria meningitidis. *J. Infect. Dis.* **127,** 56–62.

67. Mond, J. J., Vos, Q., Lees, A., and Snapper, C. M. (1995) T cell independent antigens. *Curr. Opin. Immunol.* **7,** 349–354.

68. Hougs, L., Juul, L., Ditzel, H. J., Heilmann, C., Svejgaard, A., and Barington, T. (1999) The first dose of a Haemophilus influenzae type b conjugate vaccine reactivates memory B cells: evidence for extensive clonal selection, intraclonal affinity maturation, and multiple isotype switches to IgA2. *J. Immunol.* **162,** 224–237.

69. Baxendale, H. E., Davis, Z., White, H. N., Spellerberg, M. B., Stevenson, F. K., and Goldblatt, D. (2000) Immunogenetic analysis of the immune response to pneumococcal polysaccharide. *Eur. J. Immunol.* **30,** 1214–1223.

70. MacLennan, J., Obaro, S., Deeks, J., Williams, D., Pais, L., Carlone, G., Moxon, R., and Greenwood, B. (1999) Immune response to revaccination with meningococcal A and C polysaccharides in Gambian children following repeated immunisation during early childhood. *Vaccine* **17,** 3086–3093.

71. Gold, R., Lepow, M. L., Goldschneider, I., and Gotschlich, E. C. (1977) Immune response of human infants of polysaccharide vaccines of group A and C Neisseria meningitidis. *J. Infect. Dis.* **136(Suppl.),** S31–S35.

72. Maclennan, J. M., Deeks, J. J., Obaro, S., Williams, D., Carlone, G. M., Moxon, E. R., and Greenwood, B. M. (1998) Meningococcal serogroup C conjugate vaccination in infancy induces persistent immunological memory. In: Eleventh International Pathogenic Neisseria Conference, Nice, Nassif, X., Quentin-Millet, M.-J., and Taha, M.-K. (eds.). EDK, Paris, Nice, France, pp. 151.

73. Borrow, R., Goldblatt, D., Andrews, N., Richmond, P., and Miller, E. (2000) Influence of prior meningococcal C polysaccharide vaccine on response to meningococcal C conjugate vaccine in infants. ICAAC, Toronto 2000 (Abstract).
74. Goldblatt, D., Vaz, A. R., and Miller, E. (1998) Antibody avidity as a surrogate marker of successful priming by Haemophilus influenzae type b conjugate vaccines following infant immunization. *J. Infect. Dis.* **177,** 1112–1115.
75. Richmond, P., Borrow, R., Goldblatt, D., Findlow, J., Martin, S. R. M., Cartwright, K., and Miller, E. (2000) Ability of three different meningococcal C conjugate vaccines to induce immunological memory after a single dose in UK toddlers. *J. Infect. Dis.* **183,** 160–163.
76. Anonymous (1996) Meningococcal, in *Immunisation Against Infectious Disease* (Salisbury, D. M. and Begg, N. T., eds.), HMSO, London, pp. 147–154.
77. Anonymous (1997) Control and prevention of meningococcal disease: recommendations of the Advisory Committee on Immunization Practices (ACIP). *MMWR Morb. Mortal Wkly. Rep.* **46,** 1–10.
78. Anonymous (2000) Meningococcal disease falls in vaccine recipients. *Comm. Dis. Rev. Weekly* **10,** 133, 136.
79. Devi, S. J., Zollinger, W. D., Snoy, P. J., Tai, J. Y., Costantini, P., Norelli, F., et al. (1997) Preclinical evaluation of group B Neisseria meningitidis and Escherichia coli K92 capsular polysaccharide-protein conjugate vaccines in juvenile rhesus monkeys. *Infect. Immun.* **65,** 1045–1052.
80. Finne, J., Leinonen, M., and Mäkelä, P. H. (1983) Antigenic similarities between brain components and bacteria causing meningitis. Implications for vaccine development and pathogenesis. *Lancet* **2,** 355–357.
81. Idänpään-Heikkilä, I., Høiby, E. A., Chattopadhyay, P., Airaksinen, U., Michaelsen, T. M., and Wedege, E. (1995) Antibodies to meningococcal class 1 outer-membrane protein and its variable regions in patients with systemic meningococcal disease. *J. Med.* Microbiol. *43, 335–343.*
82. Guttormsen, H. K., Wetzler, L. M., and Næss, A. (1993) Humoral immune response to the class 3 outer membrane protein during the course of meningococcal disease. *Infect. Immun.* **61,** 4734–4742.
83. Mandrell, R. E. and Zollinger, W. D. (1989) Human immune response to meningococcal outer membrane protein epitopes after natural infection or vaccination. *Infect. Immun.* **57,** 1590–1598.
84. Estabrook, M. M., Baker, C. J., and Griffiss, J. M. (1993) The immune response of children to meningococcal lipooligosaccharides during disseminated disease is directed primarily against two monoclonal antibody-defined epitopes. *J. Infect. Dis.* **167,** 966–970.
85. Brooks, G. F., Lammel, C. J., Blake, M. S., Kusecek, B., and Achtman, M. (1992) Antibodies against IgA1 protease are stimulated both by clinical disease and asymptomatic carriage of serogroup A Neisseria meningitidis. *J. Infect. Dis.* **166,** 1316–1321.
86. Farrant, J. L., Kroll, J. S., Brodeur, B. R., and Martin, D. (1998) Detection of anti-NspA antibodies in sera from pateints convalescent after meningococcal infec-

tion. In: Eleventh International Pathogenic Neisseria Conference, Nice. Nassif, X., Quentin-Millet, M.-J., and Taha, M.-K. (eds.). EDK Paris, Nice, France, pp. 208.

87. Ala'Aldeen, D. A., Stevenson, P., Griffiths, E., Gorringe, A. R., Irons, L. I., Robinson, A., et al. (1994) Immune responses in humans and animals to meningococcal transferrin-binding proteins: implications for vaccine design. *Infect. Immun.* **62,** 2984–2900.

88. Black, J. R., Black, W. J., and Cannon, J. G. (1985) Neisserial antigen H.8 is immunogenic in patients with disseminated gonococcal and meningococcal infections. *J. Infect. Dis.* **151,** 650–657.

89. Pettersson, A., Maas, A., van Wassenaar, D., van der Ley, P., and Tommassen, J. (1995) Molecular characterization of FrpB, the 70-kilodalton iron-regulated outer membrane protein of Neisseria meningitidis. *Infect. Immun.* **63,** 4181–4184.

90. Johnson, A. S., Gorringe, A. R., Mackinnon, F. G., Fox, A. J., Borrow, R., and Robinson, A. (1999) Analysis of the human Ig isotype response to lactoferrin binding protein A from Neisseria meningitidis. *FEMS Immunol. Med. Microbiol.* **25,** 349–354.

91. Wiertz, E. J., Delvig, A., Donders, E. M., Brugghe, H. F., van Unen, L. M., Timmermans, H. A., et al. (1996) T-cell responses to outer membrane proteins of Neisseria meningitidis: comparative study of the Opa, Opc, and PorA proteins. *Infect. Immun.* **64,** 298–304.

92. van der Voort, E. R., van Dijken, H., Kuipers, B., van der Biezen, J., van der Ley, P., Meylis, J., et al. (1997) Human B- and T-cell responses after immunization with a hexavalent PorA meningococcal outer membrane vesicle vaccine. *Infect. Immun.* **65,** 5184–5190.

93. Næss, L. M., Oftung, F., Aase, A., Wetzler, L. M., Sandin, R., and Michaelsen, T. E. (1998) Human T-cell responses after vaccination with the Norwegian group B meningococcal outer membrane vesicle vaccine. *Infect. Immun.* **66,** 959–965.

94. Pollard, A. J., Galassini, R., Rouppe van der Voort, E. M., Hibberd, M., Booy, R., Langford, P., et al. (1999) Cellular immune responses to Neisseria meningitidis in children. *Infect. Immun.* **67,** 2452–2463.

95. Wiertz, E. J., van Gaans-van den Brink, J. A., Schreuder, G. M., Termijtelen, A. A., Hoogerhout, P., and Poolman, J. T. (1991) T cell recognition of Neisseria meningitidis class 1 outer membrane proteins. Identification of T cell epitopes with selected synthetic peptides and determination of HLA restriction elements. *J. Immunol.* **147,** 2012–2018.

96. Wiertz, E. J., van Gaans-van den Brink, J. A., Gausepohl, H., Prochnicka-Chalufour, A., Hoogerhout, P., and Poolman, J. T. (1992) Identification of T cell epitopes occurring in a meningococcal class 1 outer membrane protein using overlapping peptides assembled with simultaneous multiple peptide synthesis. *J. Exp. Med.* **176,** 79–88.

97. Wiertz, E., van Gaans-van den Brink, J., Hoogerhout, P., and Poolman, J. (1993) Microheterogeneity in the recognition of a HLA-DR2-restricted T cell epitope from a meningococcal outer membrane protein. *Eur. J. Immunol.* **23,** 232–239.

3

Purification of Capsular Polysaccharide

Qingling Yang and Harold Jennings

1. Introduction

Meningococcus is an aerobic, fastidious, Gram-negative diplococcus that is found only in humans. Its cell wall has a cytoplasmic membrane, a peptidoglycan layer, and an outer membrane. Meningococci isolated from the bloodstream or the spinal fluid are almost always encapsulated. The capsules are polysaccharides, which consist of repeating sugar units *(1,2)*. The capsular polysaccharide can be isolated, purified, and chemically and physically defined. Based on the chemical and immunological specificity of its capsular polysaccharides, *Neisseria meningitidis* has been classified serologically into groups A, B, C, 29E, H, I, K, L, W135, X, Y and Z *(2)*. Of these, groups A, B, and C are responsible for approx 90% of meningococcal meningitis, and group B meningococcus is responsible for the majority of meningococcal disease in industrialized countries *(1,2)*. The structures of the repeating units of the meningococcal polysaccharides have been elucidated and are shown in **Table 1**.

The capsular polysaccharides of *Neisseria meningitidis* are attractive vaccine candidates because they constitute the most highly conserved and most exposed bacterial-surface antigens. The use of capsular polysaccharides as immunoprophylactic agents against human disease caused by encapsulated bacteria is now firmly established *(2)*. The capsular polysaccharides of the meningococcus are negatively charged and can be obtained in a high molecular-weight immunogenic form by precipitation from the culture medium by Cetavlon *(3,4)*. The procedure used in our laboratory is adaptable to isolation of capsular polysaccharide from culture medium of *N. meningitis* (serogroups A, B, C, H, L, X, Y, W135, Z, and 29E) in both good yields and a high degree of purity.

From: *Methods in Molecular Medicine, vol. 66: Meningococcal Vaccines: Methods and Protocols*
Edited by: A. J. Pollard and M. C. J. Maiden © Humana Press Inc., Totowa, NJ

Table 1
Structures of the Capsular Polysaccharides of *N. meningitidis*

Group	Structure of repeating unit	Reference
A	→6)α-D-ManNAc(1-PO4→	*(8)*
	3	
	↑	
	OAc	
B	→8)α-D-NeuNAc(2→	*(5)*
C	→9)α-D-NeuNAc(2→	*(5)*
	7/8	
	↑	
	OAc	
H	→4)α-D-Gal (1→2) glycerol 3-PO$_4$→	*(6)*
L	→3)α-D-GlcNAc (1→3) β-D-GlcNAc (1→3) α-D-GlcNAc-1-PO$_4$→	
		(7)
X	→4)α-D-GlcNAc-1-PO$_4$→	*(4)*
Y	→6)α-D-Glc (1→4) α-D-NeuNAc (2→ (OAc)	*(9)*
W135	→6)α-D-Gal (1→4) α-D-NeuNAc (2→	*(9)*
Z	→3)α-D-GalNAc (1→1) glycerol 3-PO$_4$→	*(10)*
29E	→7)β-D-KDO (1→3) α-D-GalNAc (1→	*(11)*

2. Materials

2.1. Media

1. 250-mL flask, 4-L flask (Fernbach or baffled Erlenmeyer).
2. Proteose Peptone medium (GC medium): dissolve 15 g Bacto Proteose Peptone No. 3. (Difco Lab., Detroit, MI), 4 g K$_2$HPO$_4$, 1 g KH$_2$PO$_4$, 5 g NaCl in about 250 mL of dH$_2$O by stirring for 30 min and add dH$_2$O to 1 L.
3. Isovitalex (Becton Dickinson Microbiology Systems, Cockeysville, MD).
4. GC Agar for plates: 10 g agar (Difco Lab., Detroit, MI) added to GC medium. Store plates at room temperature until used.

2.2. Bacteria Growth

1. Gloves, masks, loop, and sterile cotton swab.
2. Freezing solution: 65% (v/v) glycerol, 0.1 *M* MgSO$_4$ and 0.025 *M* Tris-HCl, pH 8.0. Store at room temperature.
3. Biohood, shaker and CO$_2$ incubator.
4. Formaldehyde (36.5–38%).

2.3. Isolation of Capsular Polysaccharides

1. 10% (w/v) Cetavlon (hexadecyltrimethylammonium bromide, Sigma, St. Louis, MO). A cationic detergent for precipitating the polyanionic polysaccharides from

solution. Dissolve 10 g Cetavlon in 80 mL dH$_2$O and make up to 100 mL with dH$_2$O.

2. 0.9 M CaCl$_2$: dissolve 132.3 g CaCl$_2$ in 200 mL dH$_2$O and make up volume to 1 L.
3. 100% Ethanol.
4. 0.2 M Na$_2$HPO$_4$-NaH$_2$PO$_4$: dissolve 4.42 g NaH$_2$PO$_4$, 23.85 g Na$_2$HPO$_4$ in dH$_2$O and make up to 1 L.
5. Phosphate-buffered saline (PBS): 10 mM Na-phosphate buffer, 150 mM NaCl, pH 7.4.
6. Phenol: add 200 mL 0.2 M phosphate buffer, pH 7.0, to 500 g phenol. Dissolve phenol completely in water bath at 50°C.

2.4. Purification of Polysaccharide

1. DNAse (Sigma).
2. RNAse A (Sigma).
3. Proteinase (Sigma).
4. Bio-Gel A 0.5 (Bio-Rad, Richmond, CA).

2.5. Quality Analysis

1. 4% Resorcinol (Aldrich Chemical Co., Inc): 4 g resorcinol is dissolved in 100 mL deionized water. The reagent is stable for months at 4°C.
2. 0.1 M CuSO$_4$: 2.5 g of CuSO$_4$.5H$_2$O is dissolved in 100 mL of dH$_2$O.
3. Resorcinol reagent: 5 mL of 4% resorcinol is added to 80 mL of concentrated HCl, then add 0.25 mL of 0.1 M CuSO$_4$. The final volume is made up to 100 mL with deionized water. The resorcinol reagent should be prepared at least 1 h before use and is stable for about 2 wk at room temperature when stored in an amber (brown glass) bottle.
4. Extraction solvent: *n*-butyl acetate: *n*-butanol (85:15 [v/v]).
5. Sialic acid (JM Science, Grand Island, NY) standard solution, (100 µg/100 µL water).

3. Methods
3.1. Media

1. Prepare GC medium (2 L), or other growth media (*see* **Note 1**), and put two 50-mL aliquots into 250-mL baffled flasks and two 1-L aliquots into 4-L baffled flasks. Autoclave at 121°C (20 lb/in^2) for 20 min, then cool to room temperature. Before use, add Isovitalex (1:100 diluted) to a final concentration of 1%.
2. Prepare 1 L of GC agar, and autoclave at 121°C for 30 min. Cool to about 45–50°C in a water bath, and then pour plates (1 L agar medium can pour about 30–40 plates). Other plates can also be used (*see* **Note 2**).

3.2. Growth of Meningococci

1. The stocks of *N. meningitidis* are kept frozen in glycerol solution (or as lyophilizates) at –80°C. Thaw the stock tube (or suspend stock lyophilizate) and

using a loop place butterfly streak of meningococcus on two GC agar plates. Incubate plates overnight at 37°C in an atmosphere of 5% CO_2.

2. Scrape bacteria from two agar GC plates with a sterile cotton swab and suspend the bacterial cells in two 5-mL aliquots of GC media in separate 15-mL centrifuge tubes (*see* **Note 3**).

3. Pour each 5-mL bacterium suspension into 50 mL media contained in a 250-mL flask. Allow the bacteria to grow at 37°C under normal atmospheric pressure shaking the flask at 125 rpm for about 2.5 h.

4. Transfer 50 mL of each of the broth cultures from the small flasks into one 4-L flask containing 1 L media, which is prewarmed at 37°C to avoid cold-shocking the organisms.

5. Shake overnight (about 16 h) at 125 rpm, at which time the culture of bacteria is in stationary phase and the $O.D_{600}$ of the culture should be over 1.0.

6. To kill the meningococcus, cool the culture at room temperature, then add formaldehyde (36.5–38%) to a final concentration of 1% (v/v) and shake for about 30 min at 200 rpm.

3.3. Preparation of Group-Specific Meningococcal Capsular Polysaccharides

1. Harvest the supernatant of the flask culture in 500-mL centrifuge bottles (Nalgene Labware, Rochester, NY) by centrifuging them at 5000 rpm (Sorvall RC2-B, GS3 Rotor, Du Pont, DE) for 20 min at 4°C. To precipitate the capsular polysaccharide complex, add 10% Cetavlon to final concentration of 0.1% (w/v) in the supernate, and leave at 4°C overnight. Aspirate off the bulk of the supernate and collect the complex as a pellet by centrifugation at 5000 rpm for 40 min.

2. Dissolve the Cetavlon pellet in 50 mL 0.9 M $CaCl_2$ at 4°C, and stir for 2 h. Collect the supernatant by centrifuging at 9000 rpm (Sorvall RC2-B, Rotor SS34, Du Pont, DE) for 40 min.

3. Add cold ethanol to the aforementioned supernatant to a final concentration of 25% and let stand at 4°C for 2 h. Collect supernatant by centrifuging at 5000 rpm for 40 min.

4. Add 100% ethanol to a final concentration of 80% and let stand at 4°C for 2 h.

5. Discard excess ethanol solution and collect precipitate in 50-mL centrifuge tubes with screw closure, by centrifuging them at 9000 rpm for 40 min.

6. Dissolve the pellet in 50 mL 0.2 M sodium phosphate buffer, pH 7.0, and collect the supernatant by centrifugation at 5000 rpm for 40 min.

7. Transfer the aforementioned supernate to a phenol resistant centrifuge tube (Teflon or polypropylene screw closure). Add the same volume of phenol, and vigorously shake in a vortex mixer for about 1 min or stir at 4°C for 1 h.

8. Centrifuge at 5000 rpm for 30 min. Remove the top aqueous phase carefully and then extract the phenol phase again using the same volume of 0.2 M phosphate buffer.

9. Combine the two aqueous phases and dialyse against distilled water overnight. Lyophilize the aqueous solution to yield the crude capsular polysaccharide.

3.4. Purification of Polysaccharide

1. Dissolve the lyophilized polysaccharide in 10 mL PBS. Add 30 µL RNAse (10 mg/mL) and 30 µL DNAse (10 mg/mL) and digest overnight at 37°C. Then add 30 µL proteinase (10 mg/mL) and digest overnight at 37°C.
2. Separate polysaccharide from the mixture by gel filtration on a Bio-Gel A 0.5 column (1.6 × 100 cm, Bio-Rad, Richmond, CA). Elute with PBS buffer, pH 7.4, at 24 mL/h (LKB BROMMA 2132 Microperpex Peristaltic Pump).
3. Collect fractions of 7 mL (about 150 drops) using an LKB BROMMA 2111 Multirac collector and monitor the elution using a Waters' Differential Refractometer R403.
4. Assay for polysaccharide content (*see* **Subheading 3.5.**).
5. Pool fractions containing polysaccharides in the high molecular-weight peak, dialyze against dH$_2$O and lyophilize. The yield varies according to strain and is about 40 mg/L for group B stain 992.
6. Check sample for purity by ^{1}HNMR spectroscopy.

3.5. Quality Analysis

3.5.1. Sialic Acid

1. Place a sample (containing 10–70 µg of sialic acid) in a 16 × 150 mm glass tube (Pyrex test tube is recommended), and make the sample volume up to 500 µL (volume can be varied up to 2 mL). Standard solutions of sialic acid are prepared using 20, 40, 60, 80, and 100 µg, and each is made up to 500 µL (or to an equal volume with the sample). Add 500 µL resorcinol reagent.
2. Place the tubes in a boiling water bath for 15 min. If the tube shows blue/purple/brown color, it indicates that the sample contains sialic acid. No blue color means that sialic acid is absent. A dark brown color indicates that the sample has either too high a concentration of sialic acid or that it is not pure enough.
3. Cool the tubes to room temperature (20–25°C) in a cold water bath. Add 1 mL (2×-sample volume) extraction organic solvent into each test tube and shake the tubes vigorously. Leave at room temperature until the organic-solvent layer separates completely from the aqueous phase (*see* **Note 4**). Transfer the top organic phase to a cuvet and determine the absorbence against pure organic solvent in a spectrophotometer at 580 nm. Compare with standard curve for quantification.

3.5.2. HPLC Analysis

1. Check the molecular size of polysaccharides, and the presence of protein and DNA/RNA contamination by high-performance liquid chromatography (HPLC) (using a Superose-12 column, Pharmacia Biotech, Uppsala, Sweden).

3.5.3. ^{1}HNMR Analysis

1. Dissolve 2–3 mg lyophilized sample in 700 µL of D$_2$O, transfer into a nuclear magnetic resonance (NMR) tube. Check the NMR spectra of the sample using a 500 MHz NMR spectrometer.

4. Notes

1. In addition to GC medium, Mueller Hinton broth (MHB; Difco, Detroit, MI) or Bacto Todd Hewitt Broth (THB; Difco) can also be used.
2. Mueller Hinton agar plates (MHA+HS; Difco), Chocolate agar plates Quelab, Montreal, Que) or Columbia sheep Blood Agar plates (Quelab, Montreal, Quebec) can also be used.
3. Small quantities (μg level) of crude polysaccharide can be obtained directly at this stage by suspending the scraped bacteria in PBS containing 1% (v/v) formaldehyde, gently stirring the solution for 1 h or longer at 4°C, and then performing the Cetavlon precipitation.
4. In cases where the organic layer is turbid, centrifugation should be applied to separate the two layers.

References

1. Gotschlich, E. C. (1984) Meningococcal meningitis, in *Bacterial Vaccines* (Germanier, E., ed.), Academic Press, New York, pp. 237–255.
2. Jennings, H. J. (1990) Capsular polysaccharides as vaccine candidates. *Curr. Top. Microbiol. Immunol.* **150,** 97–127.
3. Gotschlich, E. C., Liu, T-Y, and Artenstein, M. S. (1969) Human immunity to the meningococcus. III. Preparation and immunochemical properties of the group A, group B and group C meningococcal polysaccharides. *J. Exp. Med.* **129,** 1349–1365.
4. Bundle, D. R., Jennings, H. J., and Kenny, C. P. (1974) Studies on the group-specific polysaccharide of *Neisseria meningitidis* serogroup X and an improved procedure for its isolation. *J. Biol. Chem.* **249,** 4797–4801.
5. Bhattacharjee, A. K., Jennings, H. J., Kenny, C. P., Martin, A., and Smith, I. C. P. (1975) Structural determination of the sialic acid polysaccharide antigens of *Neisseria meningitidis* serogroup B and serogroup C with carbon 13 nuclear magnetic resonance. *J. Biol. Chem.* **250,** 1926–1932.
6. Michon, F., Roy, R., Jennings, H. J., and Ashton, F. E. (1984) Structural elucidation of the capsular polysaccharide of *Neisseria meningitidis* group H. *Can. J. Chem.* **62,** 1519–1524.
7. Ashton, F. E., Ryan, A., Diena, B., and Jennings, H. J. (1983) A new serogroup (L) of *Neisseria meningitidis*. *J. Clin. Microbiol.* **17,** 722–727.
8. Bundle, D. R., Smith, I. C. P., and Jennings, H. J. (1974) Determination of the structure and conformation of bacterial polysaccharides by carbon-13 nuclear magnetic resonance. *J. Biol. Chem.* **249,** 2275–2281.
9. Bhattacharjee, A. K., Jennings, H. J., Kenny, C. P., Matin, A., and Smith, I. C. P. (1976) Structure determination of the polysaccharide antigens of *Neisseria meningitidis* serogroups Y, W-135 and BO1. *Can. J. Biochem.* **54,** 1–8.

10. Jennings, H. J., Rosell, K. G., and Kenny, C. P. (1979) Structural elucidation of the capsular polysaccharide antigen of *Neisseria meningitidis* serogroup Z using ^{13}C nuclear magnetic resonance. *Can. J. Chem.* **57,** 2902–2907.
11. Bhattacharjee, A. K., Jennings, H. J., and Kenny, C. P. (1978) Strutural elucidation of the 3-deoxy-D-mannooctulosonic acid containing meningococcal 29e capsular polysaccharide antigen using carbon-13 nuclear magnetic resonance. *Biochemistry.* **17,** 645–651.

4

Protein–Polysaccharide Conjugation

Zhongwu Guo and Harold Jennings

1. Introduction

The use of bacterial capsular polysaccharides as immunoprophylactic agents in human diseases caused by encapsulated bacteria is now firmly established *(1)*. However, despite their many advantages, they do have serious limitations. First, they induce an inadequate immune response in infants *(2)*, the section of the population most vulnerable to bacterial meningitis, and second, some polysaccharides are only weakly immunogenic in adults. To overcome these deficiencies, a new generation of semisynthetic vaccines have been developed based on the conjugation of polysaccharide to protein carriers.

Several different chemical approaches to the synthesis of conjugate vaccines have been developed *(3)*. Important criteria associated with the utility of the different procedures is that they should be generally applicable, and that the covalent linkage between the saccharide and protein components should be stable. In addition, the reaction conditions should be mild enough to maintain the structural integrity of the individual components. Based on such criteria, the coupling of saccharides and proteins by reductive amination is one of the best methods *(4)*. The mechanism of such coupling is that the reaction between the carbonyl group of a saccharide and the amino groups of the carrier protein can form corresponding Schiffs' base, which can be then selectively reduced in the presence of sodium cyanoborohydride (NaBH$_3$CN) to a very stable saturated carbon-nitrogen bond as shown in **Fig. 1** *(5)*. Also reductive amination is a one-pot reaction, which can be carried out in aqueous solution under conditions mild enough to preserve not only the saccharide and protein components, but even labile substituents such as *O*-acetyl *(4)*.

Although small oligosaccharides can be conjugated by reductive amination to proteins via their hemiactetal reducing ends *(5)*, this aldehydic form is too

From: *Methods in Molecular Medicine, vol. 66: Meningococcal Vaccines: Methods and Protocols*
Edited by: A. J. Pollard and M. C. J. Maiden © Humana Press Inc., Totowa, NJ

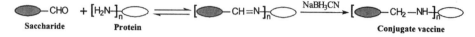

Fig. 1. Conjugation of saccharide with carrier protein by reductive amination.

inactive to be used to conjugate polysaccharides or larger oligosaccharides by the same procedure *(4)*. Therefore, to ensure the successful conjugation of large saccharides by reductive amination, it is necessary to generate within the saccharide more reactive free aldehydes. Fortunately this can be achieved easily by selective periodate oxidation of vicinal diol functionalities within polysaccharides or larger oligosaccharides *(4)*. This reaction can be used to introduce terminal aldehydes into intact polysaccharides or oligosaccharides or alternatively, with unique structures such as the group C meningococcal polysaccharide, it can be used to depolymerize the polysaccharide, and simultaneously activate the fragments with terminal aldehydes *(6)*. The native group C meningococcal polysaccharide exists in both *O*-acetylated (GCMP.OAc⁺) and unacetylated (GCMP) forms and by treating the former with mild base it can easily be transformed into the latter (**Fig. 2**). This chapter describes the depolymerization and activation of the GCMP (**Fig. 2**) prior to its conjugation to tetanus toxoid (TT), although the GCMP.OAc⁺ can also be conjugated directly using the same strategy *(6)*, because it still contains sufficient unacetylated internal sialic-acid residues *(7)* for oxidative cleavage to occur.

2. Materials

2.1. O-Deacetylation of GCMP.OAc⁺

1. GCMP.OAc⁺.
2. 0.1 M aqueous solution of sodium hydroxide (NaOH).
3. 1 M hydrochloric acid (HCl).

2.2. Oxidative Activation of GCMP

1. 10 mM aqueous solution of sodium periodate (NaIO$_4$).
2. 0.1 M sodium acetate-acetic acid (NaOAc-HOAc) buffer, pH 6.5.
3. 10% ethylene glycol.
4. 0.1 M PBS buffer, pH 7.4.
5. Bio-Gel A 0.5 column 2.0 × 30 cm.

2.3. Conjugation of GCMP to TT

1. Monomeric TT.
2. Sodium cyanoborohydride (NaBH$_3$CN).
3. 0.1 M Sodium bicarbonate (NaHCO$_3$) solution, pH 7.5–8.0.

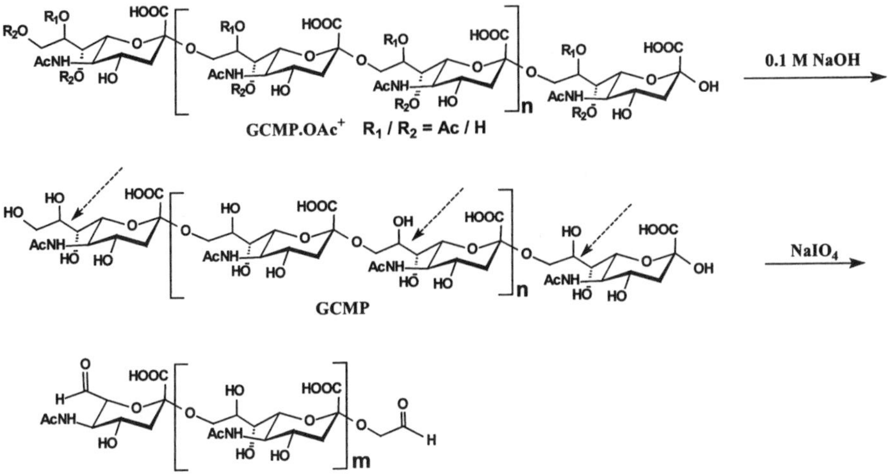

Fig. 2. Chemical structure of GCMP.OAc$^+$ and potential cleavage and activation positions of GCMP.

4. 0.1 M phosphate-buffered saline (PBS) buffer, pH 7.4.
5. Bio-Gel A 0.5 column (2.0 × 30 cm).

2.4. Analysis of the Saccharide Loading of Glycoconjugates

1. Bicinchonic acid reagent A (Pierce, Rockford, IL).
2. Bicinchonic acid reagent B (Pierce).
3. Resorcinol solution (4%).
4. 0.1 M copper sulfate ($CuSO_4$) solution.
5. Resorcinol reagent.
6. n-Butyl acetate.
7. n-Butanol.
8. Sialic-acid solution (0.1 mg/mL).
9. ^{1}HNMR analysis as described in Chapter 3, **Subheading 3.5.3.**

3. Methods

3.1. O-Deacetylation of GCMP.OAc$^+$

1. Stir a solution of GCMP.OAc$^+$ (950 mg) dissolved in 5 mL 0.1 M NaOH, pH 12~13, for 4 h at room temperature (*see* **Note 1**).
2. Neutralize solution to pH 7.0–7.5 with 1 M HCl.
3. Dialyze overnight against distilled water and lyophilize to yield the GCMP, which can be used directly in the next step.
4. Check that the product is fully O-deacetylated by ^{1}HNMR spectroscopy.

3.2. Oxidative Cleavage of GCMP

1. Add 0.25 mL of 10 mM NaIO$_4$ solution (2.5 µmol; *see* **Note 2**), to a solution of 20 mg GCMP dissolved in 0.75 mL 0.1 M NaOAc-HOAc buffer at pH 6.5. Keep in dark for 6 h.
2. Add 0.1 M 10% ethylene glycol and leave for 30 min to degrade the remaining NaIO$_4$.
3. Dialyze against distilled water and lyophilize.
4. Chromatograph product on Bio-Gel A 0.5 column (2 × 30 cm) using 0.1 M PBS buffer, pH 7.0, as eluant.
5. Collect and pool fractions (*see* Chapter 3, **Subheading 3.4.2.**) containing activated GCMP having MW 10-12kD (the major peak).
6. Lyophilize the pooled fractions to yield activated 16 mg GCMP.
7. Confirm the presence of an hydrated aldehyde signal at 5.4 ppm in the ^{1}HNMR spectrum of the product.

3.3. Conjugation of GCMP and TT (7)

1. Dissolve activated 10 mg GCMP, 5 mg monomeric TT (*see* **Note 3**) and 5 mg recrystallized NaBH$_3$CN (*see* **Note 4**) in 0.5 mL 0.1 M NaHCO$_3$ at pH 7.5–8.0.
2. Leave the solution to stand in the dark for 3–5 d with occasional shaking.
3. Apply the solution to a Bio-Gel A 0.5 column (2 × 30 cm) using 0.1 M PBS buffer, pH 7.8, as eluant.
4. Collect and pool fractions (*see* Chapter 3, **Subheading 3.4.2.**) corresponding to the first peak (*see* **Note 5**) eluted from the column.
5. Dialyze pooled fractions against distilled water overnight and lyophilize to yield the GCMP-TT conjugate (5.5–6.0 mg).

3.4. Analysis of Saccharide Loading of the Glycoconjugate

3.4.1. Protein Content

1. Add 0.1 mL of GCMP-TT solution (50 µg/mL) to one well of an enzyme-linked immunosorbent assay (ELISA) plate.
2. Add standard TT solutions (0.1 mL) containing 0–100 µg/mL TT to other wells.
3. Add BCA reagent (A : B, 50 : 1) (200 µL) to each well and incubate plate at 37°C for 30 min.
4. Determine the absorbance (540 nm) using an ELISA microplate reader and evaluate protein content from the standard TT curve.

3.4.2. Saccharide Loading

1. Dissolve an exactly weighed sampled of GCMP-TT (0.2–0.5 mg) containing about 18–25% sialic acid (*see* **Note 6**) in distilled water.
2. Determine the sialic acid content using the resorcinol method as previously described in Chapter 3, **Subheading 3.5.1.**

3. Calculate the percentage loading of saccharide in GCMP-TT using the following equation: Saccharide loading (%) = sialic acid content/(sialic-acid content + protein content) × 100.

4. Notes

1. *N*-acetyls are stable under these conditions, but *O*-acetyls can be hydrolyzed. In order to obtain partially *O*-deacetylated GCMP, either shorter reaction times or milder basic conditions can be used.
2. Calculated amount of periodate that is needed to oxidize and degrade GCMP to fragments having an average molecular weight of 10 kD plus a 25% excess (0.5 μmole).
3. To prepare monomeric TT, 4 mL of the crude TT vaccine solution (2.5 mg/mL) is passed through a Bio-Gel A 0.5 column (2.0 × 30 cm) using 0.1 *M* PBS buffer, pH 7.8, as eluant. The first peak eluted from the column is dimeric TT while the second eluted peak is the monomeric TT. Monomeric TT solution is dialyzed against distilled water overnight and then lyophilized to give a white powder of monomeric TT (55% recovery).
4. Commercial NaBH₃CN (>98%) is dissolved in minimum volume of tetrahydrofuran (THF) and the solution is filtered. Then, the THF solution is dropped into two volumes of dioxane and the mixture is kept at room temperature overnight. The crystals are filtered off, washed with dioxane, and dried under vacuum. Recrystalization of NaBH₃CN is absolutely necessary to remove trace amounts of NaBH₄, which reduces aldehydes very fast, thus preventing them from participating in the slower conjugation reaction.
5. The conjugate is usually eluted at the void volume and is easily separable from the unreacted saccharide.
6. The saccharide loading of glycoconjugates produced by this method is usually 20% but varies a little from preparation to preparation.

References

1. Jennings, H. J. (1990) Capsular polysaccharides as vaccine candidates. *Curr. Top. Microbiol. Immunol.* **150**, 97–127.
2. Gotschlich, E. C., Lepow, M. L., and Gold, R. (1977) The immune response to bacterial polysaccharides in man, in *Antibodies in Human Diagnostics and Therapy* (Haber, E. and Krause, R. M., eds.), Raven Press, New York, pp. 391–402.
3. Jennings, H. J. and Sood, R. K. (1994) Synthetic glycoconjugates as human vaccines, in *Neoglycoconjugates: Preparation and Applications* (Lee, Y. C. and Lee, R. T., eds.), Academic Press, San Diego, pp. 325–371.
4. Jennings, H. J. and Lugowski, C. (1981) Immunochemistry of group A, B and C meningococcal polysaccharide-tetanus toxoid conjugates. *J. Immunol.* **127**, 1011–1018.

5. Schwartz, B. A. and Gray, G. R. (1977) Proteins containing reductively animated disaccharides. Synthesis and chemical characterization. *Arch. Biochem. Biophy.* **181,** 542–549.

6. Beuvery, E. C., Roy, R., Kanhai, V., and Jennings, H. J. (1986) Characteristics of two types of meningococcal group C polysaccharide conjugates using tetanus toxoid as carrier protein. *Dev. Biol. Stand.* **65,** 197–204.

7. Bhattacharjee, A. K., Jennings, H. J., Kenny, C. P., Martin, A., and Smith, I. C. P. (1975) Structural determination of the sialic acid polysaccharide antigens of *Neisseria mentingitis* serogroups B and C with carbon 13 nuclear magnetic resonance. *J. Biol. Chem.* **250,** 1926–1932.

5

N-Propionylation

Zhongwu Guo and Harold Jennings

1. Introduction

Serogroup B *Neisseria meningitidis* remains a major world health problem and currently there is no fully efficacious vaccine available. The poor immunogenicity of the group B meningococcal polysaccharide both in adults and infants prevents the formulation of a comprehensive polysaccharide-based vaccine *(1)*. Although, as discussed in Chapter 4, conjugation technology can overcome the limitation of the poor immunogenicity of most capsular polysaccharides, the serogroup B meningococcal polysaccharide when conjugated to a protein carrier still failed to give a significant immune response *(2,3)*. This phenomenon is probably attributed to the molecular mimicry between the polysaccharide and human-tissue antigens. As shown in **Fig. 1**, the serogroup B polysaccharide is a homopolymer of α(2-8)-linked sialic-acid residues *(4)* and similar structures have also been identified in the human-tissue antigens, from short trimeric fragments found in mammalian gangliosides *(5)* to long decameric fragments observed in the glycoproteins of neural-cell adhesion molecules (N-CAMs) *(6)*.

Because of the above phenomenon, research efforts to develop effective serogroup B vaccines have mainly focused on alternative surface-exposed components, such as outer membrane proteins (OMPs) and lipopolysaccharides (LPSs) *(7,8)*. However, many problems associated with the development of vaccines based on these components have been identified, especially those related to the diversified serotypes and immunogenicities of these components, and so far no fully efficacious vaccine has been developed. Because the serogroup B polysaccharide is the only conserved antigenic structure on the surface of these meningococci, a polysaccharide-based vaccine would be the vaccine of

From: *Methods in Molecular Medicine, vol. 66: Meningococcal Vaccines: Methods and Protocols*
Edited by: A. J. Pollard and M. C. J. Maiden © Humana Press Inc., Totowa, NJ

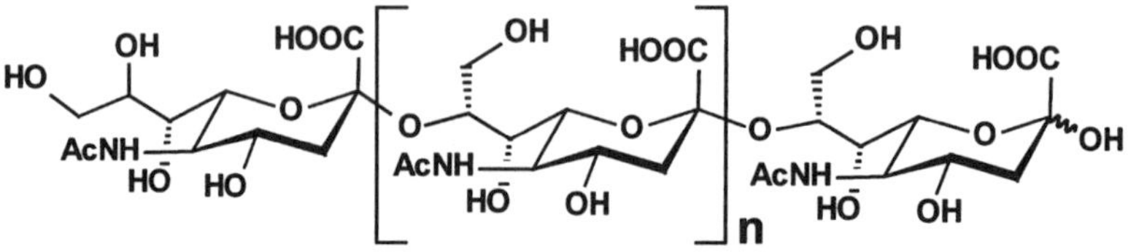

Fig. 1. Chemical structure of GBMP.

choice, provided that its poor immunogenicity could be overcome. One approach to achieve this goal is to chemically modify the polysaccharide prior to its conjugation to a protein carrier, to form a synthetic vaccine with enhanced immunogenicity of its glyco component *(9,10)*. Investigations have revealed that replacing the *N*-acetyl group of the sialic acid residues of the polysaccharide with the *N*-propionyl groups did not alter the tertiary structure of its polysaccharide backbone *(11)*, and that the tetanus toxoid (TT) conjugate of the resultant *N*-propionylated polysaccharide, when administered with strong adjuvants (Freunds' complete adjuvant or monophosphoryl lipid A RIBI adjuvant), was able to induce high titers of N-propionylated serogroup B meningococcal polysaccharide-specific bactericidal IgG antibodies in mice *(12–14)*. These antibodies were also opsonophagocytic for *Escherichia coli* K1 *(13)* because the latter has a capsule of identical structure to that of serogroup B polysaccharide *(4)*. Interestingly, antibodies specific for the propionylated form induced by the propionylated serogroup B polysaccharide-TT conjugate consist of two distinct populations, the larger of which contains most of the protective antibodies but does not cross-react with the $\alpha(2\text{-}8)$ polysialic acid *(14,15)*. This indicates that the conjugated polysaccharide mimics a unique capsular epitope on the bacterial cell surface of serogroup B meningococci and *E. coli* K1 *(14,15)* and that the protein conjugates are excellent vaccine candidates against both these organisms. One of these conjugates in which the modified serogroup B polysaccharide is conjugated to recombinant porin (rPorB) *(16)*, where the porin functions not only as a carrier but also as an adjuvant, is soon to undergo human trials. In this chapter, we describe the chemical modification of serogroup B polysaccharide and its conjugation with TT and the reaction schemes are shown in **Fig. 2**.

2. Materials

2.1. Chemical Modification of Serogroup B Meningococcal Polysaccharide: Preparation of Propionylated Polysaccharide

1. Serogroup B meningococcal polysaccharide or Colominic Acid (JM Science Inc., Grand Island, NY).
2. Sodium borohydride ($NaBH_4$).

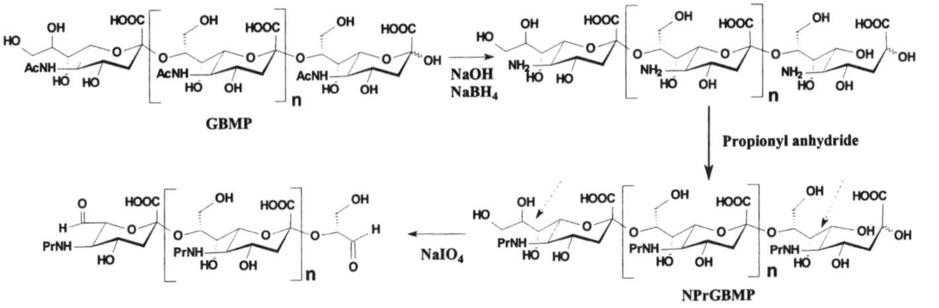

Fig. 2. Chemical modification of GBMP and potential cleavage and activation positions of NPrGBMP.

3. 2 *M* Aqueous solution of sodium hydroxide (NaOH).
4. 2 *M* Hydrochloric acid (HCl).
5. 0.1 *M* Aqueous solution of NaOH.
6. Propionic anhydride.
7. 0.1 *M* Phosphate-buffered saline (PBS) buffer, pH 7.4.
8. Bio-gel A 0.5 column (2.0 × 30 cm).

2.2. Oxidative Activation of Propionylated Serogroup B Polysaccharide

1. Propionylated serogroup B polysaccharide.
2. Sodium metaperiodate (NaIO$_4$).
3. 0.1 *M* Sodium acetate-acetic acid (NaOAc-HOAc), pH 6.5.
4. 10% Ethylene glycol.

2.3. Conjugation of Propionylated Serogroup B Polysaccharide to TT

1. Monomeric TT.
2. Sodium cyanoborohydride (NaBH$_3$CN).
3. 0.1 *M* Sodium bicarbonate (NaHCO$_3$) solution, pH 7.5–8.0.
4. 0.1 *M* PBS buffer, pH 7.4.
5. Bio-Gel A 0.5 column (2.0 × 30 cm).

2.4. Analysis of the Saccharide Loading of Glycoconjugates

1. BCA reagent A (Pierce, Rockford, IL)
2. BCA reagent B (Pierce)
3. Resorcinol solution (4%).
4. 0.1 *M* Copper sulfate (CuSO$_4$) solution.
5. Resorcinol reagent.
6. *n*-Butyl acetate.

7. *n*-Butanol.
8. 0.1 mg/mL sialic-acid solution.
9. ^{1}HNMR analysis (*see* Chapter 3, **Subheading 3.5.3.**)

3. Methods

3.1. Chemical Modification of Serogroup B Meningococcal Polysaccharide: Preparation of Propionylated Serogroup B Meningococcal Polysaccharide

3.1.1. N-Deacetylation of Serogroup B Meningococcal Polysaccharide

1. Dissolve 100 mg serogroup B meningococcal polysaccharide (Colominic acid) and 10 mL NaBH$_4$ in 10 mL 2 *M* NaOH and heat in 20-mL sealed Pyrex tube at 105°C for 7 h (*see* **Note 1**).
2. Cool the solution to room temperature and neutralize with 2 *M* HCl to ca. pH 8.0.
3. Dialyze against distilled water and lyophilize.
4. Chromatograph product on Bio-Gel A 0.5 column (2 × 30 cm) using 0.1 *M* PBS buffer, pH 7.8, as eluant.
5. Collect and pool (*see* Chapter 3, **Subheading 3.4.2.**) fractions containing sialic acid and dialyze and lyophilize to give *N*-deacetylated serogroup B meningococcal polysaccharide (MW : 10~–1kD) as a white powder (70–85 mg).
6. Perform ^{1}HNMR on the product. *N*-Deacetylation is complete when the ^{1}H signal representing the acetyl groups at 2.2. ppm disappears.

3.1.2. N-Propionylation of the N-Deacylated Serogroup B Meningococcal Polysaccharide

1. Add 0.2 mL propionic anhydride, in 5 separate portions, to 100 mg of *N*-deacetylated serogroup B meningococcal polysaccharide in 4 mL 0.1 *M* NaOH. Stir for 4 h while 2 *M* NaOH is added as required to maintain the pH between 7.0 and 8.5 (*see* **Note 2**).
2. Adjust to pH 11.0–12.0 with 2 *M* NaOH and stir for 1 h (*see* **Note 3**).
3. Neutralize the solution (pH 7.0–8.0) with 2 *M* HCl and *N*-propionylated serogroup B meningococcal polysaccharide (95–100 mg) is obtained as in **Subheading 3.1.1., steps 3–6**.
4. Perform ^{1}HNMR spectroscopy on the product to confirm that *N*-propionylation is complete.

3.2. Oxidative Activation of N-Propionylated Serogroup B Meningococcal Polysaccharide

1. Add 5 mg NaIO$_4$ to a 2 mg solution N-propionylated serogroup B meningococcal polysaccharide in 1.0 mL 0.1 *M* NaOAc-HOAc buffer at pH 6.5 (*see* **Note 4**). Keep in the dark for 30 min.
2. Add 0.1 mL 10% ethylene glycol and leave for 30 min to degrade the remaining NaIO$_4$.

3. Purify the activated *N*-propionylated serogroup B meningococcal polysaccharide as described in **Subheading 3.1.1., steps 3–6**. Yield is 16–17 mg.

3.3. Conjugation of N-Propionylated Serogroup B Meningococcal Polysaccharide and TT

1. Conjugate 10 mg activated N-propionylated serogroup B meningococcal polysaccharide to monomeric TT by reductive amination, and isolate the 6 mg *N*-propionylated serogroup B meningococcal polysaccharide-TT conjugate by methods previously described in Chapter 4, **Subheading 3.3.**

3.4. Saccharide Loading of Glycoconjugate

1. Analyze the N-propionylated serogroup B meningococcal polysaccharide-TT conjugate using procedures described in Chapter 4, **Subheading 3.4.**

4. Notes

1. The serogroup B meningococcal polysaccharide is relatively stable under these conditions. However, some degradation, such as the base-catalyzed elimination, is observed. The addition of $NaBH_4$ minimizes this degradation by reducing the carbonyl group at the reducing end of the serogroup B meningococcal polysaccharide.

2. Saccharide linkages and especially sialyl linkages are usually stable to basic conditions, however, during propionylation of *N*-deacetylated serogroup B meningococcal polysaccharide with propionic anhydride, propionic acid is released and the pH of the reaction mixture becomes acidic. Therefore, it is very important to add the anhydride in small portions and to carefully monitor and maintain the pH of the reaction mixture in the range of 7.0–8.5 by titration with 2 *M* NaOH. Addition of anhydride in small portions also reduces the risk of local heating during propionylation.

3. The strong basic conditions used during the *N*-propionylation process, ensure that there is no *O*-propionylation of the resultant *N*-propionylated serogroup B meningococcal polysaccharide.

4. The backbone structure of *N*-propionylated serogroup B meningococcal polysaccharide is stable to oxidation. Therefore, a large excess of $NaIO_4$ is used in this case and the oxidation finishes within 15 min.

References

1. Wyle, F. A., Artenstein, M. S., Brandt, B. L., Tramont, D. L., Kasper, D. L., Altieri, P.L., et al. (1972) Immunological response of man to group B meningococcal polysaccharide vaccines. *J. Infect. Dis.* **126,** 514–522.
2. Jennings, H. J. and Lugowski, C. (1981) Immunochemistry of groups A, B, and C meningococcal polysaccharide-tetanus toxoid conjugates. *J. Immunol.* **127,** 1011–1018.

3. Bartolini, A., Norelli, F., Ceccarini, C., Rappuoli, R., and Constantino, P. (1995) Immunogenicity of meningococcal B polysaccharide conjugated to tetanus toxoid or CRM197 via adipic acid dihydrazine. *Vaccine* **13,** 463–470.

4. Bhattacharjee, A. K., Jennings, H. J., Kenny, C. P., Martin, A., and Smith, I. C. P. (1975) Structural determination of the sialic acid polysaccharide antigens of *Neisseria meningitis* serogroups B and C with carbon 13 nuclear magnetic resonance. *J. Biol. Chem.* **250,** 1926–1932.

5. Ando, S. and Yu, K. K. (1979) Isolation and characterization of two isomers of brain tetrasialogangliosides. *J. Biol. Chem.* **254,** 12,224–12,229.

6. Troy, F. A. (1992) Polysialylation: from bacteria to brains. *Glycobiology* **2,** 5–23.

7. Diaz-Romero, J. and Outschoorn, I. M. (1994) Current status of meningococcal group B vaccine candidates: capsular or non-capsular. *Clin. Microbiol. Rev.* **7,** 559–575.

8. Poolman, J. T. (1995) Development of a meningococcal vaccine. *Infect. Agent Dis.* **4,** 13–28.

9. Jennings, H. J. (1990) Capsular polysaccharides as a vaccine candidates. *Curr. Top. Microbiol. Immunol.* **150,** 97–127.

10. Jennings, H. J. (1997) N-Propionylated group B meningococcal polysaccharide glycoconjugate vaccine against group B meningococcal meningitis. *Int. J. Infect Dis.* **1,** 158–164.

11. Baumann, H., Brisson, J.-R., Michon, F., Pon, R., and Jennings, H. J. (1993) Comparison of the conformation of the epitope of $\alpha(2\text{-}8)$ polysialic acid with its reduced and N-acyl derivatives. *Biochemistry* **32,** 4007–4013.

12. Jennings, H. J., Roy, R., and Gamian, A. (1986) Induction of group B meningococcal polysaccharide-specific IgG antibodies in mice by using an *N*-propionylated B polysaccharide-tetanus toxoid conjugate vaccine. *J. Immunol.* **137,** 1708–1713.

13. Ashton, F. E., Ryan, J. A., Michon, F., and Jennings, H. J. (1989) Protective efficacy of mouse serum to the *N*-propionyl derivative of meningococcal group B polysaccharide. *Microb. Pathog.* **6,** 455–458.

14. Jennings, H. J., Gamian, A., and Ashton, F. E. (1987) *N*-Propionylated group B meningococcal polysaccharide mimics a unique epitope on group B *Neisseria meningitidis*. *J. Exp. Med.* **165,** 1207–1211.

15. Pon, R. A., Lussier, M., Yang, Q-L., and Jennings, H. J. (1997) *N*-Propionylated group B meningococcal polysaccharide mimics a unique bactericidal capsular epitope in group B *Neisseria meningitidis*. *J. Exp. Med.* **185,** 1929–1938.

16. Tai, J. Y., Michon, F., Fusco, P. C., and Blake, M. S. (1997) Preclinical evaluation of a novel group B meningococcal conjugate vaccine that elicits bactericidal activity in both mice and non-human primates. *J. Infect. Dis.* **175,** 364–372.

6

Outer Membrane Protein Purification

Carmen Arigita, Wim Jiskoot, Matthijs R. Graaf, and Gideon F. A. Kersten

1. Introduction

1.1. Meningococcal Outer Membrane Proteins, Function, and Characteristics

The major outer membrane proteins (OMPs) from *Neisseria meningitidis*, which are expressed at high levels, are subdivided in five classes based on molecular weight *(1,2)* (*see* **Table 1**).

The class 1 (also mentioned PorA), class 2, and class 3 (PorB2 and PorB3, respectively) OMPs are porins. Class 1 OMPs are cation selective porins and induce formation of bactericidal antibodies. Class 2 and class 3 are anion-selective porins and are self-exclusive, so never expressed simultaneously *(2)*. Antibodies against class 2/3 are only occasionally protective and bactericidal *(3)*.

Class 4 OMPs can be reduced with mercaptoethanol. Their function is unknown but they may have pore-forming properties. Antibodies against class 4 OMPs can block the bactericidal activity of class 1 and class 2/3 OMP-specific antibodies, rendering the bacteria less immunogenic *(2)*. For this reason, class 4 OMPs are not interesting to isolate for vaccine purposes. However, it is important to eliminate these proteins from other OMP isolates.

Two types of class 5 OMPs or opacity proteins are discerned: Opa and Opc. They play a role in bacterial adhesion to and invasion of host cells *(1)*. Meningococci can change the nature and level of expression of Opa and the expression level of Opc. The opacity proteins are not suitable as vaccine candidates because of the high variability of the exposed (i.e., immunogenic) regions.

Another group of OMPs is only expressed by meningococci when they suffer from iron exhaustion. These iron-regulated proteins serve to capture and

From: *Methods in Molecular Medicine, vol. 66: Meningococcal Vaccines: Methods and Protocols*
Edited by: A. J. Pollard and M. C. J. Maiden © Humana Press Inc., Totowa, NJ

Table 1
Major Meningococcal Outer-Membrane Proteins

Outer-membrane proteins	Name	Molecular mass	Function/characteristics
Class 1	PorA	44–47 kDa	*Por*in
Class 2/3	PorB	37–42 kDa	*Por*in
Class 4	Rmp		Reduction *m*odifiable *p*rotein, unknown
Class 5	Opa	26–30 kDa	Adhesion, *opa*city protein
	Opc	25 kDa	Invasion, opacity protein
Iron-regulated proteins	Mirp	37 kDa	Iron acquisition (?); *m*ajor *i*ron-*r*egulated *p*rotein
	FrpB	70 kDa	Ferric enterobactin receptor (also FetA)

Adapted from ref. *(1)*.

internalize bound iron from the host. The bactericidal activity of antibodies elicited against these proteins is comparable to those against class 1 OMPs. Therefore, the iron-regulated proteins have attracted considerable attention as vaccine candidates *(4)*.

The isolation and purification of some meningococcal OMPs have not been described as yet. Instead, the isolation and purification of comparable proteins of other Gram-negative bacteria has been described and can be used as a starting point. In this chapter, this approach is followed for class 5 proteins and fimbriae.

This chapter deals with general methods for the isolation of OMPs. A general approach for the isolation of OMPs from meningococci or other Gram-negative bacteria is not available. Most authors first disrupt the bacterial cells, followed by the isolation of the outer membrane. The OMPs are purified from this outer-membrane preparation. A general technique for the isolation of porins (class 1, 2, and 3 OMP) is extraction of an outer-membrane preparation with a detergent in combination with ethylenediamonetetraacetic acid (EDTA) or NaCl, followed by gel-filtration chromatography *(5)*. Also ethanol precipitation followed by anion-exchange and gel-filtration chromatography has been used for porins and for class 5 OMPs *(6,7)*. In this section, special attention will be paid to the depletion of lipooligosaccharide (LOS) from the outer membrane.

In **Subheading 3.**, alternative isolation methods are dealt with. An alternative method for the production of OMPs is the cloning and expression of OMPs as inclusion bodies in Gram-positive *(8)* or Gram-negative *(9)* bacteria. During solubilization of inclusion bodies, the use of guanidinium chloride or detergents such as sodium dodecyl sulfate (SDS) causes unfolding of the OMPs. Refolding procedures involve the use of liposomes *(10)* or mild detergents *(11)*. An alternative method for LOS depletion is described as well in this section.

The purification of fimbriae will be discussed in **Subheading 4.** Although not strictly OMP, these filamentous structures from the meningococcal cell surface are involved in bacterial adhesion to tissues and therefore of interest for vaccine development.

2. Materials

2.1. Isolation of Outer Membrane from Whole Cells

2.1.1. Cell Disruption

1. Suspension buffer A: 0.75 M sucrose, 10 mM Tris-HCl, pH 7.8.
2. EDTA solution: 1.5 mM EDTA, pH 7.5.
3. Branson sonifier: 20 KC.
4. Suspension buffer B: 3.3 mM Tris-HCl, 1 mM EDTA, 0.25 M sucrose.
5. Suspension buffer C: 5 mM EDTA, 25% (w/v) sucrose.
6. Electrophoresis buffer: 5 mM Tris-HCl, 5 mM EDTA, 5% (w/v) sucrose, pH 7.7.

2.1.2. Isolation of Outer-Membrane Preparation Without Use of Mechanical Force

1. DOC buffer: 100 mM Tris-HCl, 10 mM EDTA, 0.5% (w/v) DOC, pH 8.6.
2. Sucrose buffer: 50 mM Tris-HCl, 2 mM EDTA, 1.2% DOC(w/v), 20% (w/v) sucrose, pH 8.6.
3. EDTA buffer: 50 mM Na$_2$HPO$_4$, 150 mM NaCl, 10 mM EDTA, pH 7.4.
4. Sarkosyl buffer: 0.01 M HEPES, 1% (w/v) sarkosyl.

2.1.3. Protein Purification

2.1.3.1. Class 1 And 2/3

1. Extraction buffer: 1% (w/v) Zwittergent® 3,14, 0.5 M CaCl$_2$, 0.14 M NaCl, pH 4.0.
2. Buffer A: 0.1 M sodim acetate, 25 mM EDTA, 0.05% (w/v) Zwittergent 3,14, pH 6.0. This buffer can be replaced by 50 mM Tris-HCl, 10 mM EDTA, 0.05% (w/v) Zwittergent 3,14, pH 8.0.
3. DEAE-Sepharose (Pharmacia, Uppsala, Sweden).
4. Buffer B: 50 mM Tris-HCl, 200 mM NaCl, 20 mM EDTA, 0.05% (w/v) Zwittergent 3,14, pH 7.2.
5. Sephacryl S-300 (Pharmacia).

2.1.3.2. Class 5

1. Suspension buffer A: 1 M Sodium acetate, 1 mM 2,3-dimercaptopropanol, 5% (w/v) Zwittergent 3,14, 0.5 M CaCl$_2$, pH 4.0.

2. Suspension buffer B: 50 mM Tris-HCl, 10 mM EDTA.
3. DEAE-Sepharose (Pharmacia).
4. CM-Sepharose (Pharmacia).
5. Sephacryl S-200 (Pharmacia).
6. Buffer C: 10 mM Tris-HCl, 20 mM NaCl, 10 mM EDTA, 0.05% Zwittergent 3,14, pH 8.0.
7. Trizma buffer: 50 mM Trizma, 5% Zwittergent 3,14, pH 7.2.
8. MonoQ HR 10/10 (Pharmacia).
9. MonoS HR 10/10 (Pharmacia).
10. Polybuffer exchanger: PBE 118 (Pharmacia).
11. Chromatofocussing buffer: 25 M Triethylamine, 1% (w/v) Triton X-100, pH 11.0.
12. Pharmalyte buffer (Pharmacia), 1% Triton X-100, pH 8.0.
13. Acetate buffer: 50 mM sodium acetate, 1% (w/v) Zwittergent 3,14, pH 5.6.

2.1.3.3. IRON-REGULATED PROTEINS

1. CTB buffer: 10 mM Tris, 0.05% (w/v) CTB, pH 8.0.

2.2. Isolation of Cloned Membrane Proteins from Inclusion Bodies

2.2.1. Isolation of IBs

2.2.1.1. NURMINEN METHOD

1. DNase buffer: 50 mM Tris-HCl, pH 8.0, containing 5 mg/mL Dnase.
2. NP-40 buffer: 50 mM Tris-HCl, 1% NP-40, pH 8.0.

2.2.1.2. Qi METHOD

1. TEN: 50 mM Tris-HCl, 1 mM EDTA, 10 mM NaCl, pH 8.0.
2. Lysozyme solution: 10 mg/mL water.

2.2.1.3. WARD METHOD

1. MSE Soniprep 150 sonicator.

2.2.2. Refolding of Cloned Proteins in Liposomes

1. Detergent buffer: 10 mM HEPES, 10% octyl glucoside, pH 7.2.
2. PBS, pH 7.2.
3. Sephadex G-50 (Pharmacia).
4. Dilution buffer: 10 mM Tris, 0.9% (w/v) NaCl, pH 7.4.

2.2.3. Refolding of Cloned Proteins by Use of Detergents

1. Buffer A: 20 mM Na$_2$HPO$_4$/NaH$_2$PO$_4$, 14.8 mM Zwittergent 3,12, pH 7.0.
2. SP-Sepharose HP (Pharmacia).
3. Buffer B: 20 mM Na$_2$HPO$_4$/NaH$_2$PO$_4$, 10 mM Zwittergent 3,12, pH 7.0.
4. Dialysis buffer: 10 mM Tris-HCL, 3 mM Zwittergent 3,12.

5. Buffer C: 20 m*M* Ethanolamine, 14.8 m*M* Zwittergent 3,12, pH 10.8.
6. Anion exchanger: Q-sepharose HP (Pharmacia).
7. Buffer D: 20 m*M* Ethanolamine, 10 m*M* Zwittergent 3,12, pH 10.8.
8. Neutralization buffer: 20 m*M* Tris-HCl, pH 7.8.

2.3. Purification of Fimbriae

1. Ethanolamine buffer: 0.15 *M* ethanolamine-HCl, pH 10.2.
2. Tris-saline: 50 m*M* Tris-HCl, 150 m*M* NaCl, pH 8.0.
3. Urea buffer: 5.5 *M* urea, 0.5% (w/v) DOC, 0.15 *M* NaCl, 0.05 M sodium acetate, pH 7.0.
4. Sephacryl s-1000 (Pharmacia).
5. Octyl-Sepharose CL-4B (Pharmacia).

3. Methods
3.1. Isolation of OMPs from Whole Cells
3.1.1. Cell Disruption

In order to isolate the outer membrane, it is necessary to disrupt the cells of interest. The most applied method for the isolation of outer membrane consist of a EDTA-lysozyme treatment (spheroplast formation) followed by sonication or osmotic shock for cell disruption *(12,13)*. In other methods mechanical forces are directly applied to bacterial cells (*see* **Subheadings 3.1.1.2.** and **3.1.1.3.**).

3.1.1.1. SPHEROPLASTING

Spheroplasts are cell forms devoid of the peptidoglycan layer. The EDTA is used to obtain spheroplasts because it destabilizes the outer membrane and makes it more permeable for lysozyme. This is owing to the removal of cations (principally Ca^{2+} and Mg^{2+}), which stabilize the membrane by electrostatic interaction with negatively charged LOS. Upon removal of these ions LOS chains start to repulse each other. After destabilization, the outer membrane is detached by the action of lysozyme and a spheroplast remains. The spheroplast must be subsequently disrupted to separate the membrane fraction from other cell components.

3.1.1.1.1. Formation Of Spheroplasts

1. Harvest the cells (5×10^8 bacteria/mL) by centrifugation and resuspend them in cold cell-suspension buffer A to a final density of 7×10^9 bacteria/mL.
2. Add lysozyme to the resuspended cells to a final concentration of 100 µg/mL.
3. Incubated the mixture in ice for 2 min and subsequently, transform the cells into spheroplasts by slowly adding 2 volumes of cold EDTA solution (*see* **Note 1**).

3.1.1.1.2. Disruption Of Spheroplasts. Either sonication or osmotic shock can accomplish this. Sonication is usually sufficient.

1. Perform sonication during 15-s periods with a Branson Sonifier or equivalent instrument maintaining the spheroplast suspension temperature below 10°C.
2. Continue until the absorbance of the spheroplast suspension has decreased to approx 5% of its original value.
3. Use phase-contrast microscopy for detection of non-lysed cells.

If the protein of interest is solubilized or denatured upon sonication, osmotic shock is the method of choice for spheroplast disruption. For this purpose, pour the spheroplast suspension slowly into 4 volumes of cold water and stir the solution for 10 min.

The procedure to recover the total membrane fraction from the sonicate or the osmotic lysate is as follows:

1. Centrifuge the lysate at 1200g for 15 min at 2–4°C to remove nonlysed cells.
2. Subsequently, centrifuge the supernatant at ~300,000g for 2 h at 2–4°C. This step also removes ribosome fragments. Ribosomes are disintegrated by the combined effect of EDTA and endogenous RNases.
3. Resuspend the pellet in 2 mL cold cell suspension buffer B and homogenize it with a syringe with a needle of about 0.6 mm diameter. Fill up the volume to about 20 mL with the same sucrose solution.
4. Centrifuge the suspension as described above and resuspend the pellet, as before, in 1 mL of cold suspension buffer C (*see* **Note 2**).

Direct mechanical methods for cell rupture are French-pressure cell passage and ultrasonic treatment.

3.1.1.2. THE FRENCH-PRESSURE CELL

With a French-pressure cell, bacteria can be lysed reproducibly by pressurizing a volume up to 100 mL of a cell suspension to about 100 MPa and subsequent sudden release of the pressure. This breaks bacterial cells efficiently. The method is gentle with regard to the protein conformation. Before passage through the French-pressure cell, resuspend the cells in a buffer containing RNase and DNase. Mostly a HEPES buffer is used, but many other buffers except Tris buffer can replace it. The latter has a damaging effect on membranes, owing to its chelating effect in the absence of external Mg^{2+}. The presence of Mg^{2+} is necessary to avoid the degradation of ribosomes by RNase *(13)*. Also DNase needs Mg^{2+} to be active. After French-pressure cell lysis, the outer membrane and inner membrane are detached and ready for separation.

EDTA can be omitted, but is likely to improve the separation. Furthermore, EDTA can inhibit metal proteases, resulting in an increase in protein yield.

3.1.1.3. ULTRASONIC DISRUPTION

Bacteria can also be broken by ultrasonication. This method can be applied to very small volumes and is rather simple. Moreover, sonicators are readily available. However, prolonged sonication can lead to the formation of artificial hybrids between the outer and inner membrane that cannot be separated and is a rather violent method, which can possibly result in protein denaturation.

3.1.2. Outer-Membrane Disruption: Separation of Inner From Outer Membrane in Mixed-Membrane Preparations (Osborn Method)

A generally used method for the separation of outer and inner membrane of Gram-negative bacteria was described in 1972 by Osborn and Munson *(12)*. This method consists of sucrose gradient isopycnic centrifugation.

1. Prepare step gradients by layering 2.1 mL each of 50, 45, 40, 35, and 30% (w/w) sucrose solutions over a cushion (0.5 mL) of 55% sucrose. All sucrose solutions contain 5 mM EDTA, pH 7.5.
2. Layer 1 mL of the total membrane fraction on top of the gradient and centrifuge it at 190,000–200,000g for 12–16 h at 2–6°C. Apparent equilibrium is reached within 12 h (*see* **Note 3**).

3.1.3. Isolation of Outer-Membrane Preparations Without Use of Mechanical Force

3.1.3.1. BLEBBING STIMULATION

Blebs are vesicular fractions of the outer membrane that meningococci spontaneously produce. This feature can be induced by the use of the detergent deoxycholate (DOC) and EDTA *(14)*. EDTA removes Ca^{2+} and Mg^{2+} ions, destabilizing the outer membrane by an excess of negative charge (LOS is negatively charged). This process together with the fluidization of the membrane by DOC, stimulated the OMV formation:

1. Suspend bacteria in DOC buffer and stir them for 30 min at room temperature (RT).
2. Centrifuge at 20,000g for 30 min at 4°C.
3. Repeat the extraction with a buffer volume reduced to one third.
4. Combine the supernatants and ultracentrifuge them (125,000g; 2 h; 4°C).
5. Resuspend the outer membrane vesicle (OMV) pellet in sucrose buffer (*see* **Note 4**).

3.1.3.2. Differential Solubilization

Sarkosyl (or N-lauryl sarcosine) is a detergent that, in the absence of Mg^{2+}, selectively solubilizes the inner membrane. Mg^{2+} coprecipates Sarkosyl and the inner membrane. This detergent can be replaced by Triton X-100 to obtain similar results *(15)*.

1. Harvest the cells by centrifugation at 100,000g for 1 h at 4°C.
2. Resuspend the pellet in Sarkosyl buffer and incubate the mixture at RT for 30 min to solubilize cytoplasmic membrane proteins.
3. Centrifuge at 100,000g for 1 h at 4°C to remove the Sarkosyl insoluble fraction.

In all cases the detergent concentration has to be at least 10 times that of the total mass of proteins in the membrane.

3.1.4. Protein Purification

3.1.4.1. Class 1 And Class 2/3

The purification of PorA proteins of *Neisseria meningitidis* *(6)*, based on a method used for purification of opacity-associated proteins of *Neisseria gonorrhoeae* *(16)*. The method, which can be used to purify both class 1 and class 2/3 OMP from meningococci (*see* **Fig. 1**) consists of the following steps:

1. Extract harvested cells (fresh or lyophilized) directly by use of 100 mL extraction buffer per g of bacteria (dry weight).
2. After resuspension, bring the pH to 6.0 with NaOH and extract the suspension for 1 h at RT.
3. Remove cell debris by centrifugation (1 h, 3,000g, RT or 20 min, 10,000g) and add ethanol to the supernatant to 20% (v/v). Centrifuge it again (30 min, RT, 10,000g).
4. Concentrate the supernatant by diafiltration (Amicon hollow fiber system, cutoff 30,000 D) and replace the ethanol and $CaCl_2$ by buffer A.
5. Adjust the pH to 4.0, add 20% (v/v) ethanol and incubate for 30 min.
6. Centrifuge the solution during 30 min at 10,000g. The supernatant contains rather pure class 3 OMP. Residual LOS can be removed by gel-filtration chromatography.
7. Resuspend the pellet, containing the combined class1/3/4, in buffer A. LOS is removed by DEAE-Sepharose and Sephacryl chromatography. Equilibrate a DEAE-Sepharose column with buffer A and elute the protein with a linear gradient from 0.0–0.6 M NaCl in buffer A.
8. Pool fractions containing protein and apply them on a Sephacryl column equilibrated with buffer B to achieve further LOS-depletion.
9. Separate cass 1 OMP from other OMPs by preparative sodium dodecyl sulfate-polyacrylamide gel electrophoresis (SDS-PAGE) (*see* **Note 5**).

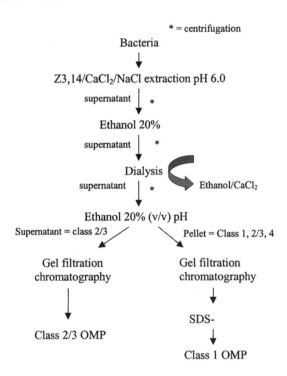

Fig. 1. Isolation of class 1 and 2/3 OMP from *Neisseria meningitidis* according to Poolman et al. *(6)*.

3.1.4.2. REMOVAL OF CLASS 4

Class 4 OMPs of *N. meningitidis* are not vaccine candidates. These proteins not only fail to elicit bactericidal antibodies against meningococci, but they also block the interaction of bactericidal antibodies against other OMPs. Thus, it is important to eliminate class 4 OMP from the proteins of interest. Most porin trimers are resistant to trypsin treatment. Because the class 4 OMP does not form trimers, it is probably cleaved by trypsin treatment *(17)*. After the trypsine cleavage of class 4 OMP, class 1 and 2/3 trimers can be separated from the tryptic fragments by gel filtration chromatography as performed in **Subheading 3.1.4.1.**

3.1.4.3. CLASS 5

The opacity associated OMPs from meningococci present structural similarities to outer membrane opacity proteins from gonococci (e.g., protein II) *(18,19)*. The same method *(16)* has been used to purify Opa proteins from

N. meningitidis and *N. gonorrhoeae*. Opa proteins can be separated from other membrane proteins by use of ion-exchange chromatography:

1. Resuspend harvested cells in suspension buffer A and stir for 1 hour at RT. Add ethanol slowly to a concentration of 20% (v/v). Remove the precipitate containing nucleic acids by centrifugation at 17,000g for 10 min. Increase the ethanol concentration to 80% (v/v) and recover the resulting precipitate by centrifugation.
2. Resuspend the precipitate containing class 5 OMP in suspension buffer B. Apply the sample onto a DEAE-Sepharose (anion exchanger) column linked to a CM-Sepharose (cation exchanger) column both equilibrated with the same suspension buffer B.
3. Wash the two columns until the 280 nm absorbance falls to baseline level. Separate the columns and apply a linear NaCl gradient between 0.0–0.5 M to the CM-sepharose column.
4. Precipitate fractions containing class 5 OMP (as monitored by absorption at 280 nm and SDS-PAGE) in 80% ethanol and resuspend them in suspension buffer B.
5. Class 5 OMP can be further purified (LOS depletion) by gel filtration with a Sephacryl S-200 column with buffer C for elution (*see* **Note 6**).

3.1.4.4. IRON-REGULATED PROTEINS

Mietzner and Morse *(20)* have first described the purification of a gonococcal protein expressed in the outer membrane as a result of the limitation in iron during bacterial growth. This method can be used as well for purification of iron-regulated proteins from meningococci *(21)*. The 37-kDa protein appeared to be the most abundant iron-regulated protein. The cationic detergent cetyltrimethylammonium bromide (CTB) selectively solubilizes the 37 kDa protein at low concentrations. At CTB concentrations between 0.025% and 0.05% (w/v), nearly all the 37 kDa protein is extracted. This characteristic is used for its purification:

1. Disrupt cells and isolate outer membranes by Sarkosyl extraction as previously described (*see* **Subheading 2.3.2.** of **Section 3.**).
2. Resuspend outer meningococcal membranes in distilled water (1 mg protein/mL) and add CTB to a final concentration of 0.05%. Incubate the mixture for 20 min at RT, and remove the insoluble material by centrifugation at 48,000g for 1 h.

Dilute the supernatant fraction to 10 mM Tris-HCl, pH 8.0, and apply it to a CM-Sepharose column with CTB buffer as eluent (equilibrated with 10 column volumes). Elution with a gradient of 0–1 M NaCl results in two peaks. The 37-kDa iron-regulated protein elutes in the second peak, as confirmed by SDS-PAGE.

3.2. Isolation of Cloned Membrane Proteins from Inclusion Bodies

Neisseria OMPs can be cloned and expressed in other Gram negative or Gram positive bacteria as inclusion bodies (IBs). IBs are aggregates of almost pure (membrane) proteins in the cytoplasm of the host cell. The proteins are not expressed in the membrane owing to its (possible) toxicity to the host cell. Among the advantages of cloning is the absence of LOS in the Gram-positive hosts and probably as well in those obtained from Gram-negative bacteria. The recovery of recombinant proteins from IBs requires the use of procedures that may lead to the (reversible) unfolding of the OMPs. A refolding step is needed in (almost) all procedures described.

3.2.1. Isolation of IBs

Three methods have been described for the isolation of IBs from genetically modified bacteria *(8,9,22)*.

3.2.1.1. NURMINEN METHOD

The method described by Nurminen et al. *(8)* for purification of recombinant *N. menigitidis* class 1 OMP from *Bacillus subtilis* contains the following steps:

1. Form spheroplasts as described in **Subheading 2.1.** of **Section 3.**
2. Collect spheroplasts by centrifugation (10,000g, 20 min) and lyse them by suspension in DNase buffer.
3. Collect IBs by centrifugation at 10,000g for 10 min and wash them in NP-40 buffer and centrifuge them again.

3.2.1.2. Qi METHOD

In 1994, Qi et al. *(9)* described another method to isolate IBs:

1. Harvest cells by centrifugation and resuspend them in 3 ml TEN buffer per g of cells. To this, add 8 µL of 50 mM phenyl methyl sulfonyl fluoride (PMSF) in anhydrous ethanol and 80 µL of lysozyme solution and stir the mixture for 20 min at RT. Subsequently, add 4 mg deoxycholate per g cells.
2. Place the mixture in a 37°C water bath and stir it with a glass rod. When the solution becomes viscous, add 20 µL of DNase I (1 mg/mL). Remove the mixture from the water bath and leave it at RT until it is no longer viscous.
3. Centrifuge the mixture at 26,892g (15,000 rpm in an SS-34 rotor) for 10 min at 4°C. Retain the pellets containing IBs and wash them thoroughly twice with TEN buffer.

3.2.1.3. WARD METHOD

The method described by Ward et al. in 1996 *(22)* is a modification of method described in **3.2.1.1.**:

1. Form spheroplasts as described in **Subheading 3.1.1.1.**
2. Disrupt the spheroplasts (10 mL) by sonication and remove cellular debris by centrifugation (230*g* for 30 min).
3. Harvest IBs at 12,000*g* for 1 h, and resuspend the resulting pellet in sterile water containing 0.05% (w/v) sodium azide, 1 m*M* PMSF and store them at –20°C.

IBs are dissolved in 6 *M* guanidine-HCl, 2% SDS, or 8 *M* urea. The high concentration of these components leads to the unfolding of the protein of interest. The reconstitution/refolding is described below.

3.2.2. Refolding of Cloned Proteins in Liposomes

Liposomes, membraneous lipid vesicles, can be used to refold Neisseria porins produced as IBs both in Gram-negative and Gram-positive hosts *(10,22)*. Because of their amphiphilicity/structure, liposomes provide the adequate environment to permit a membrane protein to regain its native structure.

The method used to obtain (proteo)liposomes consists of:

1. Dissolve the lipids forming the bilayer (e.g., L-α-phosphatidylcholine and cholesterol, molar ratio 7:2) in chloroform in a glass round-bottom flask, and remove the solvent under vacuum with rotation to produce a lipid film.
2. Add the detergent buffer, slowly to the OMP of interest (0.5 mg) dissolved in 0.1%, (w/v) SDS, to give a final concentration of 10% (w/v) OG. OG has a critical micellar concentration (CMC), i.e., the monomer concentration is high compared to the micelle concentration. Therefore, OG is dialyzable.
3. Use the detergent-protein solution to solubilize the shell dried lipid. This results in the formation of mixed lipid/protein/detergent micelles.
4. Remove the detegent by dialysis against PBS, pH 7.2 at 4°C; this will result in the formation of liposomes (*see* **Note 7**).

3.2.3. Refolding of Cloned Proteins by Use of Detergents

The protein in IBs can be refolded also by use of detergents. In this case, the folding conditions have to be determined separately for each OMP. For the class 1 OMP subtype P1.6 and P1.7,16 the folding conditions have been determined *(23)*:

1. For P1.6, the folding is initiated by a 100-fold dilution of the urea-dissolved IBs (10–20 mg protein/mL) in buffer A to a final concentration of 150–200 μg/mL protein and incubated overnight at RT. Remove aggregates, if any, by centrifuga-

tion (20 min, 8,000*g*) and purify folded protein by ion-exchange chromatography on a SP-Sepharose column equilibrated with buffer B. Elute the protein with a linear gradient of 0–2 *M* NaCl in the same buffer and pool fractions containing folded P1.6 as checked by SDS-PAGE, and dialyze them against dialysis buffer to remove NaCl.

2. Dilute the P1.7,16 porin for its folding from the urea-stock (10–20 mg/mL protein) 50–100 fold in buffer C to a final concentration of 150–200 µg/mL and incubate this overnight at RT. Purify folded protein by anion-exchange chromatography. Elute with a 0–2 *M* NaCl gradient in buffer D. Neutralize fractions immediately with neutralization buffer and pool those containing folded protein as checked by SDS-PAGE and dialyze them against dialysis buffer (*see* **Note 8**).

3.3. Purification of Fimbriae

Fimbriae or pili are filamentous protein structures consisting of repeating subunits (pilin). Analogous structures are found in gonococci. Meningococci express two classes of frimbriae-class I and class II- wich are antigenically and structurally distinct. Fimbriae are involved in adhesion and play a role in transformation (acquisition of heterologous DNA from the environment). They show a high degree of antigenic variability (*1*).

There are two methods used for the purification of fimbriae from meningococci. The "classical" method (*see* **Fig. 2**) is based on the observation that fimbriae are soluble at high pH, high ionic strength or in the presence of bivalent ions. Therefore, fimbriae can be obtained by repeated solubilization/crystallization (*25,27*):

1. Harvest the cells (typically 2*g* wet weight) and resuspend them into ethanolamine buffer (25 mL). The fimbriae are shed at this pH.
2. Centrifuged the suspension at 20,000*g* for 30 min to remove bacteria and cell debris.
3. Add saturated ammonium sulfate to the supernatant containing disaggregated fimbriae to achieve 10% saturation and stir the mixture gently for 1 h.
4. Collect the precipitated crude fimbriae by centrifugation at 15,000*g* for 10 min. Resuspend and stir the fimbriae pellet in ethanolamine buffer until dissolved.
5. Repeat the ammonium sulphate precipitation several times to achieve higher purity (*see* **Note 9**).

An alternative method has been proposed based on the separation by hydrophobic-interaction chromatography (*26*). The separation is based on the detergent-reversible interaction between fimbriae and the hydrophobic surface of a chromatographic column. This interaction is enhanced by high ionic-strength buffer, which makes it also suitable to further purify fimbriae after ammonium-

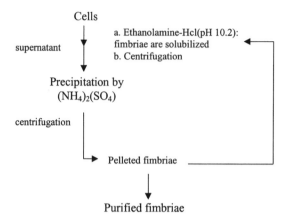

Fig. 2. Purification of fimbriae by the "classical" method.

sulfate precipitation. Although described for gonococci, this method can be used for meningococci as well:

1. Suspend cells into Tris-saline and dilute them to give an optical density at 540 nm of 0.8 AU. Sonicate 5-mL aliquots for 30 s.
2. Centrifuge at 12,500g for 30 min to remove whole cells and debris. Subsequently, pellet the fimbriae and outer membrane vesicles (OMVs) present in the supernatant by ultracentrifugation at 85,000g for 2.5 h and resuspend them in 1.0 mL Tris-saline.
3. Suspend the preparation of fimbriae and OMVs in urea buffer for 32 h before applying it to a Sephacryl S-1000 column (1.6 × 30 cm) equilibrated and eluted with urea buffer.
4. Pool fractions containing fimbriae and OMVs and apply them onto a 3 mL octyl-Sepharose column, equilibrated with urea buffer containing 0.5% deoxycholate and a 0.5–0.8% deoxycholate gradient is applied. Vesicles, being less hydrophobic than fimbriae, are eluted at lower concentrations of the detergent.

4. Notes

1. The cell suspension is continuous swirled in an ice-water bath and the diluent is added beneath the surface of the liquid to avoid local hypotonicity. In order to minimize premature lysis, vigorous agitation, and bubbling of air through the suspension should be avoided. The efficiency of spheroplast formation can be monitored by phase-contrast microscopy and should be greater than 95% in order to obtain a good separation between inner and outer membrane.
2. If sucrose-gradient electrophoresis is going to be used to separate the total membrane into an inner- and outer-membrane fraction (*see* **Subheading 3.1.1.**), the time required for sedimentation of the total membrane fraction can be shortened by addition of Mg^{2+} to the supernatant to a final concentration of 5 mM:

a. Sediment the membranes by centrifugation at 225,000g for 30 min.
b. Resuspend the pellet in cell-suspension buffer B, and add Mg^{2+} to a final concentration of 5 mM.
c. Repeat the centrifugation.
d. Suspend the washed membrane fraction in 0.5–2 mL of cold electrophoresis buffer.

On the other hand, if isopycnic centrifugation is applied to separate the inner membrane from the outer membrane, Mg^{2+} cannot be utilized because it prevents separation with this technique.

3. For larger-scale preparations, layer 6.3 mL of each sucrose solution on a cushion of 1.5 mL 55% sucrose. Two or three milliliter of the total membrane fraction can be processed. Apply centrifugation at 80,000g for 18–40 h. Although equilibrium is reached only after 30–36 h, adequate separations are achieved after 18 h already.

The bands obtained by this technique are identified by their chemical composition and specific enzymatic functions (e.g., SDS-PAGE for LOS determination [marker for the outer membrane] or NADH oxidase [marker for the inner membrane]). The outer membrane fraction shows a higher density than the inner membrane fraction.

4. A variation of this method consists of the use of EDTA and heat *(15)*. Blebs are formed after incubation with EDTA buffer for 30 min at 56°C. Cells are removed by centrifugation at 10,000g for 15 min at 4°C. The extraction is repeated and OMV are concentrated as described earlier.

5. Class 2/3 OMPs are mutually exclusive, so never expressed simultaneously. In general, the purification of class 1 OMP is a complicated task, because it is hard to separate this protein from class 2/3 OMP. However, with the described method rather pure class 1 and class 2/3 are obtained. The pH during the ethanol precipitation is critical and by varying it in the solubilization solution, specific proteins could be extracted *(16)*. Mutant strains expressing only one type of porin can be used *(17,28)* to simplify the procedure.

6. This method results in class 5 protein that still may contain LOS, because at pH values between 4.0 and 10.6, LOS is co-extracted with the protein. A variation of this method that avoids LOS contamination was described by Achtman et al. for the purification of eight class 5 OMPs variants *(7)*. The variations included in the aforementioned procedure are:
   a. The concentration of mercaptopropanol in the extraction buffer is increased to 50 mM and the pH decreased to 3.6. For class 5b OMP Empigen BB is used instead of Z3,14.
   b. After precipitation with 20% (v/v) ethanol, the pellet is resuspended in 1 M ethanolamine, pH 10.6, containing 50 mM mercaptopropanol, and then reextracted with $CaCl_2$ and Z3,14 and precipitated again with 20% ethanol.
   c. The pellets after 80% (v/v) ethanol precipitation are resuspended in Trizma buffer under stirring for 10 min at 20°C. To completely resuspend the pellet, stir the mixture at 65°C for 15 min and then cool it down to 30°C. Under these

conditions, the inhibition of protease activity with 1 mM PMSF is also necessary. After centrifugation, the supernatant is filtered through a 0.22-µm filter (Millipore Corp., Bedford, MA) and degassed.

   d. The column material used for column chromatography is Mono Q HR 10/10 and Mono S HR 10/10 in two columns in tandem.

   e. For class 5 protein a, the anion-exchange chromatography is not performed and chromatofocussing is done instead, using a poly-buffer exchanger column equilibrated with chromatofocussing buffer. The protein is eluted with a Pharmalyte buffer. The eluted protein is precipitated overnight with 80% (v/v) ethanol and resuspended in acetate buffer and applied to Mono S chromatography.

   f. The need of a DEAE-Sepharose column coupled to a CM-Sepharose column is not completely clear. Probably this step can also be done by use of only the CM-Sepharose column.

7. Detergent exchange can be accomplished by ethanol precipitation (in 80% ethanol) of the protein followed by resolubilization with the detergent of choice. Other alternatives to induce the formation of liposomes are:

   a. Gel filtration *(10)*. The lipid-protein-detergent solution is applied directly on top of a Sephadex column and eluted with PBS containing 1 mM EDTA, 0.02% NaN_3. Fractions eluting after the void volume are opalescent, which indicates the presence of liposomes.

   b. "Dilution method" *(29)*. Two milliliter of the lipid-protein detergent solution are quickly mixed in a 50 mL beaker with 20 dilution buffer, under vigorous stirring. This leads to the formation of small unilamellar vesicles with a particle size under 200 nm.

   Although the protein solubilized from inclusion bodies was not further purified by, e.g., ion-exchange chromatography or gel filtration, SDS analysis of the proteoliposomes did not show the presence of LOS from the Gram-negative host (22).

8. The purification of OMPs expressed in IBs in host cells can be simplified by adding a histidine-tag *(24)*. To accomplish this, the PorA gene is ligated to DNA encoding six histidine residues, which serve as a nickel-binding domain. This nickel-binding domain can be used as ligand in affinity chromatography. Preparations obtained in this way did not contain detectable amounts of contaminating proteins or LOS. Properly folded porin forms trimers. These can be observed with SDS-PAGE under mild conditions (e.g., without mercaptopropanol and at low SDS concentration in loading buffer, samples not heated) *(23)*.

9. This procedure, however, does not permit the removal of contaminating outer-membrane blebs. To obtain pure fimbriae, other steps such as preparative isoelectric focusing can be added. However, the solubilization/crystallization method probably results in the loss of fimbriae-associated proteins that may play a role in the immune response.

5. Concluding Remarks

A general approach for the purification of OMPs from *N. meningitidis* is not available. The characteristics of the protein of and the source of protein (meningococci, inclusion bodies, etc.) play a crucial role in the choice of the purification method. If the starting material consists of whole cells, they have first to be disrupted, generally by spheroplast formation and detergent-mediated lysis. Next, the protein-containing outer membrane has to be separated from the inner membrane. The OMP of interest can then be further separated from other components of the outer membrane (other OMPs, LOS, phospholipids) by use of chromatographic techniques. The removal of membrane components such as LOS is very difficult. LOS interacts strongly with OMPs and if not present, can affect the conformation of the purified product.

The use of recombinant DNA technology can simplify the purification of OMPs considerably. The production of large amounts of the protein of interest can be induced in various host cells, or mutations can be produced in meningococci that later on will simplify the purification procedure. A disadvantage of these techniques is the necessity to determine the refolding conditions for each separate OMP.

References

1. Poolman, J. T., van der Ley, P. A., and Tommassen, J. (1995) Surface strucutres and secreted products of menigococci, in *Meningococcal Disease* (Cartwright, K. A. V., ed.), John Wiley and Sons, New York, NY, pp. 21–34.
2. Diaz Romero, J. and Outschoorn, I.M. (1994) Current status of meningococcal group B vaccine candidates: capsular or non-capsular? *Clin. Microb. Rev.* **7,** 559–575.
3. Poolman, J. T. (1995) Development of a meningococcal vaccine. *Infect. Agents Dis.* **4,** 13–28.
4. Ala'Aldeen, D. A. A. and Cartwright, K. A. V. (1996) *Neisseria meningitidis:* vaccines and vaccine candidates. *J. Infect.* **33,** 153–157.
5. Nikaido, H. (1983) Proteins forming large channels from bacterial and mitochondrial outer membranes: porins and phage lambda receptor protein. *Methods Enzymol.* **97,** 85–100.
6. Poolman, J. T., Timmermans, H. A. M., Teerlink, T., and Seid jr., R.C. (1989) Purification, cyanogen bromide cleavage, and amino terminus sequencing of class 1 and class 3 outer membrane proteins of meningococci. *Infect. Immun.* **57,** 1005–1007.
7. Achtman, M., Neibert, M., Crowe, B. A., Strittmatter, W., Kusecek, B., Weyse, E., et al. (1988) Purification and characterization of eight class 5 outer membrane

protein variants from a clone of *Neisseria meningitidis* serogroup A. *J. Exp. Med.* **168,** 507–525.

8. Nurminen, M., Butcher, S., IdZnpään-Heikkilä, I., Wahlström, E., Muttilainen, S., Runeberg-Nyman, K., et al. (1992) The class 1 outer membrane protein of *Neisseria meningitidis* produced in *Bacillus subtilis* can give rise to protective immunity. *Mol. Microbiol.* **6,** 2499–2506.

9. Qi, H. L., Tai, J. Y., and Blake, M. S. (1994) Expression of large amounts of neisserial porin proteins in Escherichia coli and refolding of the proteins into native trimers. *Infect. Immun.* **62,** 2432–2439.

10. Muttilainen, S., Idänpään-Heikkilä, I., Wahlström, E., Nurminen, M., Mäkelä, P. H., and Sarvas, M. (1995) The *Neisseria meningitidis* outer membrane protein P1 produced in *Bacillus subtilis* and reconstituted into phospholipid vesicles elicits antibodies to native P1 epitopes. *Microb. Path.* **18,** 423–436.

11. Idänpään-Heikkilä, I., Wahlström, E., Muttilainen, S., Nurminen, M., Käyhty, H., Sarvas, M., and Mäkelä, P. H. (1996) Immunization with meningococcal class 1 outer membrane protein produced in *Bacillus subtilis* and reconstituted in the presence of Zwittergent or Triton X-100. *Vaccine* **14,** 886–891.

12. Osborn, M. J. and Munson, R. (1974) Separation of the inner (cytoplasmic) and outer membranes of gram-negative bacteria. *Methods Enzymol.* **31,** 642–653.

13. Sarvas, M. (1985) Membrane fractionation methods, in *Enterobacterial Surface Antigens: Methods for Molecular Characterization* (Korhonen, T. K., Dawes, E. A.m and Mäkelä, P. H., eds.), Elsevier, Amsterdam, The Netherlands, pp. 111–122.

14. Fredriksen, J. H., Rosenqvist, E., Wedege, E., Bryn, K., Bjune, G., Frøholm, L. O., et al. (1991) Production, characterization and control of MenB-vaccine "Folkehelsa": an outer membrane vesicle vaccine against group B meningococcal disease. *NIPH Ann.* **14,** 67–79.

15. Murphy, T. F. and Loeb, M. R. (1989) Isolation of the outer membrane of *Branhamella catarrhalis*. *Microb. Pathog.* **6,** 159–174.

16. Blake, M. S. and Gotschlich, E. C. (1984) Purification and partial characterization of the opacity associated proteins of *Neisseria gonorrhoeae*. *J. Exp. Med.* **159,** 452–462.

17. Nurminen, M. (1985) Isolation of porin trimers, in *Enterobacterial Surface Antigens: Methods for Molecular Characterization* (Korhonen, T. K., Dawes, E. A., and Mäkelä, P. H., eds.), Elsevier, Amsterdam, pp. 293–299.

18. McNeil, G., Virji, M., and Moxon, E. R. (1994) Interaction of *Neisseria meningitidis* with human monocytes. *Microb. Pathog.* **16,** 153–163.

19. Newhall, W. J., Babcock Mail, L., Wilde, C. E., and Jones, R. B. (1985) Purification and antigenic relatedness of proteins II of *Neisseria gonorrhoeae*. *Infect. Immun.* **49,** 576–580.

20. Mietzner, T. A. and Morse, S. A. (1985) Iron-regulated membrane proteins of *Neisseria gonorrhoeae*: purification and partial characterization of a 37,000-Dalton protein, in *The Pathogenic Neisseriae* (Schoolnik, G. K., Brooks, G. F.,

Falkow, S., Frasch, C. E., Knapp, J. S., McCutchan, J. A., and Morse, S. A., eds.), American Society Microbiology, Washington, DC, pp. 406–414.

21. Morse, S. A., Mietzner, T. A., Bolen, G., Le Faou, A., and Schoolnik, G. (1988) Characterization of the major iron-regulated protein of *Neisseria meningitidis*, in *Gonococci and Meningococci* (Poolman, J. T., Zanen, H. C., Meyer, T. F., Heckels, J. E., Mäkelä, P. H., Smith, H., and Beuvery, E. C., eds.), Kluwer Academic Publishers, Dordrecht, The Netherlands, pp. 405–409.

22. Ward, S. J., Scopes, D., Christodoulides, M., Clarke, I. N., and Heckels, J. E. (1996) Expression of *Neisseria meningitidis* class 1 porin as a fusion protein in *Escherichia coli*: the influence of liposomes and adjuvants on the production of a bactericidal immune response. *Microb. Pathog.* **21,** 499–512.

23. Jansen, C. M., Wiese, A., Reubsaet, L., Dekker, N., de Cock, H., Seydel, U., and Tommassen, J. (2000) Biochemical and biophysical characterization of in vitro folded outer membrane porin PorA of *Neisseria meningitidis*. *Biochim. Biophys. Acta* **1464,** 284–298.

24. Christodoulides, M., Brooks, J. L., Rattue, E., and Heckels, J. E. (1998) Immunization with recombinant class 1 outer membrane protein from *Neisseria meningitidis*: influence of liposomes as adjuvants on antibody avidity, recognition of native protein and the induction of a bactericidal immune response against meningococci. *Microbiology* **144,** 3027–3037.

25. Heckels, J. E. and Virji, M. (1988) Separation and purification of surface components, in *Bacterial Cell Surface Techniques* (Hancock, I. and Poxton, I., eds.), John Wiley and Sons, New York, NY, pp. 67–69.

26. Muir, L. L., Strugnell, R. A., and Davies, J. K. (1988) Purification of native pili and outer membrane vesicles from *Neisseria gonorrhoeae*, in *Gonococci and Meningococci* (Poolman, J. T., Zanen, H. C., Meyer, T. F., Heckels, J. E., Mäkelä, P. H., Smith, H., and Beuvery, E. C., eds.), Kluwer Academic Publishers, Dordrecht, The Netherlands, pp. 411–417.

27. Hermonson, M. A., Chen, K. C. S., and Buchanan, T. M. (1978) Neisseria pili proteins: amino-terminal amino acid sequences and identification of and unusual amino acid. *Biochemistry* **17,** 442–445.

28. Tommassen, J., Vermeij, P., Struyvé, M., Benz, R., and Poolman, J. T. (1990) Isolation of *Neisseria meningitidis* mutants deficient in class 1 (PorA) and class 3 (PorB) outer membrane proteins. *Infect. Immun.* **58,** 1355–1359.

29. Jiskoot, W., Teerlink, T., Beuvery, E. C., and Crommelin, D. J. A. (1986) Preparation of liposomes via detergent removal from mixed micelles by dilution. *Pharm. Wkbl. Sci.* **8,** 259–265.

7

Outer Membrane Protein Vesicle Vaccines for Meningococcal Disease

Carl E. Frasch, Loek van Alphen, Johan Holst, Jan T. Poolman, and Einar Rosenqvist

1. Introduction

Alternative strategies exist for prevention of group B *Neisseria meningitidis* (meningococcal) disease through vaccination (*see* Chapters 5, 8, 13, 14 in this volume). However, the most promising approach to date has been the use of outer-membrane vesicle (OMV) vaccines for induction of bactericidal antibodies against cell-surface outer-membrane proteins (OMPs).

Group B meningococcal OMV vaccines have been extensively evaluated in clinical trials. These trials have been conducted in several countries and have involved several million adults, older children, and infants *(1)*. The vaccines have shown acceptable safety (reactogenicity) profiles and induce functional antibodies as measured by induction of bactericidal antibodies. Efficacy estimates from large clinical studies *(2,3)* have been promising. However, there are some limitations with these vaccines, such as waning immunity and protection lasting about 1 yr after immunization with a two-dose schedule with no booster *(4)*, and strain/serosubtype-restricted immune responses in infants *(5)*. Induction of bactericidal antibodies was poor in young children following a two-dose immunization schedule, which correlated with the observed age-specific efficacy against group B meningococcal disease in Brazil *(6)*. More recently, studies in Chile using a three-dose immunization schedule showed good bactericidal responses in all age groups to the homologous vaccine strain, but age-related bactericidal responses to the heterologous Chilean epidemic strain was not as good, with the best responses in adults *(5)*.

The composition of various group B OMP vaccines and clinical trials using these vaccines were recently reviewed *(1,7,8)*. The PorA or class 1 protein was

From: *Methods in Molecular Medicine, vol. 66: Meningococcal Vaccines: Methods and Protocols*
Edited by: A. J. Pollard and M. C. J. Maiden © Humana Press Inc., Totowa, NJ

shown in several studies *(9,10)* to induce bactericidal antibodies and is therefore an important protein to include in group B meningococcal protein vaccines. The PorA protein is exposed on the surface of the outer membrane and exists in the membrane as trimers *(11)*, and some data suggest that its natural configuration is as a heterotrimer with the PorB porin protein *(12)*. Other proteins that induce bactericidal antibodies and should therefore be considered for inclusion in a vaccine include transferrin-binding protein tbpB and Opc, although Opc is not present in all group B meningococcal strains. Inclusion of these proteins may be important due to the antigenic diversity within PorA, because they can potentially extend vaccine coverage and protection.

Although about 80% of invasive group B and C meningococcal strains have the L3,7,9 lipooligosaccharide (LOS) immunotype *(13)*, use of LOS-based vaccines has met with limited success *(1)*. Zollinger et al. showed that Rhesus monkeys vaccinated with an OMP-B polysaccharide conjugate vaccine had high titers of L3,7,9 specific bactericidal antibodies *(14)*. Thus, the LOS could be an important vaccine component.

There are approx 20 different PorA serosubtypes based on antigenic differences in two major variable regions (VR1 and VR2) located in loops I and IV *(15)*. Although this represents broad antigenic diversity, hyperendemic levels and epidemics caused by group B meningococci tend to be clonal and of long duration. Thus, one or two PorA serosubtypes may provide broad coverage for a given geographic region and point in time. The fact that the important hyperendemic and epidemic group B strains change over time, but slowly, means that the manufacturing process for preparation of a group B OMP vaccine should be sufficiently robust to be used for various group B outbreak strains. The implication of this is that the manufacturing process, not a specific production strain, could be licensed. This concept is analogous to the influenza-virus vaccine, where the vaccine production strains may be changed from year to year as needed depending on the epidemiological situation.

Native orientation of the proteins in the outer membrane can be crucial to an effective immune response. Membrane proteins removed from the outer membrane and used as immunogens in the form of proteosomes induce large amounts of antibodies to normally buried hydrophobic determinants, but these antibodies are unreactive with native membranes *(16)*. Thus, the vaccines described in this chapter utilize LOS-depleted meningococcal outer membranes. In the future it may be possible to use native meningococcal membrane vesicles, also called NOMV, prepared from genetically modified strains containing nontoxic mutant LOS *(17)*.

Methods for production of group B OMP vaccines have been published *(18–21)*. Provided here are several detailed alternative methodologies and important quality-control tests to evaluate antigen content, purity, toxicity, potency, and consistency of manufacture. The production methodology utilized will depend on the production facilities available.

A modified Catlin medium (MC.6) was developed for large-scale fermentation of group B meningococcal strains by scientists at Merck Research Laboratories (22). This is a defined medium that works very well for growth of meningococcal strains with or without expression of iron-regulated proteins, because the iron concentration in the media can be readily controlled. It is best, however to initially test four or five strains of the same serotype and serosubtype, representative for the actual epidemic, in order to select one strain that grows best in the defined medium. This can be done in medium containing iron or in the medium with very low levels of iron, depending on whether the vaccine produced will contain increased levels of iron-regulated proteins (23).

The wild-type group B meningococci used for vaccine production will contain high molecular-weight capsular polysaccharide and about 500 µg of LOS per milligram of protein in the outer membrane (1). The polysaccharide can be depolymerized using neuraminidase and removed during further purification, while the LOS content will be greatly reduced by detergent treatment. To retain the outer-membrane bilayer conformation, a minimal amount of LOS must be retained in the membrane, but membrane-bound LOS is about 100 times less toxic compared to free LOS (24,25). The amount of LOS in the membranes will be reduced to about 5% relative to protein through solubilization with the detergent sodium deoxycholate. Although various other detergents have been used (1,20), deoxycholate is a good choice, because it is effective and is a normal breakdown product of bile metabolism. Two different strategies have been used for recovery of LOS-depleted outer membranes: 1) direct addition of deoxycholate to the resuspended cells or to the culture at the completion of fermentation and after adjustment of the pH of the culture to over 7.0, and 2) treatment of extracted outer membranes (19,21).

During purification, it is important to maintain membrane solubility and freedom from membrane aggregation. Early studies showed that visibly particulate meningococcal membrane-protein vaccines were poorly immunogenic (26). Membrane aggregation will also interfere with or prevent sterile filtration. Native nondetergent-treated membranes ("blebs" or OMV) are easily resuspended and remain soluble after pelleting in an ultracentrifuge. By contrast, detergent-treated membranes, when pelleted by ultracentrifugation, readily aggregate with some membrane fusion, as seen by electron microscopy (EM). This aggregation can be prevented by use of other methods for concentration/purification, or by centrifugation of the detergent-treated membranes onto a sucrose bed. The latter method is readily applicable to large-scale purification by continuous-flow ultracentrifugation. The presence of about 3% sucrose during purification also stabilizes the membranes, and safety of sucrose present in licensed vaccines has been shown.

**Table 1
A Modified Catlin Medium (MC.6)
Prepared in USP-Distilled Water**

Component	Gm/L of medium
NaCl	5.80
K_2HPO_4	4.00
NH_4Cl	1.00
K_2SO_4	1.00
Glucose	10.00
L-Glutamic acid	3.90
L-Arginine	0.15
Glycine	0.25
L-Serine	0.50
L Cysteine • HCl	0.10
$MgCl_2$ • $6H_2O$	0.40
$CaCl_2$ • $2H_2O$	0.03
Fe (III) citrate	0.04[a]

[a]The iron may be omitted depending on amount in medium from other sources.

The purification methods detailed in **Subheading 3.1.2.** include a number of alternative methodologies that may be used based on equipment and facilities available. Although previously published methods have used ethanol precipitation at one or more stages during purification *(19)*, use of ethanol has been avoided in the described methods owing to uncertainty of possible denaturing effects of alcohol precipitation, and possible reduced vesicle solubility.

2. Materials

2.1 Conventional OMV Vaccines

1. The liquid culture medium is the simplified Catlin medium, Catlin-6, described by Fu et al. *(22)*. The composition of this medium is shown in **Table 1**. A 100 m*M* HEPES buffer is added to the flask media to control pH to 7.0, but is not included in the fermentation MC.6 medium. If the meningococcal strains will not be grown under iron-limited conditions, the Frantz medium is an alternative partially defined medium *(27,28)*, and the composition is shown in **Table 2**. If the pH is not controlled during growth in regular Frantz medium, the final pH becomes about 5.0, whereas the modified Frantz medium does not contain glucose and the pH remains above 7.0 throughout growth.
2. Meningococcal strains: Choice of meningococcal strains will be based on prevalence found in epidemiological surveillance. One approach is to use isolates representing the two most frequent PorA serosubtypes.

Table 2
Composition of Regular and Modified Frantz Media

Component	Regular Frantz	Modified Frantz
Solution A[a]		
L-glutamic acid	1.6 gm	1.6 gm
NaCl	6.0 gm	6.0 gm
Na_2HPO_4 (anhydrous)	2.5 gm	—
Sodium glycerol phosphate	—	5.0 gm
NH_4Cl	1.25 gm	1.25 gm
KCl	0.1 gm	0.1 gm
D-cysteine hydrochloride	0.025 gm	0.025 gm
Water (WFI)	1000 mL	1000 mL
Solution B[b]		
$MgSO_4$	2.4 gm	2.4 gm
Yeast extract powder	8.0 gm	8.0 gm
Water (WFI)	100 mL	100 mL
Solution C[c]		
Glucose	20 gm	—
Water	100 mL	—

[a]Adjust pH for either to 7.4–7.5, may autoclave.
[b]Filter sterilize. (To eliminate yeast glucans this solution should first be ultrafiltered then sterile filtered.)
[c]Filter sterilize.
Regular Frantz 1000 mL solution A + 25 mL solution B + 25 mL solution C.
Modified Frantz 1000 mL solution A + 25 mL solution B.

3. Sodium deoxycholate and Benzocase (a DNase) obtained from Sigma Chemical Co. (St. Louis, MO).

2.2. Genetically Modified PorA Vaccines

1. For large-scale cultivation of meningococci, a modified Frantz medium is used (*see* **Table 2**).
2. Meningococcal strains used express various PorA proteins, but do not express a capsular polysaccharide- (CPS⁻). They include monovalent strain F91 (P1.7[h],4) and trivalent strains PL16215 (CPS⁻, P1.7,16,5,2,19,15) and PL10124 (CPS⁻, P1.5c,10,12,13,7[h],4). The strains were derived from the wild-type strain H44/76. The construction of the vaccine strains is described in Chapter 11 (*see* **refs.** *29–32*). The monovalent P1.4 strain contains two copies of the P1.4 *porA* gene, resulting in deletion of *porB*. The trivalent strains have been derived from strain HIII5, a spontaneous PorB-negative muatant of strain H44/76. Loss of capsule expression was obtained by deleting a large fragment of the *cps* locus, which resulted also in galactose-deficient lipopolysaccharide (*galE*). For the construction of strain PL16215, the P1.5,2 *porA* of strain 2996 was introduced in one of

the *opa* genes, and *porA* (P1.19,15) of strain MC51 into the *rmpM* (class 4 gene). Similarly, strain PL10124 was constructed with the *porA* genes from strains 870227 (P1.5^c,10), 870446 (P1.12,13), and 892257 (P1.7^h,4). Of both trivalent strains variants were selected not reacting with Opa-specific monoclonal antibodies (MAbs) in colony blotting.

3. Culturing is performed in 7-, 50-, 135-, or 350-L fermentors, equipped with control systems for maintaining air pressure, temperature, pH, dissolved oxygen, and mixing speed.

3. Methods

3.1. Production of OMV Bulks from Wild-Type Strains

Presented here is a general scheme for preparation of an OMP vaccine from wild-type group B meningococcal strains using alternative strategies. The exact combination of production methods used will depend on production scale as well as the facilities and equipment available (*see* **Note 1**). One method for production of an OMV vaccine containing iron-regulated proteins is shown in **Fig. 1**.

3.1.1. Growth of Meningococcal Strains

3.1.1.1. STRAIN SELECTION

To achieve maximal vaccine coverage, the strain(s) should be grown to express high molecular-weight iron-regulated proteins, and should be selected to carry the Opc protein and LOS immunotype L3,7,9 *(13,33)*. Three to five strains of the selected serotype and serosubtype should be cultivated in flasks containing the Catlin-6 medium described by Fu et al. *(22)*, except that the ferric iron citrate is reduced or omitted. Exact concentrations of ferric citrate needed will depend on levels of contaminating iron from other sources (*see* **Note 2**). Sufficient iron is often present from other sources to permit normal growth rates. Iron-regulated proteins may be induced during growth by addition of ethylenediamine dihydroxy-phenyl acetic acid (EDDA) to the media, which chelates soluble iron, then slowly releases it, permitting growth *(23)*. Each of the strains should be grown for 24 h in Catlin-6 medium containing iron plus 20, 30, 40, or 50 µ*M* EDDA. The 24 h is to allow detection and elimination of strains more prone to cell lysis with extended growth times.

An alternative method for induction of iron-regulated proteins is to grow the strains in Catlin-6 to stationary phase, then add a volume of fresh Catlin-6 equal to 50% of the initial volume containing about 0.1 m*M* Desferal for an additional 4–6 h at 37°C *(34)*. Under these conditions, the optical density (OD) will increase only slightly in presence of Desferal, but iron-regulated proteins will be induced (*see* **Notes 3** and **4**).

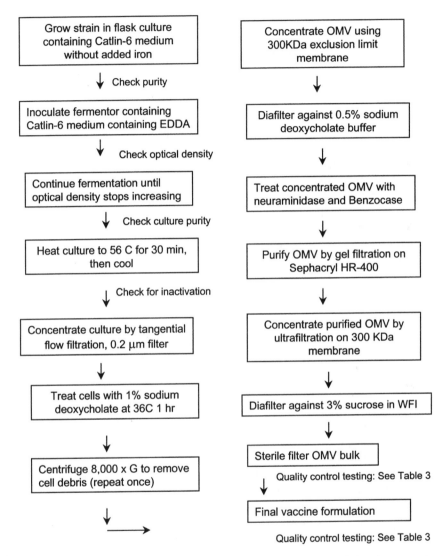

Fig. 1. One method for production of an OMV vaccine containing iron-regulated proteins.

3.1.1.2. FERMENTATION IN PRESENCE OF EDDA

1. Inoculate production strain onto solid medium, Mueller Hinton agar plates, or Tryptic soy agar containing 1% yeast extract, and grow overnight at 37°C with CO_2.
2. Check purity, then inoculate into a flask containing Catlin-6 medium without added iron, and grow on a shaker at 36°C until the OD at 600 nm reaches approx 1.0.

3. Check the purity and transfer to a larger flask containing Catlin-6 without added iron using an inoculum ratio between 1:10 and 1:20 and grow on a shaker at 36°C until the OD at 600 nm again reaches approx 1.0.
4. Check for purity and inoculate into a fermentor using the same inoculum ratio. The fermentor should contain Catlin-6 medium, iron as specified, and the predetermined concentration of EDDA.
5. The fermentation conditions are as described by Fu et al. *(22)*. The aeration should be on the surface of the medium, approx 2.5 L/min, with agitation.
6. Grow in the fermentor until the OD becomes level (remains the same for 30 min) or the dissolved oxygen level begins to rise.
7. Check culture purity using one plate that supports growth of meningococci and another that does not, such as nutrient agar (Difco), but supports growth of other bacteria including Pseudomonas and Bacillus.
8. Inactivate the culture using one of these methods:
   a. If OMV will be obtained directly from the culture broth or if deoxycholate will be added directly to the culture, then bring the temperature of the culture to 56°C for 30 min, then cool to 30–35°C.
   b. If will extract OMV from recovered cells, then add liquid phenol to 0.5% and maintain at 36°C with agitation for 2 h.
9. Proceed with OMV purification.

3.1.1.3. FERMENTATION THEN ADDITION OF DESFERAL FOR INDUCTION OF IRON-REGULATED PROTEINS

1. Inoculate production strain to solid medium, Mueller Hinton, or Tryptic soy agar containing 1% yeast extract, and grow overnight at 37°C with CO_2.
2. Check culture purity, then inoculate into a flask containing Catlin-6 medium without added iron, and grow on a shaker at 36°C until the OD at 600 nm reaches approx 1.0.
3. Check the purity and transfer to a larger flask containing Catlin-6 without iron using an inoculum ratio between 1:10 and 1:20. Grow on a shaker at 36°C until the OD at 600 nm reaches approx 1.0.
4. Prepare fermentor with a volume of Catlin-6, containing a reduced iron concentration, equal to 66% of the working volume of the fermentor (working volume is usually 80% of total volume).
5. The fermentation conditions are as described by Fu et al. *(22)*. The aeration should be on the surface of the medium, approx 2.5 L/min, with agitation.
6. Grow at 36°C until the OD levels off, then add a volume of Catlin-6 equal to 33% of the working volume of the fermentor without added iron and containing the predetermined amount of Desferal needed for iron regulated protein induction (about 0.1 mM).
7. Follow the OD and incubate an additional 6 h at 36°C.
8. Inactivate the culture using one of these methods:
   a. If OMV will be obtained directly from the culture broth or if deoxycholate will be added directly to the culture, then bring the temperature of the culture to 56°C for 30 min and cool to 30–35°C.

b. If will extract OMV from recovered cells, then add liquid phenol to 0.5% and maintain at 36°C with agitation for 2 h.
9. Proceed with OMV purification.

3.1.2. OMV Purification

Meningococcal cells contain large amounts of loosely bound outer membranes, and during normal growth meningococci release large amounts of these membranes in the form of vesicles (OMV) into the culture medium. Outer membranes, including those naturally blebbed off during growth, contain about 25–50% LOS relative to the protein. The released membrane blebs are nearly pure outer membranes, with essentially no inner-membrane contamination (*see* **Note 5**). As noted earlier, two methods for recovery of the outer membranes have used: 1) direct treatment of the bacterial cells with detergent, *(18)* or 2) purify OMV, then detergent treat to remove the LOS. Direct detergent treatment will result in some cell lysis, but assures that the bacteria are nonviable, and if done as described in **Subheading 3.1.2.1.** permits recovery of both cell extracted membranes and membranes released during growth.

3.1.2.1. Recovery of Outer Membranes by Direct Detergent Treatment

1. Concentrate culture on a 0.2-µm filter by tangential flow, then wash once with saline.
2. Add one volume of 100 mM Tris, 2 mM EDTA, pH 8.5, containing 1% sodium deoxycholate, then heat to 36°C for 1 h with continuous mixing.
3. Remove cell debris by either:
   a. Tangential flow through 0.45-µm filters, then wash bacterial cells with 50 mM Tris, 1 mM EDTA, containing 0.5% sodium deoxycholate, pH 8.5, and continue filtration. Save filtrate.
   b. Use two cycles of low speed centrifugation at 8,000g and discard cell debris, saving clear or slightly opalescent supernatant.
4. Concentrate the OMVs by ultrafiltration on a 300 KDa exclusion limit membrane, then diafilter against 50 mM Tris, 1 mM EDTA containing 0.5% sodium deoxycholate, pH 8.5.
5. The concentrate may contain large amounts of high molecular-weight group B polysaccharide, nucleic acid, and depolymerized LOS. The B polysaccharide if present may be degraded using neuraminidase and the DNA with Benzocase. Treat overnight at room temperature.
6. Purification of detergent-treated membranes may be done using either:
   a. Gel filtration on Sephacryl HR-400 or Sepharose CL-6B in 50 mM Tris, 1 mM EDTA containing 0.5% sodium deoxycholate, pH 8.5. The outer membranes will elute at the void volume of either column, well-separated from contaminants.
   b. Continuous-flow ultracentrifigation: preload the ultracentrifuge bowl with a thin layer of 60% sucrose and the remainder of bowl with 20% sucrose in high-quality water for injection (WFI). Pass the outer-membrane concentrate

through the ultra-centrifuge and the membrane vesicles will layer on top of the 60% sucrose bed.

7. Concentrate the OMVs by ultrafiltration on a 300 KDa exclusion limit membrane, then diafilter against WFI containing 3% sucrose for removal of detergent (and excess sucrose if **Subheading 3.2.1., step 6.b.** was used). The sucrose stabilizes the membrane vesicles.

8. Pass OMV through a 1.2-μm filter to remove particles, then sterile filter through a 0.2-μm filter using pressure.

3.1.2.2. RECOVERY OF OUTER MEMBRANES BY DETERGENT TREATMENT OF EXTRACTED OMV

1. Use tangential filtration on a 0.45-μm filter to concentrate cell mass.
2. Pellet cells by low-speed centrifigation, about 8,000*g*, then determine wet weight of cell mass.
3. Resuspend cell mass in 5 mL of saline per gram wet weight of cells, then extract surface membranes by shearing within a laminar flow hood using one of the following methods:
   a. Ultrasound water bath: place suspended cells in glass flasks with surface of cell mixture in flask below surface of water in the bath, treat 20–30 min.
   b. Omnimixer or blender: shear for 10 min at high setting.
   c. Passage through 20G needle; pass suspension through needle twice.
4. Pellet cells by low speed centrifigation, about 8,000*g*, then centrifuge supernatant at 12,000*g* for 30 min to further remove cellular debris.
5. Pellet outer membranes by ultracentrifugation at 100,000*g* for 2 h.
6. Resuspend outer membranes in WFI to approx 10 mg/mL. The membranes will contain both group B polysaccharide and LOS, which will be removed in the following steps.
7. Extract LOS by mixing membrane suspension with an equal volume of 100 m*M* Tris, 2 m*M* EDTA, pH 8.5, containing 2% sodium deoxycholate. Let stand at ambient temperature for 15 min.
8. Purification of detergent treated membranes may be done using either:
   a. Gel filtration on Sephacryl HR-400 or Sepharose CL-6B in 50 m*M* Tris, 1 m*M* EDTA containing 0.5% sodium deoxycholate, pH 8.5. The outer membranes will elute at the void volume of either column, well-separated from contaminants.
   b. Continuous-flow ultracentrifigation: preload the ultracentrifuge bowl with a thin layer of 60% sucrose and the remainder of bowl with 20% sucrose in high-quality water (WFI). Pass the outer-membrane concentrate through the ultracentrifuge and the membrane vesicles will layer on top of the 60% sucrose bed.
9. Concentrate the OMVs by ultrafiltration on a 300 KDa exclusion limit membrane, then diafilter against WFI containing 3% sucrose for removal of detergent. The sucrose stabilizes the membrane vesicles.
10. Pass through a 1.2-μm filter to remove particles, then sterile-filter through a 0.2-μm filter using pressure.

3.2. Production of OMV Bulks from Genetically Modified Strains Expressing PorA

3.2.1. Fermentation

1. Keep working seed lots at $-70°C$.
2. Inoculate seed into a pre-inoculation culture in two 500-mL bottles containing 150 mL modified Frantz medium, which is incubated at 36°C. From this pre-culture, the inoculum is prepared in a series of corresponding bottles with the same medium. The total quantity of 1 L is used as inoculum for the 50 L production culture of modified Frantz in the fermentor (bioreactor).
3. Cultivation of the production culture takes place in a closed system in a bioreactor. The pH is kept at 7.0, the temperature at 36°C, the dissolved oxygen concentration at 10% of the total air saturation limit. At regular intervals during cultivation a sample is taken for determination of OD, pH, dry weight, and nutrient/metabolite analysis. The cultivation is stopped when an OD (590 nm) of between 2.8 and 3.5 is reached by cooling down to below 20°C. The cultivation time is approx 24 h.

3.2.2. Production of Bulk PorA OMV (Laboratory Scale)

1. Centrifuge the culture by continuous flow centrifugation (Westphalia separator).
2. Throughout the remaining of the process Thimerosal (100 mg/L) is added as a preservative.
3. Resuspend the cells in 7.5 mL 0.1 M Tris-HCl, 10 mM EDTA, pH 8.6, per gram cells (wet weight). After resuspending, 10% desoxycholate in the same buffer is added to a final concentration of 1/20 of the buffer volume followed by 30 min extraction under stirring at room temperature.
4. Remove cell debris by centrifugation at 20,000g at 4°C for 1 h. The supernatant containing vesicles is concentrated by ultracentrifugation at 125,000g at 4°C for 2 h.
5. Wash the OMV pellet with 0.05 M Tris-HCl, 2 mM EDTA, 2.5% (w/v) DOC, pH 8.9, resuspended with 0.05 M Tris-HCl, 2 mM EDTA, 2.5% (w/v) DOC. With a 0.05 M Tris-HCl, 2 mM EDTA, 0.5% (w/v) DOC, 30% (w/v) sucrose (saccharose) buffer the DOC-content is adjusted to 1% (w/v). After homogenizing the suspention by sonication, the suspension is recentrifuged at 125,000g at 4°C for 1 h. Finally the pellet is resuspended in a 3% sucrose buffer.

3.3. Production of Aluminum Containing Adjuvants

Aluminium hydroxide (AH) and aluminium phosphate (AP) have been used widely as adjuvants, probably because of their reputation for safety in humans. A maximum amount of 0.85 mg aluminium/dose has been recommended by the U.S. Food and Drug Administration (FDA).

Meningococcal OMVs are highly immunogenic in humans *per se*, and induce bactericidal antibodies. In humans, only relatively small effects on immunogenicity were observed in when the Norwegian OMV vaccine was adsorbed to AH (protein/adjuvant ratio of 1:67 w/w); the adsorbed vaccine did induce higher bactericidal activity than the unadsorbed after two doses *(25)*. Similar results have been observed with other experimental AH-adsorbed meningococcal vaccines *(35)*.

When OMV was adsorbed to AH, the pyrogenic response in rabbits was reduced 4–10-fold *(25)*. Likewise, the limulus amoebocyte lysate (LAL) activity of OMV was reduced by adsorption on AH. However, there was also more local side effects with the adsorbed vaccines; mostly tenderness at the site of injection *(25)*. Only weak, nonspecific systemic effects, which disappeared the second day after vaccination, were observed, and no significant difference was found between adsorbed and unadsorbed vaccine *(25)*. The meningococcal group B OMV/OMP vaccines used in protection trials have all been aluminum-adjuvanted.

3.3.1. Aluminum Hydroxide

In aqueous aluminum salt solutions below pH 3.5, aluminum exists primarily as trivalent cations with six water molecules in octahedral coordination $Al(OH_2)_6^{+3}$. The first steps in the formation of AH are:

$$2\ Al(OH_2)_6^{+3} \leftrightarrow 2\ Al(OH)(OH_2)_5^{+2} \leftrightarrow Al_2(OH)_2(OH_2)_8^{+4} + 2H_3O^+$$

The form of AH used as adjuvants is a gel composed of small particles of a microcrystalline material known as boehmite and has the empirical formula $Al(O)(OH)$ *(36)*. AH adjuvant has a isoelectric point of 11.6 and a positive surface charge under physiological conditions. Because OMVs are negatively charged, they are effectively adsorbed to AH.

1. AH gels for adjuvants are formed by slowly adding 5% (w/v) sodium carbonate with rapid mixing to 3% (w/v) aluminum chloride at 60–62°C until pH of between 6.8 and 7.2 is reached.
2. Check the pH every 1–2 h and adjust as necessary using the appropriate starting solution until a stable pH is achieved.
3. The AH produced by this method will be a mixture of AH polymers of different size and anion substitution.
4. Sterilize the resulting gel by autoclaving (*see* **Note 6** and **ref. 37**).

The adsorption process are performed by slowly adding under constant stirring using a magnet bar, 0.10 mg/mL of OMV protein in 3% sucrose, to an equal volume of 6.7 mg/mL AH. The mixture is stirred over night at 4°C. This gives a final concentration of 50 µg protein and 3.33 mg AH per mL.

To minimize the variations and to avoid the nonreproducibility derived from the use of different preparations of AH, a specific commercial preparation (Alhydrogel from Superfos Biosector, Denmark) has been recommended as a scientific standard, and should be considered. Alhydrogel is a stable, viscous homogenous material retaining its properties even after storage for several years.

3.3.2. Aluminum Phosphate

1. To prepare 10 L of AP suspension, aseptically combine 0.625 L of 1.05 M $AlCl_3$ and 5.05 L of 0.14 M Na_3PO_4 with 1 L of sterile WFI with continuous mixing.
2. Adjust the pH to approx 7.0 by addition of additional WFI.
3. The $AlPO_4$ concentration will be 8 gm/L.
4. The AP adjuvant is used for vaccine formulation as described above for AH.

3.4. Vaccine Formulation

3.4.1. Conventional Wild-Type OMV Vaccines

Several different formulations of group B meningococcal OMP vaccines have been clinically evaluated in infants and young children *(1,8)*. For parenteral immunization, most clinical trials have used 25 or 50 µg/dose of protein, but up to 100 µg/dose has also been used. The Cuban vaccine contains 50 µg/dose of protein plus 50 µg/dose of group C meningococcal polysaccharide and AH adjuvant. The Norwegian vaccine contains 25 µg/dose of protein and AH adjuvant, but no polysaccharide. Because the vaccines are to be used in young children it is not recommended that group C polysaccharide be included in the formulation owing to possible induction of tolerance, whereas inclusion of a group C conjugate vaccine should be considered *(38,39)*. A recent publication describes animal studies using a meningococcal group B outer-membrane and group C conjugate vaccine *(40)*.

The adjuvants that have been used with meningococcal protein vaccines are either AH or AP, but some newer adjuvants could prove superior.

3.4.2. Genetically Modified PorA Containing Vaccines

1. Suspend the concentrated OMV for both trivalent preparations in 3% sucrose.
2. Mix the two trivalent preparations in equimolar amounts based on PorA protein content with AP as adjuvant.
3. The final formulation will contain 7.5 or 15 µg of PorA protein for each of the subtypes per dose (0.5 mL).
4. The vaccine will consist of 22.9 µmol/L $AlPO_4$ (0.3%), 241 µmol/L thiomersal (0.01% w/v), 10% (w/v) sucrose and buffer 10 mM Tris-HCl, pH 7.5.

3.5. Quality Control

The rather complex nature of OMV-based vaccines makes quality control challenging *(41,42)*. For the various formulations used to date, key antigens have been identified and well-characterized *(21,43)*. The lack of generally accepted pre-clinical tests, correlating with efficacy in humans, makes QC evaluation of different formulations difficult *(4)*.

No official requirements or guidelines have yet been established specifically for OMV vaccines. Nevertheless, based on the various formulations used in clinical trials and in vaccination programs *(44)*, our knowledge of the important characteristics for these vaccines has increased. There is certainly a need to present key quality features associated with these types of vaccine formulations. Presented below are aspects and methods applicable for all OMV vaccines. As an example of QC tests used, methods and specifications used; quality-control data are presented in **Table 3** based on data obtained with the Norwegian MenB-OMV, NIPH. All aspects of production of vaccines intended for use in humans must be done under Good Manufacturing Practices (cGMP), one set of which is described in the U.S. Code of Federal Regulations 21:210 (*see* **Notes 7–9**). **Figure 2** shows an example flow sheet with quality-control sampling points and tests for the MenB-OMV Vaccine manufactured by NIPH (Norway).

3.5.1. Quality Control of Fermentation

The fermentation should be followed by making growth curves from OD measurements (or similar). The oxygen saturation (pO_2) and pH should be monitored, but not necessarily adjusted. At the end of the growth phase, the culture must be checked for purity (Gram-staining and microscopy), no other microorganisms must be found using a rich medium such as Mueller-Hinton agar or Tryptic Soy. The inactivation step should be validated by plating the culture on a rich medium to assure that there are no viable bacteria before proceeding to OMV purification. The antigenic quality of the meningococcal strain at the end of fermentation can also be checked by "Dot-blotting" using relevant monoclonals, which are defining serotype, sero-subtype, and other important epitopes.

3.5.2. Quality Control of OMV Bulks

3.5.2.1. Quality Control of OMV Bulk from Wild-Type Strains

During production of OMV vaccines, after the final purification steps, there is a stage where OMV sub-batches can be stored (*see* **Note 10** and **ref.** *21*). Different sub-batches from other fermentor runs can be mixed, to a protein concentration of about 1–2 mg/mL. At this stage a number of the most important quality-control tests are performed. Some tests are done both on each individual sub-batch and on the pooled OMV bulk, e.g., protein concentration, antigenic pattern, LAL. Other tests, like deoxycholate and sucrose quantitation, might be done on the bulk only.

Table 3
Quality Control Data Based on NIPH-Produced MenB-OMV, 44/76 Vaccine, a "wild-type" OMV Vaccine

Ingredient/Property-Control Method	Content and Quantitative Limits
Total protein	
Modified Folin-Lowry	• 50 µg/mL + 10%
Antigen pattern	
Semi-quantitative recording	"80kD" 1–4%[a]
by scanning of SDS-PAGE	"70kD" 1–10%
(CBB-stained)	Class 1 24–35%
	Class 3 34–44%
	Class 5/Opc 9–19%
OMV and LPS immunotyping	
Immunoblotting	• Confirmed similarity with reference;
using monoclonals or other defined	specific antibodies/sera
Potency	
Immunization of mice and quantitation	• Significant dose-response between highest
of antibodies (serum IgG) by ELISA	and lowest dose. Highest dose above a
should induce median antibody level	defined level
Vesicles	
Transmission electron microscopy	• Mainly intact vesicles of 50–200 nm.
LPS	
Quantitation by HPLC	• 0.04–0.12 µg/µg protein
	(2.0–5.0 µg/mL; 4–10% relative to protein)
Group B-polysaccharide	
Quantitation by ELISA	• <0.004 µg/µg protein
	• (<0.2 µg/mL)
Deoxycholate	
Quantitation by enzyme reaction	• <0.3 µg/µg protein
and colorimetry	• (<15 µg/mL)
DNA	
Quantitation by spectrofluorometry	• <0.035 µg/µg protein
	• (<1.75 µg/mL)
Sucrose	
Quantitation by HPLC-PED	• 26–38 mg/mL
Aluminum hydroxide	
Quantitation by atomic adsorption	• 2.4–3.6 mg/mL
spectrophotometry (Aluminum)	(0.9–1.3 mg/mL)
Degree of binding to adjuvant	
Calc. from protein quant. in supernate	• >95%
Endotoxin	
Quantitation by Limulus reagent	• <20,000 EU/mL
(LAL-test on finished product)	
pH	
Determination by pH-meter	• 6.2–6.8
Sterility testing	
Membrane-filtration method (Ph. Eur.)	• Pass
Abnormal toxicity (general safety)	• Pass
Pyrogenicity	
1 µg (protein) per kg rabbit	• Pass

[a]Percentage of total protein.

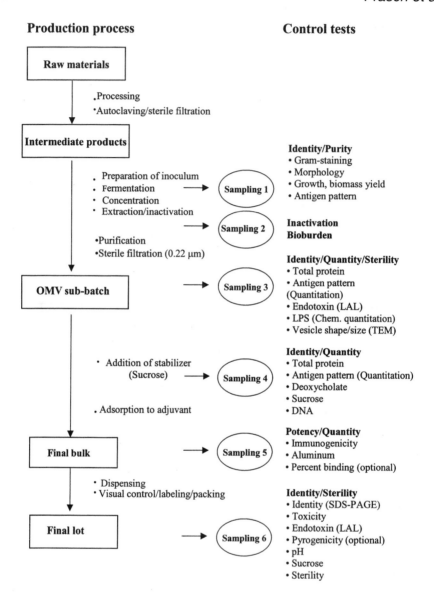

Fig. 2. A flow diagram of an actual OMV-vaccine manufacturing process as conducted at the National Institute of Public Health, Oslo, Norway, showing steps at which various quality control test samples are removed.

Total protein quantitation can be done by one of several methods, e.g., total protein nitrogen according to Kjehldahl or according to different variations of the Folin Lowry-method *(45)*.

Protein distribution/antigenic pattern in the OMV should be analyzed by sodium dodecyl sulfate-polyacrylamide gel electrophoresis (SDS-PAGE) and scanning of the Coomassie stained gel (*see* **Note 11**). The relative amounts of the various proteins can then be calculated using a suitable software program and presented as percentages of the total protein content *(21)*. For identification of the individual proteins, including the iron-regulated proteins, unstained proteins must be transferred from the SDS-PAGE gel to nitrocellulose membranes by electroblotting. Individual strips of the nitrocellulose membrane are then incubated with relevant monoclonals or sera specific for a particular component and visualized by HRP-conjugated anti-mouse antibodies or other reagents if needed, e.g., anti-rabbit HRP *(21,43)* (*see* also Chapter 19).

Evaluation of the vesicle content and structure has traditionally been done by transmission electron microscopy (TEM) *(21,37)* (*see* **Note 12**).

LPS quantitation should be done both by a chemical method and by an assay that measures the biological activity of the lipid-A moiety. For chemical quantitation, the new Purpald method is recommended *(46)*. The OMV should also be examined by silver staining of SDS-PAGE gels (*see* **Notes 13** and **14**). For quantitation of the biological activity of lipopolysaccharide (LPS), a LAL assay, using *E. coli* LPS as a reference, is recommended *(43)*.

Test for sterility should be done according to an official Pharmacopoeia method. A membrane-filtration technique is recommended owing to the possibility of increased sample volume.

Quantitation of residual deoxycholate (DOC) content is recommended and may be done using a commercially available enzyme-based colorimetric assay *(21)*. The DNA can be measured by spectrofluorometry, using *Escherichia coli* DNA as a standard *(48)*. Sucrose can be quantified by using high-performance anion-exchange chromatography, with a pulsed electrochemical detection (HPAC-PED) *(49)*.

Analysis for traces of group B capsular polysaccharide should be done on the OMV concentrated bulk. An enzyme-linked immunosorbent assay (ELISA) assay with a MAb against α(2-8) polysialic acid can be used, where the detection limit is about 0.13 µg/mL *(21)*.

3.5.2.2. QUALITY CONTROL OF OMV BULKS FROM GENETICALLY MODIFIED STRAINS

1. Examine protein composition by 10% SDS-PAGE. PorA protein is quantified after staining with Coomassie Brilliant Blue by gel scanning using Image-master (Pharmacia, Sweden) software, and given as percentage of the total protein content.

2. Determine presence of each PorA subtype antigen by immunoblotting and ELISA using MAbs as indicated in **Table 4**. The presence of PorB, class 4 OMP, Opa, and LPS is identified similarly *(43)*.
3. Determine the LPS content by scanning silver-stained SDS-PAGE *(46)*, or chemically *(46)*. The LPS may also be controlled by gas chromatography (GC).
4. Determine endotoxin biological activity by the LAL assay.
5. Do sterility testing by plating bulk products on gonococcal agar and Tryptone Soy Broth medium for 3 d at 37°C in a 5% CO_2 atmosphere. For sterility testing of the final container product 5 mL is added to 180 mL Tryptone Soy Broth and thioglycolate and incubated for 14 d at 20–25°C for Tryptone Soy Broth and at 30–32°C for thioglycolate. No growth should be observed.
6. Vesicles should be visible and intact by TEM after negative staining of ultrasonically treatment of the vaccine.
7. Examine immunogenicity of the vaccine in mice after two immunizations using ELISA and determine bactericidal activity of serum antibodies specific for each of the subtypes in the vaccine using subtype specific *N. meningitidis* strains.
8. Standard methods are used for protein, DOC, and thiomersal analysis, pH, aluminum content, and osmolality. (Additionally, *see* **Notes 15–16**.)

3.5.3. Quality Control of the Formulated Vaccines

3.5.3.1. CONVENTIONAL OMV VACCINES

Following adsorption of OMV onto the aluminum adjuvant, the vaccine can be stored as a final bulk or after filling into vials, ampoules, or syringes (*see* **Note 17**). The stage at which the tests described below are performed depends on local needs and actual process-design.

Most of the tests can be performed directly on adsorbed vaccine (immunogenicity, LAL, aluminum quantitation, etc.). However, the test for identity (antigenic pattern) requires desorbing the OMVs from the adjuvant. Sodium citrate has been used (*see* **Notes 18** and **19**).

To evaluate immunogenicity ("Potency") in mice, groups of mice are immunized subcutaneously with two doses, 3 wk apart. Sera are collected 2 wk after the last immunization. At least two different doses of adsorbed vaccine should be used. The doses will vary due to vaccine formulation, strains of mice, and so on. To determine the dose-response, doses of 0.5, 1, 2, and 4 µg protein per mouse are suggested. The difference between antibody levels in the groups of mice given the highest and lowest dose in the "potency test" should be significant and show a positive dose-response relation. Measurements of antibody levels are done by ELISA *(21)*. An "in house" standard of pooled mouse serum, designated to contain arbitrary number of units per mL, can be used (*see* **Table 3** for an example).

Table 4
**Examples of Monoclonal Antibodies Against Individual
Subtype Specific Epitopes, Different OMPs, and Mutant
Lipopolysaccharides, Used for Quality Control
of the RIVM Genetically Modified PorA Vaccine**[a]

MoAb	Protein specificity
MN14C11.6	P1.7
MN5C11G	P1.16
MN22A9.19	P1.5
MN16C13F4	P1.2
MN3C5C	P1.15
MN20F4.17	P1.10
MN20B9.34	P1.4
MN20A7.10	P1.12
MN24H10.75	P1.13
MN15A14H6	Class 3 OMP, type 15
MN3B9F or MN2D6D	Class 4 OMP
MN20E12.70	Class 5 OMP
B306	Opc
4A8B2	L3 LPS
MN31B11.22	GalE LPS

[a]*See* refs. *(43,50)*.

Quantitation of aluminum can be done by atomic adsorption spectroscopy
(21). Analysis of pH and osmolality are done by standard techniques on validated equipment. Tests for endotoxin (LAL), sucrose, and sterility are done as
for unadsorbed batches. Analyzing for the degree of binding to the adjuvant
requires slow-speed centrifugation of the AH or AP-bound proteins and a protein analysis of the supernatant. The identity test on desorbed OMV is done by
SDS-PAGE as described for unadsorbed OMV (*see* **Notes 10, 11, 18** and **19**).

The test for Thiomersal/Merthiolate (if applicable, *see* **Note 17**) can be done
by colorimetry *(51)*.

3.5.3.2. OMV Vaccines from Genetically Modified Strains

Special awareness of the genetic stability of the constructed production
strains needs to be considered. Controlling and documenting that the seed-lot
continues to be unable to produce capsule, lack of expression of PorB, and so
on, is also important. Likewise there should be quality-control testing of the
OMV for the amount of Opc and high molecular-weight proteins. Tests for the

presence of Opc should also be done in the actual bacteria used in the serum bactericidal titration used for evaluation of these vaccines.

See **Table 5** for a listing of quality-control tests on the formulated bulk and on the final filled vaccine.

4. Notes

1. The methods described here recommend that the meningococcal strains be grown in iron-deficient media, but also provide growth conditions for growth in iron-sufficient media. The recommendation for induction of iron regulated proteins is based on the observations that antibodies to some iron-regulated proteins are bactericidal and that there is broad antigenic diversity among group B and group C meningococcal strains. Thus, inclusion of iron-regulated OMPs may extend more broadly vaccine coverage.

2. The amount of iron required for normal growth of meningococci is very low. Iron will be present in the media from a variety or sources other than the iron intentionally added during media formulation. These sources include the water and other media components. It is therefore impossible to define the exact amounts of iron chelators needed for optimal induction of iron-regulated proteins. Furthermore, it is much easier to induce high levels of iron-regulated protein expression in some strains than in others, which is another reason why three to five isolates of the same serotype and serosubtype are screened for optimal growth characteristics. The iron chelator EDDA was, until recently, obtained from Sigma Chemical Company (product No. E-4135), but may no longer be available from Sigma.

3. Growing *N. meningitidis* under iron restriction induces several additional proteins. Growth of the bacteria is followed by monitoring the OD of the cultures. Outer membranes are then prepared *(28)* and examined by SDS-PAGE for presence of iron-regulated proteins with molecular weights between approx 70 and 100 KDa *(23,34)*. The production strain is selected based upon OMP yields and induction of the iron-regulated proteins. Of possibly protective potential is the TbpA and -B and the 70 kDa FrpB proteins *(16)*. To positively identify these proteins, serological reagents (monoclonals or specific sera) for use in immunoblotting, and so on, are required.

4. During characterization of a conventional OMV vaccine formulation, from a newly established fermentation and purification process, immunological reagents capable of detecting TbpA, -B, and FrpB should be used for the strain in question to assure that the strain has not been grown under Fe-limited conditions.

5. The meningococcal outer membranes are not anchored to the peptidoglycan layer as they are in the enteric Gram negative rods, and are thus easily removed from the cells by shearing without disruption of most of the cells. The shear forces may be applied in a number of ways including use of an Omnimixer (Sorval), tissue homoginizer, ultrasonic waterbath, or passage through a narrow opening under some pressure (not a French press, because this results in complete cell disruption).

Table 5
Quality-Control Testing and Limits for Formulated Genetically Modified porA Vesicle Vaccine

Final bulk
    Sterility
    Protein content
    Immunogenicity (potency) in mice: look for presence of antibodies to each PorA
      subtype included in the vaccine
    Osmolality
    Measure pH: 7.0–8.0
    Aluminum content: 19–25 mmoles/L
    Thimerosal content if multidose vaccine formulation used: 190–284 µmoles/L
Final container vaccine
    Sterility
    General safety (abnormal toxicity) test
    Endotoxin content
    Identity test for each PorA protein present
    Aluminium content: 19–25 mmoles/L

6. For the AH adjuvants, the degree of crystallinity may be increased and the protein-adsorption capacity or other important properties decreased following autoclaving.

7. Identity tests and other assays for assuring and documenting the quality of starting materials should be done according to methods described in Pharmacopoeias or equivalent. (This will not be dealt with further in this chapter.)

8. The quality of starting materials should be compatible with current requirements for parenteral medicines. Such an awareness regarding assurance of quality and documentation is highly relevant for media components in order to minimize the (legalistic) risk of using materials with the potential of being contaminated with transmissable spongiform encephalopathy (TSE). In practice one should use components that are as chemically defined as possible. However, if, e.g., bovine serum (or derivatives) might be needed, the country of origin must be declared bovine spongiform encepholopathy (BSE)-free and the actual batch supplied with certificates, traceable back to the original supplier.

9. One of the most challenging quality issues in manufacturing of OMV vaccines is the control and documentation of the production environment and the aseptic procedures. As far as possible, "open steps" should be avoided. The limited number of critical steps after harvesting and inactivation, must be done in an HEPA-Laminar-Air-Flow bench (hood) situated in a "Class 100" room or equivalent. Environmental Monitoring Programs with particle counts, settle plates, acceptance limits and warning limits, and so on, must be developed for the specific process and the actual premises.

10. The logic and basis for tests done on individual sub-batches, final bulk, and perhaps on finished product must be evaluated in the context of how the production can be best kept inside the end-product specifications. In the past the use of sub-batches, which are later pooled, has been quite common. The fermenter sizes have often been 50–100 L and the harvesting capacities have been limited. Thus, one can make pools of OMV concentrates from one single growth and purification, in order to increase the number of doses in the final batch, needing extensive quality control, stability programs, and so on.

11. It is important to establish a specification for each vaccine formulation regarding the protein profile from a SDS-PAGE, and scanning of the Coomassie Brilliant Blue stained gel. The actual specifications for the MenB-OMV vaccine from NIPH can be seen in **Table 4**.

12. A key feature of outer membrane based vaccines against meningococcal disease is believed to be that the immunogens be presented in a vesicular form. For the three different types of OMV vaccines discussed in this chapter, the various specifications demand a TEM picture documenting mainly intact vesicles with a diameter of 50–200 nm. However, whether the vesicle shape, size, or other morphological features is a prerequisite for all complex protein vaccines against meningococcal disease is not completely settled.

13. For LPS quantitation, the SDS-PAGE, silver-staining method *(47)* might be preferred for routine testing. However, this method requires a well-characterized, gravimetric determined *N. meningitidis* LPS, to be used as a standard.

14. Quantitation of the phospholipid content should also be done; at least following establishment of the production process or after process alterations such as changing production strain. One might expect amounts of phospholipid in the same range as the LPS content. The conventional OMV vaccine used in Norway during the clinical trial contained approx 3.5 µg/mL or 7% relative to protein *(5)*.

15. Special awareness of the genetic stability of the constructed production strains may be required. Controlling and documenting that the seed-lot continue to be unable to produce capsule, express PorB, and so on, will be important. Likewise there should be quality-control testing of the OMV for the amount of Opc and high molecular-weight proteins. Tests for the presence of Opc should also be done in the actual bacteria used in the SBA titration used for evaluation of these vaccines.

16. Characterization/analysis of the presentation of PorA and other membrane structures (heterotrimers with PorB; mixture of different sero-subtype PorAs, etc.), compared to wild-type OMV is an important but difficult issue.

17. Note that the trend for vaccine manufacture is to go for single dose units, thus, avoiding mercury-based preservatives. If multi-dose units and/or preservatives need to be used, then a test for efficacy of anti-microbial preservation should be done according to a standard Pharmacopoeia method.

18. For the identity test on the finished product, the OMV usually needs to be desorbed from the Al-adjuvant. Conventionally sodium citrate has been used. However, for the NIPH produced vaccine, the proteins are so tightly bound, so another method must be used (*see* **Note 19**).

19. The "NIPH desorption method" uses 0.1% ethylene diamine tetraacetic acid (EDTA) in a 0.25 *M* phosphate buffer, pH 8.6, at 37°C for approx 15 h.
    a. Mix the tetrasodium salt of EDTA (from Sigma) 11.2 mg and $Na_2HPO_4 \times 2$ H_2O 441.6 mg for a total volume of 10.0 mL (distilled water added).
    b. Spin down 1 mL of vaccine in a small tube (Eppendorf; 4.000 rpm in a table centrifuge).
    c. Take off the supernatant and add 100 µL of the EDTA-reagent, treat with ultrasound (30 s. in a bath) and incubate at 37°C over night.
    d. Carefully remove the supernatant, which then can be used for the SDS-PAGE identity test, and so on.

References

1. Zollinger, W. D. (1997) New and improved vaccines against meningococcal disease, in *New Generation Vaccines*, 2nd ed. (Levine, M. M., Woodrow, G. C., Kaper, J. B., and Cobon, G. S., eds.), Marcel Dekker, New York, 469–488.
2. Bjune, G., Hoiby, E. A., Gronnesby, J. K., Arnesen, O., Fredriksen, J. H., Halstensen, A., et al. (1991) Effect of outer membrane vesicle vaccine against group B meningococcal disease in Norway. *Lancet* **338**, 1093–1096.
3. Sierra, G. V. G., Campa, H. C., Varcacel, N. M., Izquierdo, P. L., Sotolongo, P. F., Casanueva, G. V., et al. (1991) Vaccine against group B Neisseria meningitidis: Protection trial andmass vaccination results in Cuba. *NIPH. Ann.* **14**, 195–210.
4. Perkins, B. A., Jonsdottir, K., Briem, H., Griffiths, E., Plikaytis, B. D., Høiby, E. A., et al. (1998) Immunogenicity of two efficacious outer membrane protein-based serogroup B meningococcal vaccines among young adults in Iceland. *J. Infect. Dis.* **177**, 683–669.
5. Tappero, J. W., Lagos, R., Ballesteros, A. M., Plikaytis B., Williams D., Dykes J., et al. (1999) Immunogenicity of 2 serogroup B outer-membrane protein meningococcal vaccines. A randomized controlled trial in Chile. *JAMA* **281**, 1520–1527.
6. Milagres, L. G., Ramos, S. R., Sacchi, C. T., Melles, C. E. A., Vieira, V. S. D., Sato, H., et al. (1994) Immune response of Brazilian children to a *Neisseria meningitidis* serogroup B outer membrane protein vaccine: Comparison with efficacy. *Infect. Immun.* **62**, 4419–4424.
7. Frasch, C. E. (1995) Meningococcal vaccines: past present and future, in *Meningococcal Disease* (Cartwright, K. A. V., ed.), John Wiley and Sons, New York, pp. 245–283.
8. Peltola, H. (1998) Meningococcal vaccines: current status and future possibilities. *Drugs* **55**, 347–366.
9. Van der Voort, E. M. R., Kuipers, B., Brugghe, H. F., Van Unen, L. M. A., Timmermans, H. A. M., Hoogerhout, P., and Poolman, J. T. (1997) Epitope specificity of murine and human bactericidal antibodies against PorA P1.7,16 induced with experimental meningococcal group B vaccines. *FEMS Immunol. Med. Microbiol.* **17**, 139–148.
10. Wang, J. F., Jarvis, G. A., Achtman, M., Rosenqvist, E., Michaelsen, T. E., Aase, A., and Griffiss, J. M. (2000) Functional activities and immunoglobulin variable regions

of human and murine monoclonal antibodies specific for the P1.7 PorA protein loop of *Neisseria meningitides*. *Infect. Immun.* **68**, 1871–1878.

11. Barlow, A. K., Heckels, J. E., and Clarke, I. N. (1989) The class I outer membrane protein of *Neisseria meningitidis*: Gene sequence, structural and immunological similarities to gonococcal porins. *Mol. Microbiol.* **3**, 131–139.

12. Minetti, C., Song, J., and Blake, M.S. (1998) Meningococcal PorA class 1 proteins exist in nature as a heterotrimeric proin with porB proteins, in *Eleventh International Pathogenic Neisseria Conference* (Nassif, X., Quentin-Millet, M-J., and Taha, M-K., eds.), EDK, Paris, p. 15.

13. Jones, D. M., Borrow, R., Fox, A. J., Gray, S., Cartwright, K. A., and Poolman, J. T. (1992) The lipooligosaccharide immunotype as a virulence determinant in *Neisseria meningitidis*. *Microb. Pathog.* **13**, 219–224.

14. Zollinger, W. D., Moran, E. E., Devi, S. J. N., and Frasch, C. E. (1997) Bactericidal antibody responses of juvenile rhesus monkeys immunized with group B *Neisseria meningitidis* capsular polysaccharide-protein conjugate vaccines. *Infect. Immun.* **65**, 1053–1060.

15. Sacchi, C. T. (1998) Proposed standardization of *Neisseria meningitidis* PorA variable-region typing nomenclature. *Clin. Diagn. Lab. Immunol.* **5**, 845–855.

16. Wetzler, L. M., Blake, M. S., Barry, K., and Gotschlich, E. C. (1992) Gonococcal porin vaccine evaluation: comparison of Por proteosomes, liposomes, and blebs isolated from rmp deletion mutants. *J. Infect. Dis.* **166**, 551–555.

17. Steeghs, L., Kuipers, B., Hamstra, H. J., Kersten, G., Van Alphen, L., and Van der Ley, P. (1999) Immunogenicity of outer membrane proteins in a lipopolysaccharide-deficient mutant of *Neisseria meningitidis*: influence of adjuvants on the immune response. *Infect. Immun.* **67**, 4988–4993.

18. Helting, T. B., Guthohrlein, G., Blackkolb, F., and Ronneberger, H. (1981) Serotype determinant protein of *Neisseria Meningitidis*. Large scale preparation by direct detergent treatment of the bacterial cells. *Acta Pathol. Microbiol. Scand.* *[C]* **89**, 69–78.

19. Frasch, C. E. (1990) Production and control of Neisseria meningitidis vaccines, in *Bacterial Vaccines* (Mizrahi, A., ed.), Wiley-Liss, New York, pp. 123–145.

20. Poolman, J. T. (1990) Polysaccharides and membrane vaccines, in *Bacterial Vaccines* (Mizrahi, A., ed.), Wiley-Liss, New York, pp. 58–86.

21. Holst Fredriksen, J., Rosenqvist, E., Wedege, E., Bryn, K., Bjune, G., Frøholm, L. O., et al. (1991). Production characterization and control of MenB-vaccine "Folkehelsa": an outer membrane vesicle vaccine against group B meningococcal disease. *NIPH Ann.* **14**, 67–80.

22. Fu, J., Bailey, F. J., King, J. J., Parker, C. B., Robinett, R. S. R., Kolodin, D. G., et al. (1995) Recent advances in the large scale fermentation of *Neisseria meningitidis* group B for the production of an outer membrane protein complex. *BioTechnology* **13**, 170–174.

23. Brandileone, M. C., Zanella, R. C., Vieira, V. S., Sacchi, C. T., Milagres, L. C., and Frasch, C. E. (1994) Induction of iron regulated proteins during normal growth

of *Neisseria meningitidis* in a chemically defined medium. *Rev. Inst. Med. Trop. Sao Paulo* **36**, 301–310.

24. Tsai, C. M., Frasch, C. E., Rivera, E., and Hochstein, H. D. (1989) Measurement of lipopolysaccharide (endotoxin) in meningococcal protein and polysaccharide preparations for vaccine usage. *J. Biol. Stand.* **17**, 249–258.

25. Rosenqvist, E., Hoiby, E. A., Bjune, G., Aase, A., Halstensen, A., Lehmann, A. K., et al. (1998) Effect of aluminium hydroxide and meningococcal serogroup C capsular polysaccharide on the immunogenicity and reactogenicity of a group B *Neisseria meningitidis* outer membrane vesicle vaccine. *Dev. Biol. Stand.* **92**, 323–333.

26. Frasch, C. E., Peppler, M. S., Cate, T. R., and Zahradnik, J. M. (1982) Immunogenicity and clinical evaluation of group B *Neisseria meningitidis* outer membrane protein vaccines. IN: Robbins, J. B., Hill, J. C., and Sadoff, J. C. (eds.), *Sem. Infect. Dis.* **4**, 263–267, Thieme-Stratton, NY, NY.

27. Frantz, I. D. (1942) Growth requirements of the meningococcus. *J. Bacteriol.* **43**, 757–761.

28. Frasch, C. E., McNelis, R. M., and Gotschlich, E. C. (1976) Strain-specific variation in the protein and lipopolysaccharide composition of the group B meningococcal outer membrane. *J. Bacteriol.* **127**, 973–981.

29. Van der Ley, P. A. and Poolman, J. (1992) Construction of a multivalent meningococcal vaccine strain based on the class 1 outer membrane protein. *Infect. Immun.* **60**, 3156–3161.

30. Van der Ley, P. A., van der Biezen, J., and Poolman, J. T. (1995) Construction of *Neisseria meningitidis* strains carrying multiple chromosomal copies of the porA gene for use in the production of a multivalent outer membrane protein vaccine. *Vaccine* **13**, 401–407.

31. Tommassen, J., Vermeij, P., Struyvé, M., Benz, R., and Poolman, J. T. (1990) Isolation of *Neisseria meningitidis* mutants deficient in class I (Pora) and class 3 (PorB) outer membrane proteins. *Infect. Immun.* **58**, 1355–1359.

32. Frosch, M., Schultz, E., Glenn-Clavo, E., and Meyer, T. F. (1990) Generation of capsule-deficient *Neisseria meningitidis* strains by homologous recombination. *Mol. Microbiol.* **4**, 1215–1218.

33. Rosenqvist, E., Hoiby, E. A., Wedege, E., Kusecek, B., and Achtman, M. (1993) The 5C protein of *Neisseria meningitidis* is highly immunogenic in humans and induces bactericidal antibodies. *J. Infect. Dis.* **167**, 1065–1073.

34. Banerjee-Bhatnager, N. and Frasch, C. E. (1990). Expression of ironregulated outer membrane proteins in *Neissera meningitidis* including a 70-kDa transferrin receptor and the vaccine potential of these proteins. *Infect. Immun.* **58**, 2875–2881.

35. Frasch, C. E., Zahradnik, J. M., Wang, L. Y., Mocca, L. F., and Tsai, C. M. (1988) Antibody response of adults to an aluminum hydroxide-adsorbed *Neisseria meningitidis* serotype 2b protein-group B polysaccharide vaccine. *J. Infect. Dis.* **158**, 710–718.

36. Hem, S. L. and White, J. L. (1984) Characterization of aluminum hydroxide for use as an adjuvant in parenteral vaccines. *J. Parenter. Sci. Technol.* **38**, 2–10.

37. Burrell, L. S., Lindblad, E. B., White, J. L., and Hem, S. L. (1999) Stability of aluminium-containing adjuvants to autoclaving. *Vaccine* **17,** 2599–2603.
38. MacDonald, N. E., Halperin, S. A., Law, B. J., Forrest, B., Danzig, L. E., and Granoff, D. M. (1998) Induction of immunologic memory by conjugated versus plain meningococcal C polysaccharide vaccine in toddlers: a randomized controlled trial. *JAMA* **280,** 1685–1689.
39. Lieberman, J. M., Chiu, S. S., Wong, V. K., Partridge, S., Chang, S. J., Chiu, C. Y., et al. (1996) Safety and immunogenicity of a serogroups A/C *Neisseria meningitides* oligosaccharide-protein conjugate vaccine in young children: a randomized controlled trial. *J. Amer. Med. Assoc.* **275,** 1499–1503.
40. Fukasawa, L. O., Gorla, M. C. O., Schenkman, R. P. F., Garcia, L. R., Carneiro, S. M., Rawa, I., and Tanizaki, M. M. (1999) *Neisseria meningitidis* serogroup C polysaccharide and serogroup B outer membrane vesicle conjugate as a bivalent meningococcus vaccine candidate. *Vaccine* **17,** 2951–2958.
41. Holst Fredriksen, J., Griffiths, E., Grotterød, E. M., Høiby, E. A., Rosenqvist, E., Stevenson, P., and Wedege, E. (1994) Characterization of high molecular weight components in MenB-vaccine "Folkehelsa"; An outer membrane vesicle vaccine against group B meningococcal disease, in *Pathobiology and Immunobiology of Neisseriaceae* (Conde-Glez, C. J., Morse, S., Rice, P., Sparling, F., and Calderôn, E. eds.), Instituto National de Salud Publica, Cuernovaso, Mexico, pp. 818–824.
42. Griffiths, E., Sierra, G., and Holst, J. (1994) Quality control of the Cuban and Norwegian serogroup B vaccines used in the Iceland study, in *Proceedings of the Ninth International Pathogenic Neisseria Conference* (Evans, J. S., Yost, S. E., Maiden, M. C. J., and Feavers, I. M., eds.), Winchester, UK, p. 437.
43. Claassen, I., Meylis, J., van der Ley, P., Peeters, C., Brons, H., Robert, J., et al. (1996) Production, characterization and control of a *Neisseria meningitidis* hexavalent class 1 outer membrane protein containing vesicle vaccine. *Vaccine* **14,** 1001–1008.
44. Wenger, J. D. (1999) Serogroup B meningococcal disease. New outbreaks, new strategies. *JAMA* **281,** 1541–1543.
45. Peterson, G. L. (1977) A simplification of the protein assay of Lowry et al. which is more generally applicable. *Anal. Biochem.* **83,** 346–356.
46. Lee, C-H. and Tsai, C-M. (1999) Quantification of bacterial lipopolysaccharide by the Purpald assay: measuring formaldehyde generated from 2-keto-3-deoxyoctonate and heptose at the inner core by periodate oxidation. *Anal. Biochem.* **267,** 161–168.
47. Tsai, C-M., Frasch, C. E., Rivera, E., and Hochstein, H. D. (1989) Measurement of lipopolysaccharide (endotoxin) in meningococcal protein and polysaccharide preparations for vaccine usage. *J. Biol. Stand.* **17,** 229–258.
48. Brunborg, G., Holme, J. A., Søderlund, E. G., Omichinski, J. G., and Dybing, E. (1988) An automated alkaline elution system: DNA damage induced by 1,2-dibromo-3-chloropropane in vivo and in vitro. *Anal. Biochem.* **174,** 522–536.

49. Clarke, A. J., Sarabia, V., Keenleyside, W., MacLachlan, P. R., and Whitfield, C. (1991) The compositional analysis of bacterial extracellular polysaccharides by high-performance anion-exchange chromatography. *Anal. Biochem.* **199,** 68–74.

50. Abdillahi, A. and Poolman, J. T. (1988) *Neisseria meningitidis* group B serosubtyping using monoclonal antibodies in whole cell ELISA. *Microbiol. Pathog.* **4,** 27–32.

51. Shrivastaw, K. P. and Singh, S. (1995) A new method for spectrophotometric determination of thiomersal in biologicals. *Biologicals* **23,** 65–69.

8

Methods for Manipulation of Transferrin-Binding Proteins

Leanne M. DeWinter and Anthony B. Schryvers

1. Introduction

To obtain iron, a necessary nutrient, meningococci and several other human and veterinary pathogens have iron-acquisition systems, which are expressed in vivo during infection. One target of iron-acquisition systems is transferrin (Tf), which is the major glycoprotein responsible for the transport of iron in the extracellular milieu of vertebrates. Tf-binding proteins A and B (TbpA and TbpB) function as the cell-surface Tf receptor in *Neisseria meningitidis (1)*.

TbpA is a 90–100 kDa transmembrane protein that is absolutely required for iron-acquisition from Tf *(2)*. It is proposed to serve as the transmembrane channel through which iron moves from the extracellular milieu into the periplasm *(1,3)*. Based on sequence homology and functional similarities, TbpA is thought to have a similar structure as the siderophore receptors, FhuA and FepA, which have recently been crystallized *(4–6)*. These proteins possess an N-terminal periplasmic plug domain that blocks the transmembrane channel which is formed by a C-terminal β-barrel. Conformational changes within the plug region are thought to mediate passage of iron across the outer membrane. The larger size of the homolog, TbpA, is thought to be due to larger extracellular loops that are presumed to be involved in Tf binding and iron removal.

TbpB is a 65 to 90 kDa lipoprotein *(7)* that plays an important but not essential role in iron acquisition in vitro *(2,8)*. It preferentially interacts with holo-hTf *(9)* and may be involved in initial capture of hTf. TbpB is a bilobed protein *(10,11)* anchored to the outer membrane by its acylated N-terminus *(12)*, and is largely surface-exposed.

From: *Methods in Molecular Medicine, vol. 66: Meningococcal Vaccines: Methods and Protocols*
Edited by: A. J. Pollard and M. C. J. Maiden © Humana Press Inc., Totowa, NJ

Tbps are thought to be ideal vaccine candidates because they are cell-surface exposed, essential for virulence, and expressed in vivo. Antisera from humans recovering from meningococcal disease react with Tbps *(13–15)*, indicating that Tbps are produced in vivo. Meningococci lacking Tbps have neither been reported nor identified during screening attempts *(16)*, which is indirect evidence that *N. meningitidis* Tbps are important in vivo. In a human model of urethritis, a Tbp-deficient mutant of *Neisseria gonorrhoeae* was avirulent *(17)*, indicating that Tbps are critical for survival in vivo in this species, and by inference suggests that they would also be essential for *N. meningitidis*.

Initial studies demonstrated that bactericidal and protective antibodies from mice and rabbits against purified receptor from meningococcus correlated with the presence of TbpB *(18)*, which was subsequently confirmed by studies using purified TbpB *(19)*. There is genetic and antigenic hetereogeneity among TbpBs from different meningococcal strains *(20,21)*, indicating that a polyvalent vaccine may be required, and suggesting that the hetereogeneity should be monitored once a TbpB-based vaccine is implemented. Recombinant TbpB induces a protective immune response in animals *(16)* and has been shown to be safe and potentially efficacious in humans *(22)*. Thus the prospects for development of a TbpB-based vaccine are promising. Although there are indications that TbpA may also have some potential as a vaccine antigen *(13,23)*, further studies to demonstrate feasibility are necessary. Furthermore, studies with other human pathogens such as *Haemophilus influenzae (24)* and *Moraxella catarrhalis (25)*, and animal pathogens including *Pasteurella haemolytica (26)* and *Actinobacillus pleuropneumoniae (27)* support the efficacy of TbpB as a vaccine antigen.

1.1. Purification of Native Receptor Proteins from N. meningitidis

Affinity methods were used for initial identification and characterization of the Tf receptor proteins from the pathogenic *Neisseria* species *(7,28)*, and modifications of this basic approach have been useful for experimental purposes *(15,18,23)*. However, the level of receptor protein produced under optimal expression conditions from the native locus (2 mg/L) *(12)* is insufficient for commercial vaccine purposes. Alternative expression loci could potentially yield substantially higher levels of receptor proteins but it is uncertain at what level the processing and export of the proteins would become limiting. In addition, the use of hTf as an affinity ligand has potential limitations pertaining to the cost and safety of commercial production. Native antigen produced in *Neisseria* may possess the appropriate antigenic properties, but there are many hurdles to overcome before it can be considered a viable means of commercial production of a subunit vaccine.

Because expression of the receptor proteins is iron-regulated, they are only produced during growth under iron-limiting conditions. Preparation of iron-deficient cells is usually accomplished by inclusion of an iron chelator in the standard growth medium of an overnight culture (i.e., 100 μM ethylenediamine-di(o-hydroxyphenol) acetic acid [EDDHA] in Brain-Heart Infusion [BHI] broth). It is not essential to truly iron-starve the cells; growth under conditions of iron-limitation for a number of hours is sufficient to achieve good expression levels. Expression of the receptor proteins can be simply monitored by directly spotting aliquots of the culture onto a membrane (Immobilon-nitrocellulose), and then detecting receptor with labeled hTf *(29)* (*see* **Subheading 3.3.**).

Affinity-isolation methods were initially developed using outer-membrane preparations from iron-deficient cells as a source of receptor protein to facilitate isolation of pure receptor proteins. However, the affinity methods have proven to be effective enough to purify receptor proteins from crude membrane preparations and even directly from intact cells. This provides a simple method for rapidly analyzing receptor proteins from a collection of clinical isolates.

The strength of the Tbp-hTf interaction facilitates ready purification of Tbps from complex mixtures but presents a challenge for elution of Tbps in a functional form. For analytical purposes, Tbps are eluted simply by exposing the complex to sodium dodecyl sulfate-polyacrylamide gel electrophoresis (SDS-PAGE) sample buffer and using the supernatant after low-speed centrifugation for SDS-PAGE analysis. Elution of Tbps from the affinity matrix for preparative purposes can be accomplished by inclusion of guanidine HCl in the elution buffer *(30)* or by lowering the pH *(15)*. Elution of TbpB from the affinity resin occurs at lower concentrations of guanidine HCl than TbpA, thus providing a means of separation of the two receptor proteins. Because elution of Tbps from the affinity columns essentially involves partial denaturation of the proteins, minimizing the exposure to these conditions may affect the yield of functional protein. Clearly elution at low pH is advantageous in this regard.

1.2. Purification of Recombinant Tbps from Escherichia coli.

The rationale for the choice of *E. coli* as a host for heterologous expression is that it provides a range of systems and strategies for optimizing production and purification of recombinant proteins. In addition, structural and functional analysis of the Tbps is facilitated by the wide array of genetic tools and approaches available. Although there have been extensive advances in our understanding of export and processing pathways in prokaryotes, successful production of recombinant proteins is still very much an empirical process.

Although there have been several reports on the functional expression of *Neisseria* TbpA in *E. coli* *(31,32)*, optimal production in this host species has been elusive. Studies on the expression of TbpA from the porcine pathogen, *Actinobacillus pleuropneumoniae*, revealed that even at moderate expression levels, a majority of the protein was produced in the cytoplasm but was non-functional *(33)*. There have been no published reports demonstrating production of significant quantities of recombinant TbpA using the intact *tbpA* gene *(34)*, suggesting that obtaining high-level expression of functional meningococcal TbpA will be a challenge. Expression of the *tbpA* gene without signal sequence (or as a fusion protein) can result in accumulation of recombinant TbpA in the cytoplasmic or inclusion body fraction, but this form of the protein is nonfunctional. Fortunately, this limitation need not impede vaccine development because protective efficacy has been primarily associated with TbpB *(16,25,26)*.

In contrast to TbpA, expression of a functional form of recombinant TbpB from *N. meningitidis* in *E. coli* has been fairly straightforward *(35,36)*. In studies examining overexpression of TbpB from the porcine pathogen, *Actinobacillus pleuropneumoniae*, the recombinant protein retained the ability to bind Tf, an indication of native structure, regardless of which cellular fraction it was associated with *(33)*. This indicates that appropriate folding of TbpB can occur under varying conditions. Fatty acyl groups are attached to the N-terminal cysteine of the mature, exported protein in *E. coli* *(35)*, providing a form of the protein that has some inherent adjuvant properties. Overexpression of this form of TbpB and development of nonaffinity methods for purification has provided material for Phase I trials in humans *(22)*, demonstrating that a TbpB-based vaccine for meningococcal disease is feasible.

Meningococcal TbpB has also been functionally expressed at high levels in the cytoplasm of *E. coli* fused to maltose-binding protein (Mbp), which provided a readily purified form of the protein for functional studies *(10,11,37)*. Surprisingly, production of fusion protein was more effective using the cytoplasmic expression vector, pMAL-c2, than with the periplasmic expression vector, pMAL-p2, in this system *(38)*. Initial results suggested a stable, homogeneous preparation of recombinant Mbp-TbpB was produced, but more extensive analyses have revealed that standard production conditions yields a hetereogenous preparation (data not shown). Thus alternative expression conditions or systems will have to be evaluated in order to obtain a homogeneous preparation of protein for functional, immunological, and structural studies.

2. Materials

2.1. Analytical Affinity Isolation

1. EDDHA (Ethylenediamine-di(o-hydroxyphenyl acetic acid)); Sigma: Prepare 40 mg/mL stock of EDDHA in 1 *M* NaOH and add directly to sterilized growth

medium (1 µL per mL for a 40 µg/mL stock). Alternatively Desferrioxamine (Deferoxamine mesylate) (Sigma) can be added from 10 mg/mL stock, prepared in ddH$_2$O and filter sterilized.

2. SDS-PAGE sample buffer: 125 mM Tris-HCl, pH 6.8, 0.1% SDS, 0.01% bromophenol blue, 10% glycerol.

2.2. Preparative Affinity Isolation of Tbps

1. Phenylmethylsulfonyl fluoride (PMSF); Sigma: Prepare a 10 mg/mL stock in 95% ethanol and add 100 µL to 10 mL of cell suspension. Degradation of PMSF increases at room temperature, alkaline pH, and in aqueous solutions; store stock solutions at –20°C in aliquots. Owing to its short half-life, add PMSF immediately before required and process samples in a timely fashion. PMSF is also toxic; avoid contact and inhalation.

2.3. Solid-Phase Assay for hTf Binding

1. Nitrocellulose (Immobilon-NC); Millipore.
2. TBS (Tris-buffered saline): 50 mM Tris-HCl, pH 7.5, 150 mM NaCl.
3. Blocking solution: Skim-milk powder (nonfat dry milk); BioRad, or another suitable blocking reagent dissolved to 0.5% in TBS.
4. Binding solution: Blocking solution containing a 1 : 1,000 dilution of horseradish peroxidase-conjugated hTf.
5. Horseradish peroxidase-conjugated hTf stock solution (1–2 mg/mL): Prepared by the standard periodate method *(39)* and stored frozen in 50–100 µL aliquots.
6. Colorimetric substrate (HRP color development reagent, 4-chloro-1-naphthol); BioRad: Prepared as described by manufacturer. Avoid contact and inhalation as this substance is an irritant to the skin and respiratory tract. Other colorimetric substrates are also suitable.

2.4. Preparation of an hTf Affinity Column

1. Coupling buffer: 0.1 M NaHCO$_3$, 0.5 M NaCl, 0.5% Tween 80, pH 8.3.

3. Methods
3.1. Analytical Affinity Isolation of Tbps

The following method is designed for rapid screening of receptor proteins from various meningococcal isolates. Modification of this method to individual laboratory conditions and work schedules can easily be accomplished. Receptor expression can be monitored by the simple solid-phase binding assay described below (**Subheading 3.3.**) and control Tbps can be prepared as described in the next section (**Subheading 3.2.**).

1. Inoculate isolates into BHI broth (or other rich medium) for overnight growth.
2. Inoculate 100 µL of overnight culture into 2.5 mL of prewarmed BHI broth.

After 2 h incubation, add 2.5 mL of prewarmed BHI broth containing 200 μ*M* EDDHA (*see* **Note 1**).

3. After 2–4 h incubation, take a 2 μL aliquot of the culture and spot directly onto membrane (nitrocellulose-Imobilon) for assay of hTf binding (**Subheading 3.3.**). Harvest the remaining cells by centrifugation.

4. Resuspend the cell pellet in 1 mL of 50 mm Tris-HCl, 1 *M* NaCl, 10 m*M* EDTA, pH 8.0, buffer containing 1% Sarkosyl. Incubate for 60 min with gentle agitation. Transfer to a 1.5-mL microcentrifuge tube and centrifuge for 20 min at top speed (20,000*g*) to remove cellular debris.

5. Decant supernatant and mix with 50 μL of hTf-Sepharose (**Subheading 3.4.**). After incubating for 30–60 min centrifuge at low speed (1,000*g*) for 2 min to collect the affinity matrix. Resuspend and wash the affinity resin in buffer containing 1 *M* NaCl and 0.1% Sarkosyl three times and finally once with 50 m*M* Tris-HCl, pH 8.0.

6. Resuspend the affinity resin with 50 μL of SDS-PAGE sample buffer, incubate for 30 min, and centrifuge (*see* **Note 2**).

7. Apply an aliquot of the supernatant (after boiling and addition of reducing reagent) to SDS-PAGE gel.

3.2. Preparative Affinity Isolation of Tbps

The following method describes the preparation of a moderate quantity of purified receptor complex from a wild-type strain of *N. meningitidis* and can readily be scaled up for larger culture volumes. Individual preparations of TbpA and TbpB can be obtained through the use of isogenic tbp mutants *(2)*, by additional chromatographic steps *(15)*, or by modifying elution conditions (guanidine HCl levels). The process might be simplified by directly extracting the receptor proteins from intact cells, as in the analytical procedure, but the effect on ultimate yield and purity of the receptor preparation has not been assessed.

1. Inoculate 50 mL of prewarmed BHI broth with meningococcal cells grown on chocolate agar. Grow to late log/early stationary phase of growth (6–8 h) and transfer into 1.5 L of prewarmed BHI containing 100 μ*M* EDDHA. Grow overnight (12–16 h); harvest cells by centrifugation at 10,000*g* for 10 min.

2. Resuspend the cells in cold 50 m*M* Tris-HCl, pH 8.0, add PMSF to 100 μg/mL, and pass through a chilled French-pressure cell at 16,000 psi to lyse the bacterial cells (*see* **Note 3**).

3. Centrifuge the lysate at 10,000*g* for 10 min at 4°C to remove unlysed cells and cellular debris and then collect the crude membrane pellet by centrifugation at 100,000*g* for 1 h.

4. Resuspend the membrane pellets in 40 mL of 50 m*M* Tris-HCl and then add 10 mL of 5 *M* NaCl, 1 mL of 500 m*M* EDTA and 5 mL of 30% Sarkosyl to solubilize the membranes. Incubate at 4°C for 30 min.

5. Centrifuge the solubilized membranes at 100,000g for 1 h, and apply the supernatant to a 2–5 mL hTf Sepharose column (*see* **Notes 4** and **5**). Wash the column with 10 column volumes of 50 mM Tris-HCl, pH 8, 1 M NaCl 1, 1 mM EDTA, and 0.1% Sarkosyl.
6. Elute the receptor proteins with wash buffer containing 3 M guanidine HCl (*see* **Note 6**). Individual fractions or the pooled eluant should be equilibrated in 50 mM Tris-HCl, 0.01% Sarkosyl buffer by dialysis or by passage through a desalting column.
7. Analyze the individual fractions of the pooled eluant by SDS-PAGE and with the solid-phase binding assay (**Subheading 3.3.**) or by a modification of the analytical affinity-isolation procedure (**Subheading 3.1.**) to determine the level of functional receptor protein.
8. If necessary concentrate the samples by ultrafiltration and then freeze away aliquots and store at –70°C.

3.3. Solid-Phase Assay for hTf Binding

This solid-phase binding assay was developed to accommodate a variety of receptor-containing preparations and to provide a rapid qualitative evaluation of Tf-binding activity. The assay can be semi-quantitative if dilutions of receptor are applied to the membrane and compared to dilutions of labeled Tf applied directly to a control membrane. Densitometric analysis of the colored spots can yield numerical values, but any kinetic parameters derived from this analysis should be interpreted with caution.

1. Apply 2 µL (and dilutions in 50 mM Tris-HCl) of receptor preparations onto nitrocellulose (*see* **Note 7**) in a predetermined pattern. Let the membrane dry (*see* **Note 8**).
2. Block the membrane in blocking solution with gentle rocking for 15–30 min at room temperature.
3. Wash the membrane three times in TBS buffer.
4. Incubate in binding solution with gentle rocking for 30–60 min.
5. Remove binding solution and wash the membrane three times in TBS buffer.
6. Add colorimetric substrate and incubate 15–30 min for color development.
7. Wash the membrane with double-distilled water and blot dry.

3.4. Preparation of an hTf Affinity Column

The method for preparation of the hTf affinity column is essentially as per the directions provided by the supplier of CNBr-activated Sepharose. The iron status of the bound hTf can be modified (*see* **step 8**), and the affinity resin can be reused after regeneration.

1. Use 2.86 g of freeze-dried CNBr-activated Sepharose 4B for 10 mL of resin. Swell the resin in 1 mM HCl for 15 min and transfer it to a G3 porosity sintered-

glass filter. Rinse the resin several times with 1 mM HCl to maintain a low pH for removal of resin stabilizers and preservation of reactive groups in the Sepharose.

2. Dissolve 5 mg Tf per mL of resin in coupling buffer. Working quickly to prevent the loss of reactive groups at elevated pH, wash the activated resin with a small volume of coupling buffer and then, using a spoon, add the resin to the Tf in coupling buffer.

3. Incubate on a rocking platform for 2 h at room temperature, or overnight at 4°C.

4. Load the resin into a column, drain the excess fluid containing unbound transferrin, and wash the Tf-sepharose with 10 column volumes of coupling buffer. Take care not to exceed the maximum flow rate of Sepharose 4B, which is 11.5 mL/cm^{2}h.

5. To block unoccupied sites on the Sepharose, wash the resin with 2 column volumes of 50 mM Tris-HCl, pH 8.0, 1 column volume of 50 mM Tris-HCl, 1 M ethanolamine HCl, pH 8.0, and then transfer the resin to a capped container and incubate in 50 mM Tris-HCl, 1 M ethanolamine HCl, pH 8.0 for 2 h at room temperature or overnight at 4°C.

6. Load the resin into a column, drain the blocking buffer, and wash with 3 column volumes of 50 mM Tris-HCl, pH 8.0. To remove nonspecifically adsorbed protein, wash with 3–6 column volumes of 50 mM Tris-HCl, 1 M NaCl, 6 M guanidine-HCl, pH 8.0.

7. Wash with 10 column volumes of 50 mM Tris-HCl, pH 8.0.

8. To prepare iron-loaded Tf-sepharose, apply 1 column volume of filtered 0.1 M Na citrate, 0.1 M Na bicarbonate, 10 mg/mL FeCl$_3$, pH 8.6. For apo-hTf-Sepharose, apply 1 column volume of 0.1 M Na acetate, 0.1 M Na phosphate, 25 mM EDTA, pH 5.5. In both cases, wash the resin with 5 column volumes of 50 mM Tris-HCl, 1 M NaCl, pH 8.0.

9. Regenerate hTf-Sepharose by washing with 2 column volumes of 50 mM Tris-HCl, 1 M NaCl, 10 mM EDTA, 0.05% Sarkosyl, 3 M guanidine HCl, pH 8.0, followed by 5 column volumes of 50 mM Tris-HCl, pH 8.0.

10. Store at 4°C and prevent dessication of the resin. Store for longer term in 50 mM Tris, 0.02% sodium azide, pH 8.0, at 4°C.

4. Notes

1. The first two steps for culturing the meningococci can be replaced by simply growing the isolates overnight in iron-limiting medium but may require optimization to ensure adequate growth (final OD$_{600}$ about 1).

2. The final washed affinity resin or the samples in SDS-PAGE sample buffer can safely be stored overnight at 4°C. Samples at earlier stages (cell pellets, culture supernatants, etc.) could also be stored at 4°C but may result in loss of receptor due to proteolysis and may require addition of protease inhibitors.

3. Although all procedures are preferably performed in the cold, successful purification has been attained with the chromatographic steps performed at room temperature.

4. Centrifugation of the solubilized membrane preparation prior to exposure to the affinity resin is not essential, but is advised to prolong the life of the affinity resin.

5. Although the procedure described here is in a column chromatography format, it is possible to perform part or all of the affinity procedure in batch form.

6. Alternate conditions for receptor isolation and immobilization on the affinity matrix have been described *(15)*, indicating that the affinity isolation procedure is quite robust. Although this has not been systematically evaluated, it appears that minimizing the duration and degree of denaturation during elution is critical. Thus rapidly reversing the elution buffer conditions is highly recommended if functional receptor protein is desired. The strategy of using low pH *(15)* for receptor elution, may be more amenable to optimizing production of functional protein.

7. The type of membrane used for this assay can vary, but in order to accommodate particulate receptor preparations a membrane with considerable porosity (i.e., 4.5 μM nitrocellulose) should be selected.

8. Once samples are applied to the membrane and dried, the Tf-binding activity is stable, even at room temperature, so that aliquots from cultures taken at various time points can be compared.

References

1. Gray-Owen, S. D. and Schryvers, A. B. (1996) Bacterial transferrin and lactoferrin receptors. *Trends Microbiol.* **4,** 185–191.
2. Irwin, S. W., Averill, N., Cheng, C. Y., and Schryvers, A. B. (1993) Preparation and analysis of isogenic mutants in the transferrin receptor protein genes, *tbp1* and *tbp2*, from *Neisseria meningitidis*. *Mol. Microbiol.* **8,** 1125–1133.
3. Cornelissen, C. N. and Sparling, P. F. (1994) Iron piracy: acquisition of transferrin-bound iron by bacterial pathogens. *Mol. Microbiol.* **14,** 843–850.
4. Buchanan, S. K., Smith, B. S., Venkatramani, L., et al. (1999) Crystal structure of the outer membrane active transporter FepA from *Escherichia coli*. *Nature Struct. Biol.* **6,** 56–63.
5. Ferguson, A. D., Hofmann, E., Coulton, J. W., Diederichs, K., and Welte, W. (1998) Siderophore-mediated iron transport: crystal structure of FhuA with bound lipopolysaccharide. *Science* **282,** 2215–2220.
6. Locher, K. P., Rees, B., Koebnik, R., et al. (1998) Transmembrane signaling across the ligand-gated FhuA receptor: Crystal structure of free and ferrichrome-bound states reveal allosteric changes. *Cell* **95,** 771–778.
7. Schryvers, A. B. and Lee, B. C. (1989) Comparative analysis of the transferrin and lactoferrin binding proteins in the family *Neisseriaceae*. *Can. J. Microbiol* **35,** 409–415.
8. Anderson, J. A., Sparling, P. F., and Cornelissen, C. N. (1994) Gonococcal transferrin-binding protein 2 facilitates but is not essential for transferrin utilization. *J. Bacteriol.* **176,** 3162–3170.

9. Retzer, M. D., Yu, R.-H., Zhang, Y., Gonzalez, G. C., and Schryvers, A. B. (1998) Discrimination between apo and iron-loaded forms of transferrin by transferrin binding protein B and its N-terminal subfragment. *Microb. Pathog.* **25**, 175–180.

10. Renauld-Mongénie, G., Latour, M., Poncet, D., Naville, S., and Quentin-Millet, M. J. (1998) Both the full-length and the N-terminal domain of the meningococcal transferrin-binding protein B discriminate between human iron-loaded and apo-transferrin. *FEMS Microbiol. Lett.* **169**, 171–177.

11. Retzer, M. D., Yu, R.-H., and Schryvers, A. B. (1999) Identification of sequences in human transferrin that bind to the bacterial receptor protein, transferrin-binding protein B. *Mol. Microbiol.* **32**, 111–121.

12. Lissolo, L., Dumas, P., Maitre, G., and Quentin-Millet, M. J. (1994) Preliminary biochemical characterization of transferrin binding proteins from *Neisseria meningitidis*, in *Pathobiology and Immunobiology of Neisseriaceae* (Conde-Glez, C. J., Morse, S., Rice, P., Sparling, F., and Calderon, E., eds.), proceedings of the VIII International Pathogenic Neisseria Conference. Instituto Nacional de Salud Vública, Morolos, México, pp 399–405.

13. Ala'Aldeen, D. A. A., Stevenson, P., Griffiths, E., et al. (1994) Immune responses in humans and animals to meningococcal transferrin-binding proteins: implications for vaccine design. *Infect. Immun.* **62(7)**, 2984–2990.

14. Gerlach, G. F., Anderson, C., Potter, A. A., Klashinsky, S., and Willson, P. J. (1992) Cloning and expression of a transferrin-binding protein from *Actinobacillus pleuropneumoniae. Infect. Immun.* **60**, 892–898.

15. Johnson, A. S., Gorringe, A. R., Fox, A. J., Borrow, R., and Robinson, A. (1997) Analysis of the human Ig isotype response to individual transferrin binding proteins A and B from *Neisseria meningitidis. FEMS Immunol. Med. Microbiol.* **19**, 159–167.

16. Rokbi, B., Mignon, M., Maitre-Wilmotte, G., Lissolo, L., Danve, B., Lougent, D. A., et al. (1997) Evaluation of recombinant transferrin binding protein B variants from *Neisseria meningitidis* for their ability of induce cross reactive and bactericidal antibodies against a genetically diverse collection of serogroup B strains. *Infect. Immun.* **65**, 55–63.

17. Cornelissen, C. N., Kelley, M., Hobbs, M. M., et al. (1998) The transferrin receptor expressed by gonococcal strain FA1090 is required for the experimental infection of human male volunteers. *Mol. Microbiol.* **27**, 611–616.

18. Danve, B., Lissolo, L., Mignon, M., et al. (1993) Transferrin-binding proteins isolated from *Neisseria meningitidis* elicit protective and bactericidal antibodies in laboratory animals. *Vaccine* **11**, 1214–1220.

19. Lissolo, L., Maitre-Wilmotte, G., Dumas, P., Mignon, M., Danve, B., and Quentin-Millet, M.-J. (1995) Evaluation of transferrin-binding protein 2 within the transferrin-binding protein complex as a potential antigen for future meningococcal vaccines. *Infect. Immun.* **63**, 884–890.

20. Rokbi, B., Mazarin, V., Maitre-Wilmotte, G., and Quentin-Millet, M. J. (1993) Identification of two major families of transferrin receptors among *Neisseria*

meningitidis strains based on antigenic and genomic features. *FEMS Microbiol. Lett.* **110,** 51–58.

21. Rokbi, B., Mignon, M., Caugant, D. A., Quentin-Millet, M. J. (1997) Heterogeneity of *tbpB,* the transferrin-binding protein B gene, among serogroup B from *Neisseria meningitidis* strains of the ET-5 complex. *Clin. Diagn. Lab. Immunol.* **4,** 522–529.

22. Danve, B., Lissolo, L., Guinet, F., Boutry, E., Speck, D., Cadoz, M., et al. (1998) Safety and immunogenicity of a *Neisseria meningitidis* group B transferrin binding protein vaccine in adults. Nassif, X., Quentin-Millet, M.-J., and Taha, M.-K. 53–53. Eleventh International Pathogenic Neisseria Conference. Abstracts of the Editions Médicales et Scientifiques, Paris, France.

23. Ala'Aldeen, D. A. A. and Borriello, S. P. (1996) The meningococcal transferrin-binding proteins 1 and 2 are both surface exposed and generate bactericidal antibodies capable of killing homologous and heterologous strains. *Vaccine* **14,** 49–53.

24. Webb, D. C. and Cripps, A. W. (1999) Immunization with recombinant transferrin binding protein B enhances clearance of nontypeable *Haemophilus influenzae* from the rat lung. *Infect. Immun.* **67,** 2138–2144.

25. Myers, L. E., Yang, Y.-P., Du, R.-P., et al. (1998) The transferrin binding protein B of *Moraxella catarrhalis* elicits bactericidal antibodies and is a potential vaccine antigen. *Infect. Immun.* **66,** 4183–4192.

26. Potter, A. A., Schryvers, A. B., Ogunnariwo, J. A., Lo, R. Y. C., and Watts, T. (1999) Protective capacity of *Pasteurella haemolytica* transferrin-binding proteins TbpA and TbpB in cattle. *Microb. Pathog.* **27,** 197–206.

27. Rossi-Campos, A., Anderson, C., Gerlach, G.-F., Klashinsky, S., Potter, A. A., and Willson, P. J. (1992) Immunization of pigs against *Actinobacillus pleuropneumoniae* with two recombinant protein preparations. *Vaccine* **10,** 512–518.

28. Schryvers, A. B. and Morris, L. J. (1988) Identification and characterization of the human lactoferrin-binding protein from *Neisseria meningitidis. Infect. Immun.* **56,** 1144–1149.

29. Schryvers, A. B. and Lee, B. C. (1993) Analysis of bacterial receptors for host iron binding proteins. *J. Microbiol. Methods* **18,** 255–266.

30. Ogunnariwo, J. A. and Schryvers, A. B. (1992) Correlation between the ability of *Haemophilus paragallinarum* to acquire ovotransferrin-bound iron and the expression of ovotransferrin-specific receptors. *Avian Dis.* **36,** 655–663.

31. Cornelissen, C. N., Biswas, G. D., and Sparling, P. F. (1993) Expression of gono-coccal transferrin-binding protein 1 causes *Escherichia coli* to bind human transferrin. *J. Bacteriol.* **175,** 2448–2450.

32. Palmer, H. M., Powell, N. B. L., Ala'Aldeen, D. A., Wilton, J., and Borriello, S. P. (1993) *Neisseria meningitidis* transferrin-binding protein 1 expressed in *Escherichia coli* is surface exposed and binds human transferrin. *FEMS Microbiol. Lett.* **110,** 139–146.

33. Gonzalez, G. C., Yu, R.-H., Rosteck, P., and Schryvers, A. B. (1995) Sequence, genetic analysis, and expression of *Actinobacillus pleuropneumoniae* transferrin receptor genes. *Microbiology* **141,** 2405–2416.

34. Ogunnariwo, J. A., Woo, T. K. W., Lo, R. Y. C., Gonzalez, G. C., and Schryvers, A. B. (1997) Characterization of the *Pasteurella haemolytica* transferrin receptor genes and the recombinant receptor proteins. *Microb. Pathog.* **23,** 273–284.

35. Legrain, M., Speck, D., and Jacobs, E. (1995) Production of lipidated meningococcal transferrin binding protein 2 in *Escherichia coli. Protein Exp. Purif.* **6,** 570–578.

36. Vonder Haar, R. A., Legrain, M., Kolbe, H. V. J., and Jacobs, E. (1994) Characterization of a highly structured domain in Tbp2 from *Neisseria meningitidis* involved in binding to human transferrin. *J. Bacteriol.* **176,** 6207–6213.

37. Renauld-Mongénie, G., Poncet, D., Von Olleschik-Elbheim, L., et al. (1997) Identification of human transferrin-binding sites within meningococcal transferrin-binding protein B. *J. Bacteriol.* **179,** 6400–6407.

38. Riggs, P. (1994) Expression and purification of maltose binding protein fusions, in *Current Protocols in Molecular Biology* (Ausubel, F. M., Brent, R., Kingston, R. E., et al., eds.), Wiley, New York, pp. 16-6-1–16-6-14.

39. Wilson, M. B. and Nakane, P. K. (1978) Recent developments in the periodate method of conjugating horseradish peroxidase (HRPO) to antibodies, in *Immunofluorescence and Related Staining Techniques* (Knapp, W., Holubar, K., and Wick, G., eds.), Elsevier/North Holland Biomedical Press, Amsterdam; pp. 215–224.

9

Methods for the Preparation and Crystallization of Fab Fragments in Complex with Peptide Antigens Derived from *N. meningitidis* Outer Membrane Proteins

Richard F. Collins and Jeremy P. Derrick

1. Introduction

An understanding of the molecular basis for the recognition of outer-membrane proteins (OMPs) by antibody is an important goal in the development of a more rational approach to vaccine design. X-ray crystallography has been outstandingly successful in delineating the detailed chemical interactions that are responsible for the high affinity and high selectivity of antibody-antigen interactions *(1)*. Although a number of X-ray structures of OMPs have now been reported (e.g., *2*), determination of the structure of a novel OMP is far from routine. Furthermore, it is more useful to know the structural basis for molecular recognition of a particular antigen by antibody than the structure of the cognate antigen alone. For this reason, work in this area has concentrated on studying the structures of antigen in complex with antibody Fab fragments. In practice, this requires the synthesis of a short peptide or oligosaccharide that binds to the antibody in question and then determination of the structure of the bound antigen by X-ray crystallography. Clearly, this has the limitation that only well-defined continuous epitopes can be studied in this way, but fortunately this is frequently the case with monoclonal antibodies (MAbs) that have been prepared against meningococcal OMPs. This type of approach has also been used to study the binding of the polysaccharide O-antigen from *Shigella flexneri (3)*, and in principle it could be applied to meningococcal polysaccharide antigens if suitable small oligosaccharides could be synthesised in milli-

From: *Methods in Molecular Medicine, vol. 66: Meningococcal Vaccines: Methods and Protocols*
Edited by: A. J. Pollard and M. C. J. Maiden © Humana Press Inc., Totowa, NJ

gram quantities. As always, the principal obstacle to the determination of an X-ray crystal structure is the preparation of crystals that diffract X-rays to a sufficiently high resolution. A number of technical advances have occurred in recent years that have made this easier and in this article we will describe how they can be applied to Fab-antigen crystallization. It should be emphasized, however, that some Fab-antigen complexes seem to exhaust all practicable attempts to generate suitable crystals and that the reasons for this are not always clear. The purpose of this article is to provide a practical guide to the preparation of Fab fragments from MAbs and the setting up of crystallization trials for Fab-antigen complexes.

2. Materials
2.1. Antibody Purification

1. Concentrated hybridoma cell-culture supernatant.
2. 10 mL column containing protein G coupled to Sepharose 4B (*see* **Note 1**).
3. Amicon 50 mL ultrafiltration cell (P-5121) with 43-mm YM30 ultrafiltration membrane (P-13722).
4. P1 peristaltic pump, UV-1 Optical Unit and REC 101 chart recorder (Amersham Pharmacia Biotech).
5. Column buffer: 50 mM sodium acetate/acetic acid, pH 5.5.
6. Elution buffer: 100 mM glycine pH 3.0.
7. Dialysis buffer: 50 mM sodium acetate pH 4.5.

2.2. Fab Preparation and Purification

1. 1 M DTT.
2. 0.5 M EDTA.
3. Papain (Sigma P-4762) at 1 mg/mL prepared freshly each experiment.
4. Mono S HR 10/10 or Mono Q HR 10/10 ion exchange columns (Amersham Pharmacia Biotech).
5. Buffers A and B (*see* **Table 1**).
6. Centricon 10 concentrator (Amicon No. 4205).
7. 10% (w/v) sodium azide.

2.3. Peptide Purification

1. N-acetylated peptide (produced commercially, 10 mg scale).
2. Solution A: High-purity water with 0.1% (v/v) trifluoroacetic acid (Romil H853).
3. Solution B: HPLC grade 99.93 + % acetonitrile (Sigma 27-071-7).
4. Genesis C18 4μ reverse-phase column with guard column (Jones chromatography 77112804 & 8P6975P).
5. 15-mL polypropylene tubes with lids.
6. Hewlett Packhard 1100 series high-performance liquid chromatography (HPLC).
7. 10% (w/v) sodium azide.

Table 1
Alternative Chromatographic Conditions for Purification of Murine IgG Monoclonal Fab Fragments (*see* Subheading 3.2.2.)

Column	Buffer A	Buffer B
Mono S HR 10/10[a]	50 mM sodium acetate/ acetic acid, pH 4.5	50 mM sodium acetate/ acetic acid, pH 4.5, plus 1 M NaCl
Mono Q HR 10/10	50 mM Tris-HCl, pH 8.0	50 mM Tris-HCl, pH 8.0, plus 1 M NaCl

[a]Columns are run on an FPLC System (Amersham Pharmacia Biotech) at a flow rate of 4 mL/min, using a linear gradient of 0% to 100% Buffer B over 10 column volumes.

2.4. Crystallization

1. Crystal screen (HR2-110, Hampton Research, Laguna Niguel, CA.
2. 22-mm glass coverslips No 1.5.
3. Dimethyldichlorosilane (BDH UN-2831).
4. 24-well tissue culture trays (Linbro No 76-033-05).
5. MS4 silicone compound grease (Dow Corning).
6. Leica Wild M3Z Stereo Zoom Microscope with transmission light stand.

3. Methods
3.1. Antibody Purification

The following methods for antibody purification and Fab production are based on our experience with murine MAbs. They may need to be adapted for antibodies from other sources.

1. Concentrate antibody cell-culture supernatants 12-fold at 4°C before freezing and storing at –80°C (*see* **Note 1**). Remove appropriate volumes (generally between 20 and 60 mL) for purification as required and thaw slowly at 25°C before placing on ice. Perform all antibody purification and dialysis steps in a 4°C cold room. Equilibrate a column of immobilized protein G-Sepharose 4 (10 mL) with three column volumes of column buffer (*see* **Note 2**).
2. Adjust the pH of the concentrated cell-culture supernatant to 5.5 using 0.5 M acetic acid and apply to the Protein G column at a flow rate of 2 mL/min (*see* **Note 3**). Monitor the absorption of the eluent at 280 nm continuously; the elution of unretained material can be followed from the large increase in absorbance. Continue pumping with column buffer until the absorption reading subsides to its baseline value.
3. Initiate elution of the antibody by application of elution buffer. This will be characterized by a second absorbance peak, much reduced in size compared

with the first, which may be collected manually or by using a fraction collector (*see* **Note 4**).

4. Concentrate pooled fractions containing purified MAb to 2 mg/mL (assume an absorbance coefficient of 70 mM^{-1}cm^{-1} at 280 nm) using an Amicon 50 mL capacity ultrafiltration cell fitted with a 43-mm YM30 ultrafiltration membrane at a pressure of 40 psi from a pressurized N_2 source (*see* **Note 5**).

3.2. Fab Preparation and Purification

3.2.1. Fab Preparation

1. Add DTT and EDTA to the MAb solution (giving final concentrations of 50 mM and 1 mM respectively; *see* **Note 6**) following dialysis. Add 7 μg of papain per mg of antibody and mix the solution well. Incubate the digest mixture at 37°C for 1.5–2.0 h (*see* **Note 7**).
2. Dialyse Fab digests against at least 2 L of Buffer A (*see* **Table 1**) for 2 h at 4°C to remove the DTT and EDTA.

3.2.2. Fab Purification

1. Purify Fab fragments from the digest mixture using ion-exchange chromatography. Chromatographic behavior will vary depending on the MAb sequence; details of two types of conditions that we have found successful previously are given in **Table 1**.
2. Separate Fab and Fc fragments over a linear NaCl gradient; elution conditions will vary depending on the type of antibody. Care should be taken to optimize the separation of different Fab isoforms and in some cases this may require alteration of the gradient program.
3. Dialyze the resulting purified Fab fragments at 4°C for 10 h against 2 L of a crystallization buffer, the composition of which will vary. Generally for initial crystallization trials, we recommend the use of a low ionic-strength buffer close to neutral pH, e.g., 20 mM Tris-HCl, pH 7.5.
4. Concentrate the solution of Fab fragments to 20–40 mg/mL using an Amicon 50-mL ultrafiltration cell with a 43 mm YM10 membrane. Alternatively, for final volumes of less than 1 mL, a Centricon-10 device may be used (*see* **Note 7**).
5. Prevent bacterial degradation by adding sodium azide to 0.05% (w/v) and store the Fab solution at 4°C. Sodium azide is toxic: gloves and a mask should be worn when weighing out the chemical.

3.3. Peptide Purification

1. Peptides are synthesized and obtained in a crude form from MWG- BIOTECH on a 10 mg scale, with N-acetylation. Dissolve each crude peptide powder containing 20–30 mg of peptide in 2 mL of H_2O and remove insoluble contaminants remaining from the synthesis by centrifugation in a benchtop centrifuge at 12,000 rpm for 5 min. Freeze-dry the frozen peptide solutions overnight.

2. Dissolve the lyophilized crude peptide in several mL of H_2O to give an approximate concentration of 5 mg/mL and purify the peptide using reverse-phase chromatography. Apply the sample to the column in water containing 0.1% (v/v) trifluoroacetic acid (TFA) (solution A) at a flow rate of 3 mL/min. TFA is corrosive and toxic: it should be handled with face and glove protection in a fume hood.

3. Elute the peptide by application of a linear gradient from solution A to 100% of solution B (acetonitrile) over 50 min at the same flow rate. Acetonitrile is toxic: a fume hood or extractor fan should be used to minimize exposure to the vapor. Gloves and face protection should be worn when handling this solvent. Detect peaks by absorbance at 214 nm (*see* **Note 8**).

4. Pool peak fractions containing the purified peptide, concentrate by lyophilization and make a 20 mM stock solution in water (containing 0.05% sodium azide w/v) for use in crystal trials. Sodium azide is toxic: it should be handled with gloves. A mask should be worn when weighing out the chemical. Verify the mass of the peptide by electrospray mass spectrometry.

3.4. Crystallization

3.4.1. Strategy and Identification of Initial Conditions

Initial crystallization conditions will vary depending on the Fab fragment and antigen. In order to rapidly identify the most promising conditions to pursue, sparse matrix screening methods are now commonly employed *(4)*. This involves screening the sample against a range of precipitants with different buffer compositions, pHs, and additives, which are available commercially in kit form. Sampling of a wide range of overlapping conditions permits the rapid identification of the most important components that contribute to crystallization. At this stage the crystals may be very small, but identification of even a microcrystalline precipitate can provide an important clue as to which conditions should be refined. The most convenient and widely used method for screening different crystallization conditions is the hanging-drop method *(5)*. A small volume of the protein sample is diluted 1:1 with precipitant solution and suspended over a reservoir of the same precipitant solution. Water is then slowly removed from the drop by a process of vapor diffusion, increasing the concentration of protein and precipitant within the drop over a period of several days. Trials are carried out using 24-well Linbro tissue-culture plates, which allow easy visualization of the drop using a low-magnification microscope (50×) and a transmitted light stand.

3.4.2. Crystal Preparation

1. Silanize the glass coverslips before use to reduce the contact area of the hanging drop. Place 50–100 coverslips in approx 50 mL of dimethyldichlorosilane and allow them to soak for several minutes. Remove the coverslips and wash several

times with ethanol to remove the dimethyldichlorosilane. Dry the slips in a 50°C oven for 4–6 h before use.

2. Freshly prepare a solution of Fab and peptide antigen by mixing the purified Fab from **Subheading 3.2.2.** with peptide from **Subheading 3.3.** in a molar ratio of 1:5 Fab:peptide. The final concentration of protein should between 20 and 40 mg/mL (*see* **Notes 9–11**).

3. Place 1 mL of precipitant solution in the well of a Linbro tissue-culture tray and cover the radius of the top of the well with a thin layer of vacuum grease. Application from a syringe allows neat and even coverage.

4. Mix appropriate volumes of Fab and peptide solutions together and place 0.8 µL of the mixed Fab:peptide solution in the center of a silanized coverslip. Add 0.8 µL of the well buffer to the protein solution and mix thoroughly by pipetting up and down at least 5 times.

5. Place the coverslip above the well on the ring of grease and with the drop facing downwards, seal the trial by gently pressing the coverslip down. Carry out initial trials in a constant temperature room or incubator at 20°C but results can sometimes be improved by repeating at other temperatures (and also *see* **Notes 12** and **13**).

4. Notes

1. Maintenance of the crude cell-culture supernatant at 4°C during antibody purification is important to reduce proteolysis and other post-translational modifications that can adversely effect the homogeneity of the Fab preparation. For the same reasons, repeated freeze-thaw cycles were also avoided.

2. We routinely prepare our own protein G-Sepharose, but it can be obtained commercially and will give very similar results.

3. The adhesion of some antibodies to the protein G column is improved by this adjustment to slightly acidic pH.

4. We find that some antibodies are not stable at the low pH values (~3.0) used to elute them from protein G columns, resulting in reduced recoveries. Under these circumstances, other elution strategies can be adopted, using higher ionic strength buffers at neutral pH for example.

5. After concentration, we typically find a yield of 1 mg of antibody per mL of concentrated cell-culture supernatant that was applied to the protein G column. The concentrated antibody, in volume of about 30–40 mL, is then dialyzed against 5 L of dialysis buffer for 2 h at 4°C.

6. Following the dialysis step some of the antibody preparation may precipitate: this can be removed by centrifugation at 15,000*g* for 10 min if necessary and does not usually represent a great loss of antibody.

7. These conditions are optimized for mouse IgG1 and IgG2a. These should be treated as guidelines only and we recommend that trials at different papain concentrations are conducted on a small scale first. The progress of cleavage of the 50,000 molecular-weight heavy chain into two approximately equal halves can be followed readily using standard 12.5% SDS-PAGE gels.

8. Most peptides elute between 15–30% solution B and synthesis impurities at concentrations greater than 40% solution B.
9. We typically obtain Fab yields of about 30% of theoretical from pure IgG.
10. For co-crystallization with Fab, optimal results are generally obtained with peptides of between 9 and 16 amino acids. We recommend conducting co-crystallization trials with several peptides of different lengths.
11. This is a suggested starting ratio; depending on the outcome of the initial trial, other ratios can be attempted between 1 : 1 to 1 : 20.
12. Initial conditions are refined by adjustment of precipitant concentration, buffer composition, and pH. In many cases the concentrations of precipitant used in the initial screen are too high and will generate "showers" of microcrystals. Under these circumstances, it is often useful to reduce the precipitant concentration and/or the protein concentration, to reduce the incidence of nucleation events. Micro- and macroseeding techniques have also been usefully employed in the crystallization of Fab-antigen complexes, as discussed by Wilson et al. *(6)*.
13. Another useful variant that can be introduced at this stage is Streptococcal protein G, which binds to the C_H1 domain on Fab. In the case of the MAb against the P1.7 serosubtype, addition of protein G was crucial to obtaining good-quality crystals of the Fab-antigen complex *(7,8)*.

Acknowledgment

This work was supported by a grant from the Wellcome Trust. JPD is a Fellow of the Lister Institute of Preventive Medicine.

References

1. Braden, B. C. and Poljak, R. J. (1995) Structural features of the reactions between antibodies and protein antigens. *FASEB J.* **9,** 9–16.
2. Buchanan, S. K., Smith, B. S., Ventatramani, L., Xia, D., Esser, L., Palnitkar, M., et al. (1999) Crystal structure of the outer membrane active transporter FepA from *Escherichia coli. Nature Struct. Biol.* **6,** 56–63.
3. Vyas, M. N., Vyas, N. K., Meikle, P. J., Sinnott, B., Pinto, B. M., Bundle, D. R., and Quiocho, F. A. (1993) Preliminary crystallographic analysis of a Fab specific for the O-antigen of *Shigella flexneri* cell surface lipopolysaccharide with and without bound saccharides. *J. Mol. Biol.* **231,** 133–136.
4. Jancarik, J. and Kim, S.-H. (1991) Spare matrix sampling: a screening method for crystallization of proteins. *J. Appl. Cryst.* **24,** 409–411.
5. McPherson, A. (1990) Current approaches to macromolecular crystallization. *Eur. J. Biochem.* **189,** 1–23.
6. Wilson, I. A., Rini, J. M., Fremont, D. H., Fieser, G. G., and Stura, E. A. (1991) X-Ray crystallographic analysis of free and antigen-complexed Fab fragments to investigate structural basis of immune recognition. *Methods Enzymol.* **203,** 153–176.
7. Derrick, J. P., Feavers, I., and Maiden, M. C. J. (1999) Use of streptococcal pro-

tein G in obtaining crystals of an antibody Fab fragment in complex with a meningococcal antigen. *Acta Cryst.* **D55,** 314–316.

8. Derrick, J. P., Maiden, M. C. J., and Feavers, I. (1999) Crystal structure of an Fab fragment in complex with a meningococcal serosubtype antigen and a protein G domain. *J. Mol. Biol.* **293,** 81–91.

10

Application of Optical Biosensor Techniques to the Characterization of PorA-Antibody Binding Kinetics

Janet Suker and Bambos M. Charalambous

1. Introduction

The design of novel vaccines and strategies to combat infectious disease requires an understanding of the interactions between pathogen and host. Biological interactions in vivo often rely on specific recognition mechanisms that begin with a binding step. The development of biosensor technology has allowed the real-time measurement of the binding characteristics of biomolecules and provides a powerful new tool for the analysis of molecular recognition. An optical biosensor comprises a detector linked to an optical transducer that generates a measurable signal from a biological interaction occurring at the detector surface. Evanescent optical biosensors have been available since the late 1980s, the most commonly known commercial systems being IAsys (which uses the resonant mirror sensor) *(1,2)* and BIAcore (which employs the optical phenomenon of surface plasmon resonance) *(3)*. There is a multitude of different applications of biosensor technology including measurement of concentration, kinetic analysis, structural studies, fermentation monitoring, receptor-cell interactions, and equilibrium analysis. The most widespread applications have been to protein-protein interactions, in particular receptor-ligand and antibody-antigen binding. More recent studies have been extended to protein-carbohydrate, DNA-DNA, and DNA-RNA interactions. Examples of the diverse uses of biosensors are found in the field of meningococcal research such as in the study of transferrin binding pro-

From: *Methods in Molecular Medicine, vol. 66: Meningococcal Vaccines: Methods and Protocols*
Edited by: A. J. Pollard and M. C. J. Maiden © Humana Press Inc., Totowa, NJ

teins *(4,5)*, lipo-oligosaccharide (LOS)-antibody interactions *(6)* and serum responses to experimental vaccines *(7)*.

This chapter outlines one specific application of the IAsys resonant mirror biosensor to study the binding kinetics of PorA-antibody interactions. The method describes how the IAsys technology can be used to obtain both qualitative and quantitative information about the effects of antigenic variation on PorA-antibody recognition and also highlights the benefits and pitfalls of the use of biosensors in immunology. Firstly, the principles behind the IAsys technique and a general outline of the method will be given and then background information for each of the major procedures in the method will be explained.

1.1. Principles of the IAsys Technique

The IAsys biosensor consists of a resonant mirror structure *(1)* at the base of a disposable cuvette within which the interaction in question is carried out. One of the interacting moieties (the ligand) is immobilized on to the cuvette surface and subsequent interaction with another molecule (the ligate) alters the physical characteristics at the surface. The resonant mirror structure consists of two dielectric layers on glass. A high refractive index waveguide is separated from a high refractive index glass prism by a low index coupling layer. Monochromatic light is scanned on to the device and at a particular angle, the resonant angle, some of this light energy passes from the prism, through the spacer layer, to propagate in the waveguide as an evanescent wave. The light returns via the coupling layer and is incident upon a detector. Changes in refractive index owing to interactions at the sensor surface alter the angle at which the light can be made to propagate in the waveguide. This is recorded as an arc second response that is related directly to the concentration of ligate. Furthermore, the response data can be fitted to an appropriate mathematical equation to derive 'on' and 'off' rates of ligate binding and dissociation and hence determine the strength of the interaction by calculation of equilibrium constants. This latter facility has led to kinetic interaction analysis becoming the most widespread application of biosensor technology, particularly in the field of immunology.

1.2. Kinetics Analysis Using a Biosensor

For general descriptions of the use of biosensors in immunology, the reader is directed to the reviews in references *(8)* and *(9)*. Traditional immunoassays such as enzyme-linked immunosorbent assay (ELISA) and radioimmunoassay (RIA) provide valuable information on antibody binding, but are time-consuming and have limitations such as that one of the reactants must be labeled and that the data obtained is from end-point measurements. Biosensors can overcome these restrictions and provide rapid measurements of real-time reaction kinetics. However, biosensor technology also has limitations because certain assumptions in the interpretation of response data may not be fulfilled in every case. For example, data fitting usually assumes a 1:1 stoichiometry but interactions between ligand and ligate may deviate from first-order reaction kinetics owing to re-binding, mass-transport effects, or multivalency of ligand or ligate. Different mathematical strategies can be employed to take into account these factors *(10)*, but the literature is inconsistent about the best interpretation of these data and many authors over-simplify or fail to state the model used.

In the study of antibody-binding kinetics it is important to distinguish between the 'affinity' or the 'avidity' of antibody-antigen interactions. The affinity of an antibody is the strength of binding of a monovalent ligand to a single antigen-binding site, whereas avidity (or 'functional affinity') refers to the overall strength of interaction between a complex antigen and a bi- or multivalent antibody. The strength of antibody (Ab)-antigen (Ag) interaction can be expressed as an equilibrium (or association) constant, K_A that is determined from the equation:

$$Ab + Ag \leftrightarrow Ab:Ag$$

and thus reflects the 'on' and 'off' rates of the interaction. The equilibrium constant may also be expressed as a dissociation constant (K_D). With small independent haptens binding is usually as rapid as diffusion allows, and the 'off' rates will determine differences in affinity constants. With larger haptens the interaction becomes more complex as the 'on' rate may vary as a consequence of diffusion rates. In the case of heterogeneous populations of antibodies or antigens, a combination of association constants will exist but an average equilibrium constant can be determined when 50% of the Ab:Ag complex is formed. Moreover, immunoglobulin molecules can interact via both their antigen binding sites with multiple epitopes that are present on the surface of bacterial pathogens. This increases the overall strength of binding, as both sites must be released simultaneously to dissociate. For example a decavalent IgM can have low-affinity binding sites but the avidity of the whole antibody to a bacterial surface displaying multiple identical epitopes can be very high. These considerations may make the interpretation of biosensor data more complex.

Another factor that complicates the interpretation of biosensor data is that the equations commonly used to calculate equilibrium constants assume that both binding partners are moving freely in solution. However, as the biosensor requires that the ligand is immobilized on the sensor surface, the design of experiments to measure true affinity constants must account for this, for example by using competition assays with free ligand *(11)*. It is therefore important that the limitations of biosensor technology are recognized and that caution is exercised in the interpretation of rate constants. Nevertheless, with the use of appropriate experimental design, biosensor data may be used to provide new insights into the mechanisms of molecular recognition.

1.3. Outline of the Method

In order to study antibody interactions with PorA proteins in their native conformation and to allow screening of multiple variants of PorA, this experiment is carried out with purified MAb immobilized at the biosensor surface to which outer-membrane vesicle (OMV) preparations are added. The interaction could be carried out with PorA immobilized at the surface and the antibody added as ligate but this may alter the structure of PorA and would require making a fresh cuvette for every variant to be studied.

First, purified monoclonal antibody (MAb) is bound to a dextran-coated cuvette then membrane-vesicle preparations from meningococcal strains encoding different PorA variants are added. The amount of PorA in each membrane preparation is normalized by sodium dodecyl sulfate-polyacrylamide gel electrophoresis (SDS-PAGE) densitometry and used to estimate the molar concentration of PorA protein in each preparation. The membrane vesicle suspensions are added to the biosensor cuvette and the interaction responses of different concentrations of PorA to the immobilized MAb are monitored. To show differences in the association rates and the amount of membrane vesicles bound to the immobilized MAb, the interaction profiles for each preparation of PorA at a single concentration are overlaid using the FASTplot software. This also illustrates whether or not a particular PorA variant is recognized by the MAb. The association and dissociation data at different concentrations of PorA are then collected and analyzed using the FASTfit software. From the FASTfit data, the apparent affinity constants of the different PorA-MAb interactions are calculated and reported as relative avidity.

1.4. Major Procedures Involved in the Protocol

1.4.1. Choice of Surface

The manufacturer (Labsystems Affinity Sensors) provides cuvettes with a choice of surfaces for immobilization of different ligands. If a large ligand is to be immobilized on to the cuvette surface, a thin coating matrix such as aminosilane is required to maintain the moiety within the evanescent-wave region. If a small protein ligand is used, it can be efficiently immobilized via its amino groups to a carboxymethyl-dextran surface using succinimide-ester chemistry. For nonprotein ligands, for example carbohydrates, the carbohydrate can be biotinylated and immobilized via a streptavidin bridge to a biotin-coated cuvette. In this application, the dextran surface is chosen for immobilization of antibody because: 1) the interacting ligate is the larger binding partner; 2) the chemistry of antibody immobilization to dextran is well-characterised; 3) the immobilized antibody is stable and binding activity is retained.

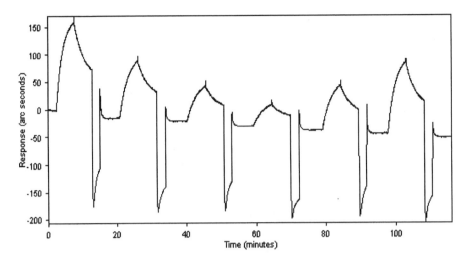

Fig. 1. Typical association and dissociation profiles at different ligate concentrations. Reproduced from IAsys tutorial software (Affinity Sensors).

1.4.2. Purification of OMVs Containing PorA and Estimation of PorA Molar Concentration

To ensure that the PorA proteins are as close as possible to their native conformation, ligate is prepared as OMVs. It is possible to carry out the interaction analysis with whole meningococcal cells and to determine which PorA variants bind to the MAb. However, for kinetic analysis, the relative concentration of PorA must be measured so that known concentrations of protein can be added to the cuvette for calculation of 'on' and 'off' rates. PorA preparations are made by a simple outer-membrane extraction procedure *(12)* and the presence of vesicles confirmed by electron microscopy (EM).

1.4.3. Interaction Analysis with MAb and Regeneration of the Sensor Surface

The cuvette coated with immobilized MAb is inserted into the IAsys instrument and aliquots of PorA vesicles are added manually. Data collection and experimental conditions are recorded using the IAsys software and the binding interaction is displayed as arc-second response plotted in real-time on the computer screen. Unbound ligate is diluted to zero concentration by washing and the dissociation is monitored in a similar manner. The surface is then regenerated before the next binding interaction by stripping any remaining bound ligate using a suitable buffer that maintains the integrity of the immobilized ligand. The cycle of binding–wash–dissociation–regeneration is repeated for different concentrations of ligate and the data is saved for analysis. **Figure 1** illustrates a typical set of data showing the association and dissociation profiles of six different ligate concentrations.

1.4.4. Data Analysis Using the FASTfit and FASTplot Software

FASTfit is a program designed to analyze, and display the data collected from the IAsys biosensor running the IAsys software. This program fits the captured digital data from the biosensor by least squares analysis to either monophasic or biphasic interaction kinetics and calculates 'on' and 'off' rates. Because immunoglobulin molecules have two identical binding sites, the binding data in this application is fitted to a biphasic curve, with the occupancy of the first binding site representing the first reaction rate. However, complications arise from measuring the interaction kinetics of membrane vesicles because particulate ligate may not be freely diffusable in the reaction and binding is likely to be multivalent. Consequently, the association and dissociation rates cannot be used to calculate true affinity constants, but comparisons can be made between the apparent avidity of the different PorA variants.

2. Materials

2.1. IAsys Biosensor Requirements

IAsys instrumentation and software is supplied by Labsystems Affinity Sensors (Saxon Way, Bar Hill, Cambridge, UK). Further information can be obtained from: iasys.support@thermobio.com or the website http://www.affinity-sensors.com

1. Manual, single-cell model of the IAsys resonant mirror biosensor. (Dual cuvettes and robotic systems are now available for more rapid screening of multiple samples).
2. Desk-top PC with minimum system requirements of a 486 processor with 66 MHz clock speed and 32 MB of RAM running Windows 95/8.
3. Instrument running and data collection software IAsys version 2.1.8.
4. IAsys help manuals: Methods Guide (basic principles and experimental design); Users Guide (use of the IAsys instrument) and FASTfit Guide (data analysis and software).

2.2. Immobilization of MAb to a Carboxymethyl Dextran (CM-Dextran) Surface

1. CM-Dextran cuvettes (Labsystems Affinity Sensors code FCD-0101). Cuvettes are stored at room temperature before immobilization of ligand.
2. NHS coupling kit containing: N-hydroxysuccinimide (NHS); 1-ethyl-3-(3-dimethylaminopropyl) carbodiimide (EDC) and 1 M ethanolamine, pH 8.5

(Labsystems Affinity Sensors). The EDC and NHS reagents are stored at –20°C and the ethanolamine at room temperature (stable for several months).

3. Purified MAb MN20F4.17 *(13)*. The MAb is available from National Institute for Biological Standards and Control (NIBSC) in the form of ascites fluid. It was purified by standard methods *(14)*: ammonium sulphate precipitation followed by affinity chromatography with protein G using a fast protein liquid chromatography (FPLC) system (Amersham Pharmacia Biotech).

4. Running buffer: Phosphate-buffered saline Tween (PBST): 138 mM sodium chloride, 2.7 mM potassium chloride, 4 mM sodium phosphate, 1.8 mM potassium phosphate, 0.05% (v/v) Tween 20.

5. Immobilization buffer: 10 mM sodium acetate, pH 4.3.

6. Regeneration buffer: 10 mM HCl.

Buffers 4, 5, and 6 are stored at room temperature and are stable for several weeks. During an experiment, the buffers are stored in the holder on top of the instrument to maintain them at the instrument running temperature.

Cuvettes with the immobilised antibody can be stored for several months at 4°C under PBST without significant deterioration. Prior to use, the cuvette must be equilibrated to the interaction temperature by placing it into the biosensor and washing once with regeneration buffer.

2.3. Purification of OMVs Containing PorA and Estimation of PorA Concentration

2.3.1. Meningococcal Strains

In this study NIBSC strains: 2151 (P1.5c,10); 2743 (P1.5c,10a); 2202 (P1.7d,10) and 2208 (P1.5c, VR2 deleted) were used. 2208 is a naturally occurring mutant containing an identical *porA* gene to the prototype P1.10 strain (2151) apart from an 87 base-pair deletion that entirely removes VR2. This was used as a negative control strain. Strains 2151, 2743, and 2202 contain different combinations of epitopes in VR1 and VR2.

2.3.2. Media and Buffers

1. 'Chocolate' agar plates: 10 % (v/v) horse blood, heated to 80°C in Blood Agar Base No. 2 (Oxoid, CM271).

2. Mueller Hinton broth (Oxoid, CM405).

3. TE buffer: 200 mM Tris-HCl/1 mM EDTA, pH 8.0.

4. TES buffer: 200 mM Tris-HCl/1 M sucrose, 1 mM EDTA.

5. Chicken egg-white lysozyme (1 mg/ml).

6. Bicinchoninic acid (BCA) protein assay kit (Pierce 23225).

7. Standard reagents and equipment for SDS-PAGE analysis *(15)*.

8. Gel-scanning software (for example LabWorks Analysis Software, Ultra Violet Products).

2.4. Interaction Analysis with MAb and Regeneration of the Biosensor Cuvette Surface

1. Prepared membrane vesicles and cuvette with immobilized ligand (*see* **Subheading 2.2.** and **2.3.**).
2. PBST wash buffer: 138 mM sodium chloride, 2.7 mM potassium chloride, 4 mM sodium phosphate, 1.8 mM potassium phosphate, 0.05 % (v/v) Tween 20.
3. Regeneration buffer: 10 mM HCl.

2.5. Data Analysis Using the FASTfit and FASTplot Software

1. FASTfit version 2.01 and FASTplot version 3.0 software for data plotting and analysis.
2. GraphPad PRISM® V2.01, (GraphPad Software Inc.) or other standard graphics packages can be used to determine the linear correlation of the 'on' rates (K_{ON}) with the estimated PorA concentration and to plot the data with their respective errors.
3. Computer file in *.RMD format containing experimental data.

3. Methods

3.1. IAsys Biosensor Analysis

Some prior knowledge is required before attempting the procedures outlined in this method (for example, the operator should be familiar with the contents of the IAsys manuals listed in **Subheading 2.1.**). Hence, where detailed instructions are provided in the IAsys guides, they are not repeated here. Where a wash step is indicated, this means three changes with 200 µL buffer.

3.2. Immobilization of MAb to a Carboxymethyl Dextran (CMD) Surface

1. Switch on the instrument, insert a fresh CMD biosensor cuvette and start the data collection software.
2. Start a new experiment, record the experimental details in the notebook and alter the data-collection parameters: temperature to 25°C and data collection to 5 s (*see* **Note 1**).
3. Wash with PBST and leave for 10–20 min to obtain a steady baseline. During this time, check the integrity of the cuvette surface by running a resonance scan to ensure that it is satisfactory prior to immobilization (*see* **Note 2**).
4. Immediately before use, mix equal volumes of the NHS and EDC solutions. Add 200 µL of the mixed NHS/EDC solution to the cuvette and leave for 7 min to activate the carboxyl groups on the CMD.
5. Wash with PBST and leave for 2 min.
6. Wash with immobilization buffer (10 mM sodium acetate, pH 4.3) and leave for 2 min.
7. Add 200 µL purified MAb MN20F4.17 at 50 µg/ml in 10 mM sodium acetate, pH 4.3, to the cuvette and leave for 10 min to allow electrostatic uptake to occur (*see* **Note 3**).

8. Remove any free MAb by washing with PBST and leave for 2 min.
9. Replace the PBST with 200 μL ethanolamine at pH 8.5 and leave for 3 min.
10. Wash with regeneration buffer and leave for 2 min (*see* **Note 4**).
11. Wash with PBST and leave for 5 min.
12. Stop the experiment and save as a *.RMD file.
13. Proceed to interaction with antibody (**Subheading 3.4.**) or remove the cuvet (still containing PBST) wrap it in parafilm and store at 4°C. Coated cuvets can be stored at 4°C for several weeks provided that the surface is not allowed to dry out.

3.3. Purification of OMVs Containing PorA and Estimation of PorA Concentration

Appropriate safety precautions should be taken when handling live meningococci. Steps involving live meningococcal cells should be carried out in a class II safety cabinet (including centrifugation of broth culture).

1. Streak out the required strains on chocolate agar plates and incubate overnight at 37°C in a 5% CO_2 atmosphere.
2. Inoculate 5 mL of Mueller-Hinton broth with a large colony from the overnight growth and incubate the broth cultures at 37°C until OD_{600} ~0.6 (approx 6 h).
3. Harvest 4 mL of each culture and either freeze the pellets overnight or continue to **step 4**.
4. Resuspend cell pellets from 4 mL broth culture in 200 μL TE buffer.
5. Add 200 μL ice-cold TES buffer and mix by inversion.
6. Add 24 μL 1 mg mL^{-1} lysozyme and mix.
7. Add 400 μL sterile distilled water.
8. Shake the mixture on a shaker for 30 min.
9. Sediment the spheroplasts at 40,000g for 20 min.
10. Resuspend spheroplasts in 800 μL ice-cold distilled water (using a needle and syringe to aid resuspension).
11. Sediment the membrane fragments at 40,000g for 20 min.
12. Resuspend the membranes in 500 μL PBS/T water. The preparation can be frozen at –20°C for several months.
13. Before interaction analysis, the membrane preparations should be brought to room temperature and mixed well.
14. Estimate the total protein concentrations of the prepared membranes using the microtiter plate protocol included in the BCA assay kit (or other protein assay).
15. Run approx 20 μg total protein for each vesicle preparation on a 12% SDS-PAGE gel, according to standard procedures (*15*).
16. Scan the gel and integrate the peaks to estimate the percentage protein in each PorA band (Mr approx 44,000). The principles of densitometry on stained bands on an SDS protein gel are described in (*16*).
17. Calculate the total amount of PorA in each vesicle preparation.

3.4. Interaction Analysis with MAb and Regeneration of the Sensor Surface

1. If the cuvette has been stored at 4°C, allow it to warm up slightly before inserting it into the IAsys equipment (to avoid condensation forming on the cuvette, which will interfere with detection).
2. Switch on the data-collection software, start a new experiment and adjust data-collection rate to 5 s (*see* **Note 1**).
3. Wash with PBST and follow the response until a steady baseline is obtained (usually 30–40 min). Check the resonance scan again during this time (*see* **Note 2**).
4. While waiting for the baseline to stabilize, make up a range of dilutions of membrane preparations in PBST. For this method, the range of PorA concentrations to use is from 10 nM to 5000 nM for each strain (*see* **Note 5**).
5. When the baseline is steady, stop the experiment and start a new one, record experimental details in the notebook, set data collection to 0.3 s, and save as a new *.RMD file (NB: save data frequently during an experiment).
6. Wash with PBST and leave for 5–10 min.
7. Add 200 µL of the first dilution of vesicles.
8. Follow the binding for 10 min (*see* **Note 6**).
9. Wash unbound membranes with PBST.
10. Follow dissociation for 5 min.
11. Wash twice with regeneration buffer and leave for 2 min.
12. Wash with PBST for 2–5 min (*see* **Note 7**).
13. Repeat **steps 7–12** for 5–10 different concentrations of each PorA variant (*see* **Note 5**).
14. Stop the experiment and save the data to *.RMD file (*see* **Note 8**).

3.5. Data Analysis Using the FASTplot and FASTfit Software

3.5.1. Data Presentation Using FASTplot

The interaction profiles of the same concentration of different PorA variants with the immobilized P1.10 MAb are captured from the IAsys file of the experiment (*.RMD) and overlaid on to the same graph.

1. Open FASTplot and import the experimental data from the *.RMD file.
2. Manually define the baseline and binding interaction regions for each interaction to be displayed. A zoom function is available to allow the interaction profiles to be seen more clearly.
3. Set the coincidence time to specify the exact time of the binding phase (zero time-point for all curves to be overlaid).
4. Transfer the selected regions to the plot.
5. Repeat **steps 2–4** for the different PorA subtypes.
6. Add a title to the overlay plot and annotate the curve by using the plot properties dialog box (*see* **Fig. 2**).

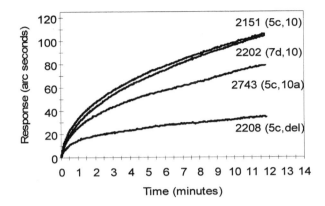

Fig. 2. Overlay plots of the interaction profiles of membrane preparations of differ-ent PorA subtypes with the P.10 specific MAb, MN20F4.17. The concentration of PorA is 100 nM for all the interaction profiles displayed. A single amino acid substitu-tion present (R→P) in the VR2 domain of subtype 10a compared to 10 appeared to reduce the binding interaction of the mAb. In contrast, differences in the VR1 of strains 2151 and 2202 did not appear to alter the interaction profile of the MAb, suggesting that the interaction is VR2 specific. Figures are the strain number and figures in brack-ets are the PorA subtype.

3.5.2. Kinetics Analysis Using FASTfit

Data must be fitted in turn for each concentration of membrane vesicles added to the biosensor cuvette. A zoom function is available to enlarge the region of interest.

1. Open FASTfit and load the data file (*.RMD) generated by the IAsys software.
2. Correct the baseline drift if present.
3. Set the start marker of the first association data region at the point of addition of the membrane vesicles to the cuvette.
4. Set the start marker of the first dissociation region at the point of evacuating and filling the cuvette with wash buffer (dilution to zero concentration).
5. Specify the analysis regions for the baseline, association, and dissociation of the first interaction profile using the color-coded range selectors. Set the baseline range selec-tor for approx 1 min of data before the association starts. Set the beginning of the association data range 5 s after the start of the association start marker (*see* **Note 9**) and the end of the association range for 10s from that point. Set the dissociation range for 5 min of data starting just after the dissociation start marker.
6. Choose the analysis required (*see* **Note 10**) and fit the data.
7. Record the association rates (k_{ON}) and dissociation rates (k_{OFF}) with their error values, and whether the data is fitted best to a monophasic or biphasic exponen-tial (*see* **Note 10**). Also record the R_{max} value.

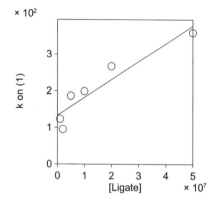
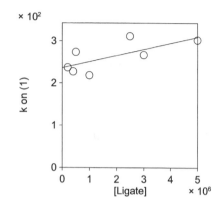

Fig. 3. The 'on' rates of two meningococcal PorA variants interacting with the immobilized MAb MN20F4.17. K_{ON} rates for the monophasic binding of meningo-coccal-membrane vesicles containing two PorA variants; left panel is P1.10, the right panel is P1.10a. The 'on' rates are fitted by least squares and the slope is the associa-tion constant (k_{ass}). However, because of the particulate nature of the ligate, these are only relative measurements and should not be considered as true rate constants. The P1.10 PorA variant has approx 60-fold greater relative avidity for MAb MN20F4.17 than the P1.10a variant.

8. Repeat **steps 5–7** using total association data ranges of 25s, 50s, 100s, 300s, and 600s and record the association rates (k_{ON}) with their error value for each data range (keep the dissociation range to 5 min).
9. Repeat **steps 3–8** for each interaction profile and for each different ligate.
10. Plot the association rate (k_{ON}) for each PorA concentration and perform a linear correlation on the data points (*see* **Note 11** for values to be excluded from this plot). The gradient of this line is the association rate constant (k_{ass}) (*see* **Fig. 3**).
11. The dissociation rate constant (k_{diss}) is calculated from the mean and standard deviation of the dissociation rates obtained from PorA concentrations from 200 nM to 5000 nM and should be close to the value of the intercept of the plot of k_{ON} versus ligate concentration (*see* **Note 12**).
12. The dissociation equilibrium constants of the different PorA proteins are calcu-lated from the ratio of k_{diss}/k_{ass} (*see* **Note 12**).

4. Notes

1. During the association and dissociation stages the data should be collected as rapidly as possible (0.3 s intervals). Conversely, during the buffer or reagent incubations or ligand immobilization, the data-collection rate should be decreased to 5 s intervals. It is also important to save data files frequently during the experi-mental runs.
2. The resonance scan before immobilization and between bindings should show a single symmetrical peak indicating homogeneous coating of the surface. If the

scan is atypical at this stage, it may indicate a faulty cuvette and a fresh cuvette should be tested. The resonance scan can be checked at any stage during an experiment. However, the shape of the peak may change during binding and asymmetrical scans obtained during an experiment should recover after washing.

3. For efficient immobilization of the ligand, the pH and buffer conditions are optimized to obtain maximum interaction with the surface prior to coupling. The optimum pH for the immobilization buffer will vary depending on the pI of the biomolecule to be immobilized. This must be determined empirically by measuring the arc second response due to electrostatic interaction of the ligand in buffers of different pH.

4. The regeneration conditions must preserve ligate-binding activity and must be optimized for specific applications.

5. The ideal concentrations of ligate to use for calculations of equilibrium constants are from $10 \times K_D$ to $0.01 \times K_D$. However, in most cases, the K_D is not known in advance so the appropriate range of concentrations to use must be determined empirically. Dilutions can be made either by adding an appropriate amount of a concentrated stock solution to the correct amount of buffer in the cuvette or by making up the dilutions in advance and adding 200 µL of the pre-diluted solution to the cuvette. It is preferable to add the different dilutions of ligate in a random order and to repeat the first dilution again at the end of an experiment. This allows verification of the reproducibility of the cuvette surface.

6. The interaction data should be collected until binding is approaching saturation, i.e., when the interaction profiles are observed to be entering the plateau phase. The data can be analyzed in the FASTfit program while an experiment is running to check the progress of binding.

7. Allow at least 1–2 min for baseline between each interaction to facilitate setting data ranges within FASTfit.

8. It is possible to merge data from different data files during FASTfit analysis and it is a good idea to include data points repeated on different days.

9. Data for analysis by FAStfit is not captured immediately after the addition of membrane vesicles to the cuvette as changes in bulk refractive index give a biosensor response. Also data should not be captured and analyzed when the interaction profile begins to plateau. At this point the immobilized MAb is reaching saturation with the PorA antigen, which results in a reduction of the association rate.

10. The first stage is to decide whether the data is fitted best to a single exponential (monophasic) or a biphasic exponential. Most reactions, whether mono- or biphasic, can be fitted to a biphasic exponential because reaction velocities decrease with time as the reaction becomes limited by reactant depletion or product accumulation. The limiting factor in this experiment is the saturation of the MAb immobilized on the surface of the biosensor cuvette. Consequently, the data to be included for the calculation of the association rate constant should be from the early part of the binding-interaction profile, which is best fitted by a monophasic exponential.

The fit for the association data from the longest time periods (up to 600 s) will be poor initially because the software will be attempting to best fit the data to a monophasic exponential. At these time-points, the ligand is approaching the saturation of the immobilized MAb and consequently the binding kinetics are biphasic. The range of data to analyze at each concentration of ligate will depend on the association or dissociation rates. The object is to reduce the data range to be analyzed until good single-phase fits are obtained with small errors. This will become evident, as the errors will decrease dramatically as the range of data selected becomes monophasic. Several different ranges are selected and a record made of the rate constants and errors. You will find that as you decrease the data range the rate constant will increase without significant increases in error. If you continue to decrease the data range, the errors will increase and the rate constant becomes erratic.

Alternatively, the data can be fitted to a biphasic exponential and the software will determine the initial (k_{ON1}) and subsequent (k_{ON2}) rate constants. However, in our experience the more accurate method is to reduce the time period over which the data is captured so that it is best fitted by a monophasic exponential.

11. The plot of k_{ON} values against the PorA concentration to derive the association rate constant (k_{ass}) should not include concentrations of PorA that are approaching the saturation of the binding sites of the immobilized MAb. This will result in reduced association rates that deviate from linearity.

12. The affinity of a molecular interaction may be expressed as a K_D (dissociation equilibrium constant), which is the reciprocal of the association equilibrium (K_A) or affinity constant. The k_{diss} can be derived from the direct measurement of dissociation data ($k_{diss} = k_{OFF}$), or from the intercept of the plot of K_{ON} vs PorA concentration. However, as the k_{diss} approaches zero (slow off rates) the less accurate the value derived from the intercept of the k_{ON} vs ligate concentration becomes, and experimentally derived data is preferred. An approximate K_D can also be obtained from a plot of the total extent of binding vs ligate concentration and is used to confirm the values obtained.

Acknowledgment

The authors would like to thank Tim Kinning of Labsystems Affinity Sensors for critical reading of the manuscript.

References

1. Cush, R., Cronin, J. M., Stewart, W. J., Maule, C. H., Molloy, J., and Goddard, N. J. (1993) The resonant mirror: a novel optical biosensor for direct sensing of biomolecular interactions. Part 1: Principle of operation and associated instrumentation. *Biosensors Bioelectron.* **8,** 347–353.
2. Lowe, P. A., Clark, T. J., Davies, R. J., Edwards, P. R., Kinning, T., and Yeung, D. (1998) New approaches for the analysis of molecular recognition using the IAsys evanescent wave biosensor. *J. Mol. Recog.* **11,** 194–199.

3. Jonsson, U., Fagerstam, L., Ivarsson, B., Johnsson, B., Karlsson, R., Lundh, K., et al. (1991) Real-time biospecific interaction analysis using surface plasmon resonance and a sensor chip technology. *Biotechniques* **11**, 620–627.
4. Boulton, I. C., Gorringe, A. R., Gorinsky, B., Retzer, M. D., Schryvers, A. B., Joannou, C. L., and Evans, R. W. (1999) Purified meningococcal transferrin-binding protein B interacts with a secondary, strain-specific, binding site in the N-terminal lobe of human transferrin. *Biochem. J.* **339(1)**, 143–149.
5. Renauld-Mongenie, G., Latour, M., Poncet, D., Naville, S., and Quentin-Millet, M. J. (1998) Both the full-length and the N-terminal domain of the meningococcal transferrin-binding protein B discriminate between human iron-loaded and apo-transferrin. *FEMS Microbiol. Lett.* **169**, 171–177.
6. Charalambous, B. M., Evans, J., Feavers, I. M., and Maiden, M. C. (1999) Comparative analysis of two meningococcal immunotyping monoclonal antibodies by resonant mirror biosensor and antibody gene sequencing. *Clin. Diagn. Lab Immunol.* **6**, 838–843.
7. Christodoulides, M., Brooks, J. L., Rattue, E., and Heckels, J. E. (1998) Immunization with recombinant class 1 outer-membrane protein from *Neisseria meningitidis*: influence of liposomes and adjuvants on antibody avidity, recognition of native protein and the induction of a bactericidal immune response against meningococci. *Microbiology* **144(11)**, 3027–3037.
8. Pathak, S. S. and Savelkoul, H. F. (1997) Biosensors in immunology: the story so far. *Immunol. Today* **18**, 464–467.
9. Morgan, C. L., Newman, D. J., and Price, C. P. (1996) Immunosensors: technology and opportunities in laboratory medicine. *Clin. Chem.* **42(2)**, 193–209.
10. Saunal, H., Karlsson, R., and Van Regenmortel, M. H. V. (1997) Antibody affinity measurements, in *Immunochemistry 2* (Johnstone, A. P. and Turner, M. W., eds.), Oxford University Press, Oxford, pp. 1–30.
11. Nieba, L., Krebber, A., and Pluckthun, A. (1996) Competition BIAcore for measuring true affinities: large differences from values determined from binding kinetics. *Anal. Biochem.* **234**, 155–165.
12. Witholt, B., Boekhout, M., Brock, M., Kingma, J., van Heerikhuizen, H., and de Leij, L. (1976) An efficient and reproducible procedure for the formation of spheroplasts from variously grown *Escherichia coli. Anal. Biochem.* **74**, 160–170.
13. Poolman, J. T., Kriz Kuzemenska, P., Ashton, F., Bibb, W., Dankert, J., Demina, A., et al. (1995) Serotypes and subtypes of *Neisseria meningitidis*: results of an international study comparing sensitivities and specificities of monoclonal antibodies. *Clin. Diagn. Lab. Immunol.* **2**, 69–72.
14. Harlow, E. and Lane, D. (1988) *Antibodies: A Laboratory Manual.* Cold Spring Harbor Laboratory Press, Cold Spring Harbor, NY.
15. Laemmli, U. K. (1970) Cleavage of structural proteins during the assembly of the head of bacteriophage T4. *Nature* **227**, 680–685.
16. Hames, B. D. and Rickwood, D. (eds.) (1998) *Gel Electrophoresis of Proteins a Practical Approach* Oxford University Press, Oxford.

11

Construction of *porA* Mutants

Peter van der Ley and Loek van Alphen

1. Introduction

The PorA or class 1 protein is one of the major meningococcal outer-membrane proteins (OMPs). It is one of the two porins found in this organism, the other one being the PorB or class 2/3 protein. It folds into a 16-stranded β-barrel structure, which is now well-established for bacterial porins, in which seven loops are exposed at the cell surface and the remaining one forms the constriction of the pore *(1,2)*. There are approx 20 different serosubtypes of PorA *(3)*, based on sequence variability in the longest surface-exposed loops 1 and 4 (*see* **Fig. 1**). In addition, minor sequence variations within individual subtypes have been observed. As a result, some subtypes such as P1.10 actually constitute a family of variants differing by single amino acid substitutions, which may affect antibody recognition; for other subtypes such as P1.4 the number of variants is more limited *(4,5)*. Several studies with experimental outer membrane-derived vaccines have shown that PorA is a major inducer of bactericidal antibodies *(6–8)*, making it a crucial component of any meningococcal vaccine. These antibodies are highly subtype-specific. Epidemic strains tend to be clonal and mainly express a single PorA subtype that changes only slowly over time *(9)*. In hyperendemic situations, more variation is found but it is generally still possible to select a limited number of PorA subtypes that will cover most of the strains *(10)*. However, PorA variation in both time and geography means that it is unlikely that a universal once-and-for-all meningococcal vaccine based on this protein alone can ever be made. This necessitates the use of vaccine strains with flexible PorA composition, in which new variants can be inserted into established production strains when required by new epidemiological circumstances. This chapter will describe methods to construct

From: *Methods in Molecular Medicine, vol. 66: Meningococcal Vaccines: Methods and Protocols*
Edited by: A. J. Pollard and M. C. J. Maiden © Humana Press Inc., Totowa, NJ

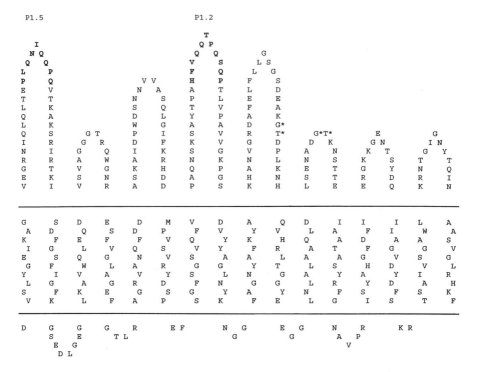

Fig. 1. Topology model for PorA protein. Residues shown in boldface represent the surface-exposed P1.5 and P1.2 epitopes in loop 1 and 4. Residues marked with an asterisk represent the points of insertion into the *KpnI* site in loop 5 or 6.

isogenic meningococcal strains with altered *porA* genes, which can be used both for vaccine production and as test strains to determine the precise epitope specificity of bactericidal antibodies directed against the various loops of PorA.

2. Materials

2.1. Cultivation of Meningococci

1. GC agar base (Difco) supplemented with 1% IsoVitaleX (Becton Dickinson).
2. Meningococcal medium (MM): to 1000 mL of dH_2O add 1.3 g glutamic acid, 0.02 g cysteine, 2.5 g $Na_2HPO_4.2H_2O$, 0.09 g KCl, 6.0 g NaCl, 1.25 g NH_4Cl, 0.6 g $MgSO_4.7H_2O$, 5.0 g glucose, 2.0 g yeast extract. Dissolve, adjust pH to 7.8, and sterilize by 0.2-μm filtration.

2.2. Colony Blot

1. Protran BA 85 nitrocellulose filters, 82-mm diameter and 0.45-μm pore size (Schleicher & Schuell).

2. Phosphate-buffered saline (PBS) (0.9% NaCl in 10 mM sodiumphosphate buffer, pH 7.2) with 0.1% Tween 80.
3. Casein hydrolysate (ICN biochemicals).
4. Monoclonal antibodies (MAbs): subtype-specific MAbs used for the constructions described here are MN14C11.6 (P1.7), MN5C11G (P1.16), MN22A9.19 (P1.5), MN16C13F4 (P1.2); these are available from NIBSC (Potters Bar, UK).
5. Protein A conjugated to horseradish peroxidase.
6. TMB/DONS substrate solution. A: mix 0.02 M Na_2HPO_4 and 0.01 M citric acid 1:1, and adjust to pH 5.5 by adding extra of either solution. B: dissolve 24 mg tetramethylbenzidine and 80 mg dioctylsulfosuccinate in 10 mL 96% ethanol. Mix 30 mL of A with 10 mL of B and add 20 µL of 30% H_2O_2; use immediately.

3. Methods

3.1. porA Gene Replacement

Neisseria meningitidis is naturally competent for DNA uptake (*see* **Note 1**), and the frequency of transformation can be high enough to directly select *porA* transformants in a colony-blot procedure as described below. This method is based on the introduction of a new subtype epitope into the recipient strain. We have used it to construct a set of isogenic derivatives from strain H44/76, each one expressing a different PorA subtype present in a hexavalent outer-membrane vesicle (OMV) vaccine.

1. Grow the bacteria overnight at 37°C in a humid atmosphere with 5% CO_2, on GC agar plates with 1% IsoVitaleX. Resuspend bacteria with cotton swabs in MM + 10 mM $MgCl_2$, to an optical density (OD) at 600 nm in the range 0.2–0.5.
2. To 2.0 mL of bacterial suspension, add DNA to a final concentration of 1 µg/mL or higher (*see* **Note 2**).
3. After incubation at 37°C for 1–3 h, prepare 10^{-3}, 10^{-4}, and 10^{-5} dilutions in PBS (*see* **Note 3**). Plate 4× 0.25 mL of each dilution and incubate overnight at 37°C.
4. Place a sterile nitrocellulose filter with its grid pattern on the agar surface, wait until it has become completely wet, and then carefully remove it without disturbing the colony pattern. Plates and filters should be marked for later orientation. Transfer the filters to PBS + 0.1% Tween 80, and inactivate at 56°C for 1 h with gentle shaking. Return the plates to the 37°C incubator for at least 6 h in order to regenerate the colonies.
5. Wash the filters 2 times in fresh PBS + 0.1% Tween 80 at room temperature (*see* **Note 4**).
6. Incubate for 30 min in blocking solution PBS + 0.1% Tween 80 + 0.3% casein. This and all following incubation steps should be done at room temperature and with shaking.
7. Incubate for 1 h in PBS + 0.1% Tween 80 + 0.3% casein containing an appropriate dilution of MAb directed against the incoming PorA subtype.

8. Wash 3 × 10 min with PBS + 0.1% Tween 80.
9. Incubate for 1 h in PBS + 0.1% Tween 80 + 0.3% casein containing an appropriate dilution of protein A × peroxidase conjugate.
10. Wash 3 × 10 min with PBS + 0.1% Tween 80, and 1× briefly in water.
11. Place the filters in TMB/DONS substrate solution, and incubate (without shaking) for several minutes until some green colonies become visible. Wash the filters with water to stop the color reaction.
12. Identify the positive colonies on the regenerated plates using the grid pattern, pick them up, and streak out on fresh plates.
13. Repeat the colony blot (**steps 4–11**) on putative transformants until no more negative colonies of the untransformed parent strain are present.

The method described previously has some limitations. First, it requires that a MAb specific for the *porA* gene used in the transformation is available, as negative selection is not feasible. Second, although in our experience it works very well for strain H44/76, for other strains with lower transformation efficiency, it can become very cumbersome. In such cases, an alternative is the use of plasmid pCO14K in combination with selection for kanamycin resistance. This plasmid contains the complete *porA* gene of strain 2996 (subtype P1.5,2), with the *kanR* gene inserted into the *XhoI* site located ca. 0.6 kb downstream of *porA* (*see* **Fig. 2**). Another *porA* subtype can easily be inserted into pCO14K by replacing the 0.75 kb *EclXI-KpnI* fragment with the corresponding part derived from another strain, encoding the N-terminal ca. 250 amino acids including loops 1–5. Transformation with *SphI*-linearized pCO14K and selection for kanamycin resistance will result in *porA* exchange in approx 5% of the transformants. Replacement of the entire *porA* gene of strain H44/76 can be verified by loss of reaction in colony blot with P1.7 and P1.16 specific MAbs MN14C11.6 and MN5C11G recognizing VR1 and VR2 (loops 1 and 4), respectively. If required, previous digestion with EcoRI will ensure that only VR2 can be exchanged (*see* **Fig. 2**). The expression of the newly constructed PorA protein can be monitored on Western blot using MAb MN23G2.38 which recognizes a conserved sequence located in loop 3. In this way, even *porA* genes that are not recognized by any of the available subtype-specific antibodies can be used.

1. Grow the bacteria overnight at 37°C in a humid atmosphere with 5% CO_2, on GC agar plates with 1% IsoVitaleX. Resuspend bacteria with cotton swabs in MM + 10 mM $MgCl_2$, to an OD at 600 nm in the range 0.2–0.5.
2. To 2.0 mL of bacterial suspension, add DNA to a final concentration of 1 µg/mL or higher (*see* **Note 2**). Include a negative control without DNA.
3. After incubation at 37°C for 1–3 h, plate 4 × 0.25 mL on GC agar plates with 1% IsoVitaleX and 100 µg/ml kanamycin, and incubate overnight at 37°C. Restreak

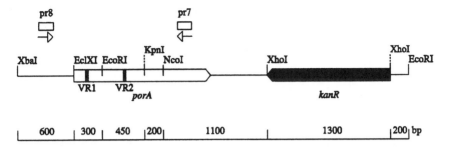

Fig. 2. Restriction map of the insert in plasmid pCO14K, carrying the *porA* gene from strain 2996 and a downstream *kanR* marker. The pTZ19R vector backbone is not shown.

kanamycin-resistant colonies on selective plates. Spontaneous kanamycin-resistant mutants can also occur, but generally at a much lower frequency and after longer incubation compared to transformants.

4. Verify expression of the desired combination of PorA epitopes in a colony blot as described earlier.

3.2. Insertions in PorA Surface Loops

We have used the more conserved loops 5 and 6 of PorA for the insertion of additional sequences up to 26 amino acid residues *(11)*. The additional epitopes were accessible at the cell surface and did not interfere with PorA expression. In frame insertions were made into the unique *KpnI* site of plasmid pCO20 located in loop 5 of PorA, and into the *KpnI* site of plasmid pPH204 specifically created in loop 6 instead of 5 (*see* **Fig. 1** for the insertion points). Upon induction with IPTG, *Escherichia coli* carrying these plasmids will produce a LacZ-PorA fusion protein, which can be used to monitor binding of antibodies to the inserted epitope in a Western blot, thus verifying its correct insertion. When transforming back into meningococci, selection can be for the newly inserted epitope or for the epitope present in loop 4, as the short distance separating these regions will ensure efficient co-transformation. In this way, multivalent PorA proteins carrying additional P1.7, P1.16, P1.4, or P1.9 epitopes in loop 5 or 6 have been constructed. In all cases, the new epitopes could be detected in whole-cell enzyme-linked immunosorbent assay (ELISA).

1. Ligate a double-stranded, nonphosphorylated oligonucleotide with *KpnI*-compatible sticky ends in a 30-fold molar excess to *KpnI*-digested plasmid pCO20 or pPH204. After ligation, digest again with *KpnI* in order to linearize plasmid molecules without an insert. As linear DNA is far less efficient in transforming *E. coli*, this will enrich for the right constructs.

2. Isolate plasmid DNA from the ampicillin-resistant *E. coli* transformants, and use *KpnI* digestion to check for oligonucleotide insertion.

3. Induce the *E. coli* transformants by growing them in the presence of 1 mM IPTG, and test cell lysates by sodium dodecyl sulfate-polyacrylamide gel electrophoresis (SDS-PAGE) and Western blotting for the presence of a LacZ-PorA fusion protein reactive with P1.2 MAb MN16C13F4 and with antibody specific for the inserted epitope. Pellet the cells from a culture with OD at 600 nm of 1.0, resuspend in 200 μL sample buffer and use 10 μL per lane.

4. Transform into meningococci with colony-blot selection as described earlier.

3.3. Deletions in PorA Surface Loops

Specific deletions of the VR1 or VR2 regions from loop 1 and 4 have been constructed by polymerase chain reaction (PCR) mutagenesis *(12)*. By using two complementary primers corresponding to the sequence 5′-GGCAGG AACTACCAG-(deletion)-AGCCGCATCAGGACG-3′ a 78 bp deletion has been made in the VR1 region of P1.7,16 PorA. The primers, which span the region to be deleted, were used in combination with either an upstream (5′GGAAGCTTGGTTGCGGCATTTATCAGATATTTGTTCTG-3′) or downstream (5′-CGTCAGGCGGTGTACCTGATGGTT-3′) *porA* primer to generate two PCR products. These were purified from agarose gel, mixed, and used as template in a second PCR with only the outside primers. The PCR was performed with AmpliTaq for 30 cycles of 1 min at 95°C, 1 min at 55°C, and 2 min at 72°C in a PCR buffer containing as 10X stock 100 m*M* Tris-HCl, pH 8.3, 500 m*M* KCl, 15 m*M* MgCl$_2$ and 0.1% gelatin. The final PCR product was digested with *EclXI-KpnI* and ligated into pCO14K digested with the same enzymes (*see* **Fig. 2**). For construction of a similar 26-residue deletion in VR2 the *porA* gene from strain 2208 was used, which has acquired this loop 4 deletion spontaneously. Transformation of the constructs into meningococcal strain H44/76 was done as described above for pCO14K. The resulting strains can be used to determine the fine specificity of PorA-directed bactericidal antibodies generated after vaccination.

3.4. Additional Chromosomal Copies of porA

For use in the production of multivalent OMV vaccines, derivatives of strain H44/76 carrying multiple chromosomal copies of *porA* have been constructed *(13)*. One extra *porA* gene has been inserted into an *opa* gene, by ligating a 2.6 kb fragment carrying the complete P1.5,2 *porA* gene of strain 2996 into one of the H44/76 *opa* genes and isolating a transformant simultaneously expressing P1.16 and P1.2 PorA proteins by colony-blot selection as described earlier. The advantages of using *opa* genes for this purpose are that expression is not required for cell viability or vaccine production, and because of the presence of four copies the chance of recombination is increased. Another *porA* gene has been inserted into the *rmpM* gene encoding the class 4 protein, also encoding an OMP that is not required for viability or vaccine composition; in this case, a 3.5 kb fragment consisting of *kanR* and *porA* in tandem was inserted into the *SnaBI* site located in the presumed periplasmic domain of *rmpM*. Transformation and selection for kanamycin-resistance resulted in a strain with simultaneous expression of three distinct PorA subtypes and without expression of any immunologically detectable class 4 protein (*see* **Note 5**).

3.5. Constitutive Expression of Other OMPs Using the porA Promoter

The *porA* gene has a unique *EclXI* site located within the region encoding the signal sequence, at amino acid position –3 relative to the start of the mature protein. This can be used for constitutive expression of other OMPs, such as the normally iron-regulated FrpB protein. A PCR primer was designed that introduces an *EclXI* site at the homologous position of the *frpB* signal sequence, and used in combination with a second primer that introduces an *NcoI* site directly after the stop codon. The resulting PCR product was then used to replace the *EclXI-NcoI* fragment from *porA* in plasmid pCO14K (*see* **Fig. 2**). Transformation into strain H44/76, with selection for kanamycin resistance and loss of PorA expression as described earlier, then resulted in constitutive high-level expression of FrpB. In this way, immunogenicity studies can be performed with outer-membrane complexes containing FrpB, without simultaneous expression of other iron-regulated proteins that would confuse interpretation. The method can also be used for high-level expression of other OMPs that are normally present in minor amounts or that require special growth conditions for expression.

3.6. Combined Mutations in PorA and Other Major OMPs

Spontaneous PorA-negative variants are found at relatively high frequency, resulting from mutation in a polyG-tract of the promoter region or from deletion of the complete gene via recombination between repeat regions (*14,15*). Inactivation can be also achieved by transformation with a construct in which the *kanR* gene has been inserted into the *KpnI* site of *porA*, resulting in complete loss of PorA from outer-membrane preparations. Mutant strains lacking PorA show no obvious in vitro growth defects, presumably because the PorB porin can take over its function (*16*). However, PorB-deficient mutants have a slightly lower growth rate, and *porA porB* double mutants could not be constructed and are thus probably not viable. A mutant *porA* gene with 26-residue deletions in both loops 1 and 4 was compatible with a *porB* knockout mutation, suggesting that these loops are not essential for pore functioning. Either *porA* or *porB* knockout mutations can be made in combination with *rmpM* inactivation without loss of viability, despite the fact that both porins were shown to form complexes with class 4 protein.

4. Notes

1. For transformation into *N. meningitidis*, it is essential that the construct contains a copy of the neisserial uptake sequence *(17)*. Many genes, such as *porA*, contain this as part of the transcriptional terminator located after the stop codon; in some cases it is also found within coding regions. If neither is the case, it should be inserted into the construct; for this purpose, we have used the following two oligonucleotides: 5'-TTCAGACGGCTGTAC-3' and 5'-AGCCGTCTGAAGTAC-3'. After annealing, they form a double-stranded oligonucleotide with *Kpn*I-compatible sticky ends. The particular position relative to the gene used for transformation is not important.

2. As vectors containing only the ColE1 origin of replication (e.g., pTZ19R, pUC18, pBluescript II SK) cannot replicate in *Neisseria*, the transformants found will result from recombination with the chromosomal *porA* gene. Linearized plasmid DNA can be used directly from the restriction-enzyme digestion, without change of buffer. There is no particular requirement for DNA purification, and most commercially available plasmid DNA isolation kits will do (e.g., Wizard Plus SV Minipreps DNA Purification System, Promega).

3. To maximize the chance of identifying transformants, it is important to have plates with as many well-separated colonies as possible. This is usually found with the 10^{-4} dilution, but the other dilutions should be included as well as the number of viable bacteria in the suspension may vary.

4. It is important to remove all bacteria not directly bound to the nitrocellulose, as they might otherwise fall off during later incubation steps and lead to an irregular staining pattern; with some strains that have a strong tendency to clump, it may be necessary to wipe them off directly wearing gloves.

5. There is no requirement for very long flanking homologous sequences in order to get efficient recombination; for instance, pCO14K transforms efficiently with only 0.2 kb of chromosomal DNA downstream of *kanR*. Also, insertion of at least 3.5 kb of additional DNA is no problem.

References

1. van der Ley, P., Heckels, J. E., Virji, M., Hoogerhout, P., and Poolman, J. T. (1991) Topology of outer membrane porins in pathogenic *Neisseria* spp. *Infect. Immun.* **59,** 2963–2971.
2. Derrick, J. P., Urwin, R., Suker, J., Feavers, I. M., and Maiden, M. C. J. (1999) Structural and evolutionary inference from molecular variation in *Neisseria* porins. *Infect. Immun.* **67,** 2406–2413.

3. Sacchi, C. T., Lemos, A. P. S., Brandt, M. E., Whitney, A. M., Melles, C. E. A., Solari, C. A., et al. (1998) Proposed standardization of *Neisseria meningitidis* PorA variable-region typing nomenclature. *Clin. Diagn. Lab. Immunol.* **5**, 845–855.
4. Suker, J., Feavers, I. M., and Maiden, M. C. J. (1996) Monoclonal antibody recognition of members of the meningococcal P1.10 variable region family: implications for serological typing and vaccine design. *Microbiology* **142**, 63–69.
5. Bart, A., Dankert, J., and van der Ende, A. (1999) Antigenic variation of the class 1 outer membrane protein in hyperendemic *Neisseria meningitidis* strains in The Netherlands. *Infect. Immun.* **67**, 3842–3846.
6. Rosenqvist, E., Høiby, E. A., Wedege, E., Bryn, K., Kolberg, J., Klem, A., et al. (1995) Human antibody responses to meningococcal outer membrane antigens after three doses of the Norwegian group B meningococcal vaccine. *Infect. Immun.* **63**, 4642–4652.
7. Tappero, J., Lagos, R., Ballesteros, A. M., Plikaytis, B., Williams, D., Dykes, J., et al. (1999) Immunogenicity of 2 serogroup B outer-membrane protein meningococcal vaccines. A randomized controlled trial in Chile. *JAMA* **281**, 1520–1527.
8. Cartwright, K., Morris, R., Rümke, H., Fox, A., Borrow, R., Begg, N., et al. (1999) Immunogenicity and reactogenicity in UK infants of a novel meningococcal vesicle vaccine containing multiple class 1 (PorA) outer membrane proteins. *Vaccine* **17**, 2612–2619.
9. Suker, J., Feavers, I. M., Achtman, M., Morelli, G., Wang, J.-F., and Maiden, M. C. J. (1994) The *porA* gene in serogroup A meningococci: evolutionary stability and mechanism of genetic variation. *Mol. Microbiol.* **12**, 253–265.
10. Scholten, R. J. P. M., Bijlmer, H. A., Poolman, J. T., Kuipers, B., Caugant, D. A., van Alphen, L., et al. (1993) Meningococcal disease in the Netherlands, 1958–1990: A steady increase in the incidence sinds 1982 partially caused by new serotypes and subtypes of *Neisseria meningitidis*. *Clin. Infect. Dis.* **16**, 237–246.
11. van der Ley, P., van der Biezen, J., Hohenstein, P., Peeters, C., and Poolman, J. T. (1993) Use of transformation to construct antigenic hybrids of the class 1 outer membrane protein in *Neisseria meningitidis*. *Infect. Immun.* **61**, 4217–4224.
12. Rouppe van der Voort, E., van der Ley, P., van der Biezen, J., George, S., Tunnela, O., van Dijken, H., et al. (1996) Specificity of human bactericidal antibodies against PorA P1.7,16 induced with a hexavalent meningococcal outer membrane vesicle vaccine. *Infect. Immun.* **64**, 2745–2751.
13. van der Ley, P., van der Biezen, J., and Poolman, J. T. (1995) Construction of *Neisseria meningitidis* strains carrying multiple chromosomal copies of the *porA* gene for use in the production of a multivalent outer mebrane vesivle vaccine. *Vaccine* **13**, 401–407.
14. van der Ende, A., Hopman, C. T. P., Zaat, B., Oude Essink, B., Berkhout, B., and Dankert, J. (1995) Variable expression of class 1 outer membrane protein in *Neisseria meningitidis* strains is caused by variation in the spacing between –10 and –35 regions of the promoter. *J. Bacteriol.* **177**, 2475–2480.

15. van der Ende, A., Hopman, C. T. P., and Dankert, J. (1999) Deletion of *porA* by recombination between clusters of repetitive extragenic palindromic sequences in *Neisseria meningitidis*. *Infect. Immun.* **67,** 2928–2934.
16. Tommassen, J., Vermeij, P., Struyvé, M., Benz, R., and Poolman, J. T. (1990) Isolation of *Neisseria meningitidis* mutants deficient in class 1 (PorA) and class 3 (PorB) outer membrane proteins. *Infect. Immun.* **58,** 1355–1359.
17. Goodman, S.D. and Scocca, J. J. (1988) Identification and arrangement of the DNA sequence recognized in specific transformation of *Neisseria gonorrhoeae*. *Proc. Natl. Acad. Sci. USA* **85,** 6982–6986.

12

Construction of LPS Mutants

Peter van der Ley and Liana Steeghs

1. Introduction

Lipopolysaccharide (LPS) is a major component of the meningococcal outer membrane. It consists of a hexa-acylated glucosamine disaccharide substituted at both ends with diphosphoethanolamine, to which an oligosaccharide chain of up to 10 sugar residues is attached *(1,2)*. It lacks a long repeating O-antigen side chain, as is typically found in many *Enterobacteriaceae*, and is therefore also sometimes referred to as lipooligosaccharide or LOS. The oligosaccharide part shows structural variation among strains, which forms the basis for division into the different immunotypes L1 to L12 *(3)*. In addition, individual strains can vary their LPS structure through high-frequency phase variation of several genes encoding glycosyltransferases *(4)*. This can affect virulence-related properties such as invasion of host cells and serum resistance *(5)*. In the context of vaccine development, meningococcal LPS is relevant in several ways. First, the cell surface-exposed oligosaccharide part may contain epitopes recognized by bactericidal or otherwise protective antibodies; however, the presence of host-identical structures such as the terminal lacto-*N*-neotetraose means that the possibility of inducing autoimmune pathology should also be considered *(6)*. Second, the membrane-anchoring lipid A part has strong endotoxin activity, by inducing the synthesis of proinflammatory cytokines in a variety of host cells *(7)*. This plays a major role in the pathological manifestations of meningococcal sepsis, and is also responsible for most of the reactogenicity found with outer membrane vesicle (OMV)-based vaccines.

Most of the genes required for meningococcal LPS biosynthesis have now been identified. Through their insertional inactivation, a variety of well-defined mutants with truncated oligosaccharide or altered lipid A can be con-

From: *Methods in Molecular Medicine, vol. 66: Meningococcal Vaccines: Methods and Protocols*
Edited by: A. J. Pollard and M. C. J. Maiden © Humana Press Inc., Totowa, NJ

structed, as described in this chapter. Such mutants can include novel LPS species that are more suitable for inclusion in human vaccines. An unexpected outcome of this work has been the isolation of mutants completely devoid of LPS, something that was previously considered to be impossible on the basis of work done on lipid A biosynthesis in *Escherichia coli (8)*.

2. Materials
2.1. Cultivation of Meningococci

1. GC agar base (Difco) supplemented with 1% IsoVitaleX (Becton Dickinson).
2. Meningococcal medium (MM): to 1000 mL of dH_2O add 1.3 g glutamic acid, 0.02 g cysteine, 2.5 g $Na_2HPO_4.2H_2O$, 0.09 g KCl, 6.0 g NaCl, 1.25 g NH_4Cl, 0.6 g $MgSO_4.7H_2O$, 5.0 g glucose, 2.0 g yeast extract. Dissolve, adjust pH to 7.8, and sterilize by 0.2-µm filtration.

2.2. Colony Blot

1. Protran BA 85 nitrocellulose filters, 82-mm diameter and 0.45-µm pore size (Schleicher & Schuell).
2. (PBS) (0.9% NaCl in 10 mM sodiumphosphate buffer, pH 7.2) with 0.1% Tween 80.
3. Casein hydrolysate (ICN biochemicals).
4. Monoclonal antibodies (MAbs): L3-specific MN4A8B2 and L8-specific MN14F20-11.
5. Protein A conjugated to horseradish peroxidase.
6. TMB/DONS substrate solution. A: mix 0.02 M Na_2HPO_4 and 0.01 M citric acid 1:1, and adjust to pH 5.5 by adding extra of either solution. B: dissolve 24 mg tetramethylbenzidine and 80 mg dioctylsulfosuccinate in 10 mL 96% ethanol. Mix 30 mL of A with 10 mL of B and add 20 µL of 30% H_2O_2; use immediately.

2.3. LPS Gel Electrophoresis

1. Running gel: 5.5 mL of dH_2O, 5.5 mL of gel buffer (3.0 M Tris-HCl, 0.3% SDS, pH 8.4), 5.5 mL of acryl-/bisacryl-amide solution (46 g acrylamide + 3 g bisacrylamide per 100 mL), 35 µL of ammonium persulfate (100 mg/mL), 3.5 µL of TEMED.
2. Stacking gel: 8.4 mL of dH_2O, 3.1 mL of gel buffer, 1.0 mL of acryl-/bisacryl-amide solution (23.75 g acrylamide + 0.75 g bisacrylamide per 50 mL), 150 µL of ammonium persulfate (100 mg/mL), 15 µL of TEMED.
3. Cathode buffer: 0.1 M Tris, 0.1 M Tricine, 0.1% sodium dodecyl sulfate [SDS]
4. Anode buffer: 0.2 M Tris-HCl, pH 8.9, with ca. 5 mL of 6 N HCl per L.
5. Sample buffer: 0.5 M Tris-HCl pH 6.8, 30% glycerol, 6% SDS.

3. Methods
3.1. Spontaneous LPS Phase Variants

Several LPS mutants can be readily isolated as spontaneous phase variants. For instance, phase variation between the common immunotypes L3 and L8 results

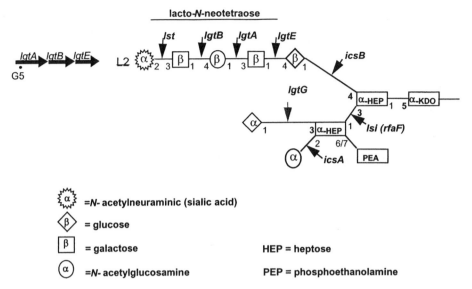

Fig. 1. Primary structure of the oligosaccharide chain of immunotype L2 LPS. Shown are the genes encoding the various glycosyltransferases and their corresponding additions. Immunotype L3 LPS has the same structure except for the additional Glc residue added by LgtG. The arabic numbers indicate the positions of the binding sites; α and β indicate the anomeric configuration.

from high-frequency mutation in the homopolymeric tract of G residues in the *lgtA* gene, encoding the glycosyltransferase required for adding GlcNAc to Gal within the terminal lacto-*N*-neotetraose (*see* **Fig. 1**). Such variants can be isolated from L3 strains by colony blot as negative colonies with the L3-specific MAb MN4A8B2 or positive colonies with the L8-specific MAb MN14F20-11 (*see* also **Note 1**).

1. Grow the bacteria overnight at 37°C in a humid atmosphere with 5% CO_2, on GC agar plates with 1% IsoVitaleX. Resuspend bacteria with cotton swabs in MM + 10 m*M* $MgCl_2$, to an optical density (OD) at 600 nm in the range 0.2–0.5.
2. Prepare 10^{-3}, 10^{-4}, and 10^{-5} dilutions in PBS. Plate 4×0.25 mL of each dilution and incubate overnight at 37°C. To maximize the chance of identifying variants, it is important to have plates with as many well-separated colonies as possible. This is usually found with the 10^{-4} dilution, but the other dilutions should be included as well as the number of viable bacteria in the suspension may vary.
3. Place a sterile nitrocellulose filter with its grid pattern on the agar surface, wait until it has become completely wet and then carefully remove it without disturbing the colony pattern. Plates and filters should be marked for later orientation. Transfer the filters to PBS + 0.1% Tween 80, and inactivate at 56°C for 1 h with gentle shaking. Return the plates to the 37°C incubator for at least 6 h in order to regenerate the colonies.

4. Wash the filters 2 times in fresh PBS + 0.1% Tween 80 at room temperature. It is important to remove all bacteria not directly bound to the nitrocellulose, as they might otherwise fall off during later incubation steps and lead to an irregular staining pattern; with some strains that have a strong tendency to clump, it may be necessary to wipe them off directly wearing gloves.

5. Incubate for 30 min in blocking solution PBS + 0.1% Tween 80 + 0.3% casein. This and all following incubation steps should be done at room temperature and with shaking.

6. Incubate for 1 h in PBS + 0.1% Tween 80 + 0.3% casein containing an appropriate dilution of MAb specific for immunotype L3 or L8.

7. Wash 3 × 10 min with PBS + 0.1% Tween 80.

8. Incubate for 1 h in PBS + 0.1% Tween 80 + 0.3% casein containing an appropriate dilution of protein A – peroxidase conjugate.

9. Wash 3 × 10 min with PBS + 0.1% Tween 80, and 1 × briefly in water.

10. Place the filters in TMB/DONS substrate solution, and incubate (without shaking) for several minutes until green colonies become visible. Wash the filters with water to stop the color reaction.

11. Identify the positive (or negative, depending on the antibody used and the direction of the switch) colonies on the regenerated plates using the grid pattern, pick them up, and streak out on fresh plates.

12. Repeat the colony blot (**steps 3–10**) until the majority of the colonies has the required immunotype. As phase variation is reversible, it is not possible to obtain 100% pure variants of immuntype L3 or L8.

3.2. Mutants with a Truncated Oligosaccharide Chain

Specific removal of the lacto-*N*-neotetraose chain from meningococcal LPS is possible by mutation in the *icsBA* locus *(9)*. This operon encodes the glycosyltransferases required for chain elongation from the lipid A-$(KDO)_2$-$(Hep)_2$ basal structure, with IcsA first adding GlcNAc to Hep-II and IcsB subsequently adding Glc to HepI (*see* **Fig. 1**). The specific order in which these enzymes work means that an *icsB* knockout mutant will only lack the lacto-*N*-neotetraose, but still contains an intact HepII-GlcNAc branch, which is shortened to just HepII in an *icsA* mutant. These mutants have an exposed inner core HepI-HepII region, which contains some epitopes cross-reactive with wild-type LPS, for instance for the MAb MN31G9.19. For their construction, the *kanR* gene can be inserted into unique restriction sites located within *icsB* (*BsiWI*) or *icsA* (*ClaI*), followed by transformation with selection for kanamycin-resistance (*see* **Note 2**).

1. Grow the bacteria overnight at 37°C in a humid atmosphere with 5% CO_2, on GC agar plates with 1% IsoVitaleX. Resuspend bacteria with cotton swabs in MM + 10 mM $MgCl_2$, to an OD at 600 nm in the range 0.2–0.5.

2. To 2.0 mL of bacterial suspension, add DNA to a final concentration of 1 µg/mL or higher. Include a negative control without added DNA. Linearized plasmid

DNA can be used directly from the restriction enzyme digestion, without change of buffer. There is no particular requirement for DNA purification, and most commercially available plasmid DNA isolation kits will do.

3. After incubation at 37°C for 1–3 h, plate 4 × 0.25 mL on GC agar plates with 1% IsoVitaleX and 100 µg/mL kanamycin, and incubate overnight at 37°C. Restreak kanamycin-resistant colonies on selective plates. Spontaneous kanamycin-resistant mutants can also occur, but generally at a much lower frequency and after longer incubation compared to transformants.

4. Verify expression of truncated LPS by Tricine-SDS-PAGE (*see* below) or colony blot.

Partial removal of the lacto-*N*-neotetraose chain is possible by constructing similar *kanR*-insertion mutants in the *lgtA-E* locus (*see* **Note 3**). The resulting mutant LPS lacks the terminal Gal in the case of *lgtB* mutation, Gal-GlcNAc for *lgtA* and Gal-GlcNAc-Gal for *lgtE* (*see* **Fig. 1** and ref. *4*). The same galactose-deficient LPS is also made by mutants with an inactivated *galE* gene, which is required for synthesis of the activated precursor UDP-Gal. By inserting *kanR* in the *ClaI* site of *galE*, subsequent chromosomal recombination will only occur with the active copy located in the *cps* capsular biosynthesis locus and not with the truncated, inactive second copy elsewhere on the chromosome *(10)*. Although *lgtE* and *galE* mutants are expected to make the same LPS, the presence of minor components with additional Glc residues has been reported in the case of *galE* mutants, presumably resulting from the somewhat relaxed sugar specificity of the remaining LgtE glycosyltransferase *(11)*. Finally, it should be noted that *lgtA* insertion mutants make a "frozen L8" type of LPS, because in contrast to natural L8 variants, they can no longer revert to L3. This may be important for certain applications where homogeneous cell suspensions or LPS preparations are required.

Further truncation of the LPS oligosaccharide chain, extending into the inner-core region, is possible through insertional inactivation of the *rfaC* and *rfaF* genes encoding the meningococcal heptosyltransferases *(12,13)*. In *rfaF* mutants, a single heptose residue is still present, while in an *rfaC* mutant only lipid A-$(KDO)_2$ is made (*see* **Fig. 1**). These mutations do not affect in vitro viability of the bacteria. Also, expression levels of the major outer membrane proteins (OMPs) remain the same, in contrast to *E. coli* and other *Enterobacteriaceae* where similar heptose-deficient "deep rough" mutants have strongly reduced amounts of porins *(14)*.

3.3. Mutants with Altered Lipid A Biosynthesis

The *lpxD-fabZ-lpxA* gene cluster is required for the first steps in the lipid A biosynthesis pathway *(15)*. Surprisingly, it turned out that insertional inactivation of meningococcal *lpxA* is possible without compromising cell viability *(8)*. The encoded enzyme is responsible for adding the *O*-linked 3-OH fatty

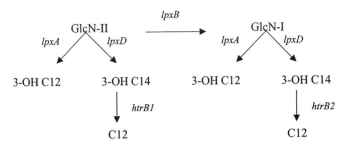

Fig. 2. Schematic representation of the meningococcal lipid A biosynthesis pathway. After acylation of UDP-GlcNAc by LpxA and LpxD, dimerization by LpxB takes place. Secondary acylation by HtrB2 and HtrB1 (in that order) follows later, presumably after addition of KDO to GlcN-II.

acid to UDP-*N*-acetylglucosamine, which is the first step in the lipid A biosynthesis pathway (*see* **Fig. 2**). An *lpxA* knockout mutant can be constructed by transformation with plasmid pLAK33, in which *kanR* has been inserted into the *BstEII* site located within *lpxA* on a 2.1 kb *lpxD-fabZ-lpxA* fragment. The kanamycin-resistant transformants should be passed several times on selective plates to make sure that no cells of the parent strain remain. The resulting LPS-deficient mutant grows more slowly than the parent strain, requiring at least 24 h to form normal-sized colonies, but for the rest has no special growth requirements. The outer membrane containing the major proteins PorA, PorB, RmpM, and Opa is still present. Also, the group B capsular polysaccharide is still made; indeed, its presence seems to be essential for viability of an LPS-deficient mutant as *lpxA* inactivation is not possible in capsule-deficient strains.

Later steps in lipid A biosynthesis can be blocked by insertional inactivation of the two *htrB/msbB* homologs found in *N. meningitidis*, termed *htrB1* and *htrB2*. These genes encode the acyloxyacyltransferases required for addition of the secondary lauroyl chains to lipid A (*see* **Fig. 2**). Insertion of *kanR* into *htrB1* results in LPS with penta- instead of hexa-acylated lipid A, in which the secondary lauroyl chain is specifically missing from the nonreducing end of the GlcN disaccharide (*see* **Note 4**). Insertion of *kanR* into *htrB2* is not possible in wild-type strain H44/76 expressing full-length immunotype L3 LPS, but can be readily achieved in a *galE* mutant expressing a truncated oligosaccharide chain (*see* **Note 5**). In this case, the major lipid A species lacks both secondary lauroyl chains. These mutants do not require a lower growth temperature than normal, in contrast to, for instance, *E. coli*, where *htrB* mutants do not grow above 33°C *(16)*. Both *htrB1* and *htrB2* mutant LPS have reduced endotoxin activity, as measured for example in their ability to induce synthesis of tumor necrosis factor (TNF)-α by leucocytes.

3.4. Isolation and Characterization of Mutant LPS

The following method for isolation of meningococcal LPS is a modification of the hot phenol-water extraction method originally described by Westphal and Jann (*17*).

1. Grow the bacteria overnight at 37°C, in 0.5 L bottles with each 200 mL of meningococcal medium, in a rotary shaker at 160 rpm.
2. Inactivate the bacteria for 30 min at 56°C.
3. Centrifuge for 15 min at 5000 rpm. The total yield for 16 bottles is 3–4 g of cells (wet weight).
4. Resuspend the cells in 40 mM Na$_2$HPO$_4$, 5 mM EDTA, pH 7.0, using 15 mL of buffer per 1 g wet weight.
5. Add 6 mg of lysozyme per 1 g wet weight, and incubate overnight at 4°C while mixing.
6. Transfer the suspension to a 0.5-L bottle. Heat to 70°C, and add the same volume of phenol also pre-heated to 70°C. Mix thoroughly, and incubate for 30 min in a 70°C waterbath while mixing.
7. Cool the bottle first in a 30°C waterbath, and subsequently in an ice bath to ca. 10°C.
8. Centrifuge the mixture for 30 min at 3500 rpm and decant the water phase. This fraction contains the LPS.
9. Re-extract the phenol phase with the same volume of 70°C-preheated water (**steps 6–8**).
10. Combine the water phases and dialyze against tap water for 2 d in order to remove the phenol.
11. Lyophilize the dialyzed preparation.
12. Resuspend the powder in ca. 30 mL of water with 10 mM MgCl$_2$.
13. Add DNase and RNase to a concentration of 50 µg/mL each, and incubate 4 h at 37°C while mixing. Continue incubation overnight at 37°C after the addition of 50 µg/mL of proteinase K.
14. Ultracentrifuge the mixture for 3 h at 105,000g and resuspend the pellet in 20 mL of water. Let it dissolve at 4°C and lyophilize again. Repeating this step will increase purity.
15. Check the resulting LPS preparation by SDS-PAGE and silver staining (*see* below).

The lipid A moiety can be isolated from purified LPS as a water-insoluble product after mild acid hydrolysis.

1. In a 2-mL eppendorf tube, suspend 5.5 mg of LPS in 0.7 mL deionized water + 0.7 mL 2% acetic acid. Mix thoroughly and heat to 100°C for 4 h.
2. Cool the vial, and spin in a microfuge for 30 min at 13,000 rpm (4°C).
3. Discard the supernatant, resuspend the pellet in 1.6 mL of deionized water, and centrifuge again. Repeat this step.

4. To the washed pellet, add 0.3 mL of dH_2O and 0.75 mL of a 1:2 (v/v) methanol-chloroform mixture and mix thoroughly. The lipid A will go to the methanol-chloroform phase.

5. Remove the (top) water layer, add 0.3 mL of fresh dH_2O, and repeat the extraction.

6. The final chloroform-methanol phase contains lipid A suitable for analysis by mass spectrometry.

Analysis of LPS by Tricine-SDS-PAGE and silver staining *(18)*; this method can resolve mutant LPS species differing by only a single sugar residue.

1. Prepare the running gel and pour the gel between 17×15 cm glass plates. After polymerization, prepare the stacking gel on top of it.

2. Sample preparation: 0.2 mg of purified LPS in 1.0 mL sample buffer, incubate 10 min at 100°C, and load 5–10 µL per well.

3. Run the gel overnight (16–17 h) at a constant current of 20 mA; the voltage should rise from 20–30 V at the start to 75–125 V at the end.

4. Fix the gel for 20 min in 40% ethanol –5% acetic acid; perform this and all subsequent steps at room temperature.

5. Oxidize with 0.77% sodiummetaperiodate ($NaIO_4$) in 40% ethanol — 5% acetic acid.

6. Wash 3 times with dH_2O for 10 min.

7. Stain for 15 min in staining solution: 150 mL of deionized water to which is added 1.4 mL 2 *N* NaOH, 2.0 mL concentrated ammonium hydroxide (NH_4OH) solution, 1.0 g of silver nitrate ($AgNO_3$).

8. Wash 3 times with deionized water for 10 min.

9. Develop with 200 mL of deionized water containing 10 mg of citric acid and 0.1 mL of 37% formaldehyde.

10. Stop the staining reaction after 2–15 min with 10% acetic acid for 1 min followed by repeated washing in deionized water.

4. Notes

1. Phase variation between immunotypes is only found for certain LPS epitope combinations, depending on the particular gene repertoire of the strain *(19)*. For instance, L3 strains can switch to L8 and vice versa through *lgtA* mutation, but only those strains that contain the *lgtC* gene can switch between L1 and L8 through addition of an extra Gal, as detected by using the L1-specific MAb 17-1-L1. Phase variation between L3 and L2, resulting from the absence or presence of an additional Glc residue attached to the second heptose (*see* **Fig. 1**), can be detected in for example strain H44/76 by using the L2-specific MAb MN42F12.32. In this case, frameshift mutation in the polyC tract of *lgtG* is responsible; as many L3 strains lack *lgtG* this particular switch is not common.

2. The *kanR* marker used by us is derived from pUC4K; it contains a promoter active in *N. meningitidis*, and has no significant polar effect on downstream genes

in the same operon. However, when used for insertional inactivation its orientation relative to the gene is important: in the opposite orientation kanamycin-resistant transformants are found at very low frequency or not at all. Apparently, in that case its expression is reduced due to simultaneous transcription from two directions.

3. For transformation into *N. meningitidis*, it is essential that the DNA construct contains a copy of the neisserial uptake sequence *(20)*. Many genes, such as *icsA* and *lpxA*, contain this as part of the transcriptional terminator located after the stop codon; in some cases it is also found within coding regions. If neither is the case, it should be inserted into the construct; for this purpose, we have used the following two oligonucleotides: 5′-TTCAGACGGCTGTAC-3′ and 5′-AGCCGT CTGAAGTAC-3′. After annealing they form a double-stranded oligonucleotide with *KpnI*-compatible sticky ends. The particular position relative to the gene used for transformation is not important.

4. There is no requirement for very long flanking homologous sequences in order to get efficient recombination; for instance, we have made the *htrB1* knockout mutant using *kanR* insertion into the middle of a fragment of only 0.5 kb. Also, insertion of at least 3.5 kb of additional DNA is no problem.

5. As an additional marker we have used the *ermC* gene from plasmid pIM13 *(21)*, which confers resistance to erythromycin. We have inserted it as a 1.2 kb *HindIII-ClaI* fragment into the multiple cloning site of pBluescript II SK, resulting in plasmid pER2. This fragment contains both a promoter active in *N. meningitidis* and a transcriptional terminator. Selective plates should contain 5 µg/mL of erythromycin for *N. meningitidis*, and 200 µg/mL for *E. coli*.

References

1. Kulshin, V. A., Zähringer, U., Lindner, B., Frasch, C. E., Tsai, C.-M., Dmitriev, B. A., and Rietschel, E. T. (1992) Structural characterization of the lipid A component of pathogenic *Neisseria meningitidis. J. Bacteriol.* **174,** 1793–1800.

2. Pavliak, V., Brisson, J.-R., Michon, F., Uhrin, D., and Jennings, H. J. (1993) Structure of the sialylated L3 lipopolysaccharide of *Neisseria meningitidis. J. Biol. Chem.* **268,** 14146–14152.

3. Scholten, R. J. P. M., Kuipers, B., Valkenburg, H. A., Dankert, J., Zollinger, W. D., and Poolman, J. T. (1994) Lipo-oligosaccharide immunotyping of *Neisseria meningitidis* by a whole-cell ELISA with monoclonal antibodies. *J. Med. Microbiol.* **41,** 236–243.

4. Jennings, M. P., Hood, D. W., Peak, I. R. A., Virji, M., and Moxon, E. R. (1995) Molecular analysis of a locus for the biosynthesis and phase-variable expression of the lacto-*N*-neotetraose terminal lipopolysaccharide structure in *Neisseria meningitidis. Mol. Microbiol.* **18,** 729–740.

5. van Putten, J. P. M. and Robertson, B. D. (1995) Molecular mechanisms and implications for infection of lipopolysaccharide variation in *Neisseria. Mol. Microbiol.* **16,** 847–853.

6. Tsai, C.-M. and Civin, C. I. (1991) Eight lipooligosaccharides of *Neisseria meningitidis* react with a monoclonal antibody which binds lacto-*N*-neotetraose (Galβ1-4GlcNAcβ1-3Galβ1-4Glc). *Infect. Immun.* **59**, 3604–3609.

7. Zähringer, U., Lindner, B., and Rietschel, E. T. (1994) Molecular structure of lipid A, the endotoxic center of bacterial lipopolysaccharides, in *Advances in Carbohydrate Chemistry and Biochemistry*, vol. 50 (Horton, D., ed.), Academic Press, Inc., San Diego, pp. 211–276.

8. Steeghs, L., den Hartog, R., den Boer, A., Zomer, B., Roholl, P., and van der Ley, P. (1998) Meningitis bacterium is viable without endotoxin. *Nature* **392**, 449–450.

9. van der Ley, P., Kramer, M., Martin, A., Richards, J. C., and Poolman, J. T. (1997) Analysis of the *icsBA* locus required for biosynthesis of the inner core region from *Neisseria meningitidis* lipopolysaccharide. *FEMS Microbiol. Lett.* **146**, 247–253.

10. Jennings, M. P., van der Ley, P., Wilks, K. E., Maskell, D. J., Poolman, J. T., and Moxon, E. R. (1993) Cloning and molecular analysis of the *galE* gene of *Neisseria meningitidis* and its role in lipopolysaccharide biosynthesis. *Mol. Microbiol.* **10**, 361–369.

11. Lee, F. K. N., Stephens, D. S., Gibson, B. W., Engstrom, J. J., Zhou, D., and Apicella, M. A. (1995) Microheterogeneity of *Neisseria* lipooligosaccharide: analysis of a UDP-glucose 4-epimerase mutant of *Neisseria meningitidis* NMB. *Infect. Immun.* **63**, 2508–2515.

12. Stojiljkovic, I., Hwa, V., Larson, J., Lin, L., So, M., and Nassif, X. (1997) Cloning and characterization of the *Neisseria meningitidis rfaC* gene encoding α-1,5 heptosyltransferase I. *FEMS Microbiol. Lett.* **151**, 41–49.

13. Jennings, M. P., Bisercic, M., Dunn, K. L. R., Virji, M., Martin, A., Wilks, K. E., et al. (1995) Cloning and molecular analysis of the *lsi1* (*rfaF*) gene of *Neisseria meningitidis* which encodes a heptosyl-2-transferase involved in LPS biosynthesis: evaluation of surface exposed carbohydrates in LPS mediated toxicity for human endothelial cells. *Microb. Pathog.* **19**, 391–407.

14. Koplow, J. and Goldfine, H. (1974) Alterations in the outer membrane of the cell envelope of heptose-deficient mutants of *Escherichia coli*. *J. Bacteriol.* **117**, 527–543.

15. Steeghs, L., Jennings, M. P., Poolman, J. T., and van der Ley, P. (1997) Isolation and characterization of the *Neisseria meningitidis lpxD-fabZ-lpxA* gene cluster involved in lipid A biosynthesis. *Gene* **190**, 263–270.

16. Karow, M., Fayet, O., Cegielska, A., Ziegelhoffer, T., and Georgopoulos, C. (1991) Isolation and characterization of the *Escherichia coli htrB* gene, whose product is essential for bacterial viability above 33°C in rich media. *J. Bacteriol.* **173**, 741–750.

17. Westphal, O. and Jann, J. K. (1965) Bacterial lipopolysaccharide extraction with phenol-water and further application of the procedure. *Methods Carbohydr. Chem.* **5**, 83–91.

18. Tsai, C. M. and Frasch, C. E. (1982) A sensitive silver stain for detecting lipopolysaccharides in polyacrylamide gels. *Anal. Biochem.* **119**, 115–119.

19. Jennings, M. P., Srikhanta, Y. N., Moxon, E. R., Kramer, M., Poolman, J. T., Kuipers, B., and van der Ley, P. (1999) The genetic basis of the phase variation repertoire of lipopolysaccharide immunotypes in *Neisseria meningitidis*. *Microbiology* **145,** 3013–3021.

20. Goodman, S. D. and Scocca, J. J. (1988) Identification and arrangement of the DNA sequence recognized in specific transformation of *Neisseria gonorrhoeae*. *Proc. Natl. Acad. Sci. USA* **85,** 6982–6986.

21. Monod, M., Denoya, C., and Dubnau, D. (1986) Sequence and properties of pIM13, a macrolide-lincosamide-streptogramin B resistance plasmid from *Bacillus subtilis. J. Bacteriol.* **167,** 138–147.

13

Recombinant Proteins in Vaccine Development

Myron Christodoulides, Keith A. Jolley, and John E. Heckels

1. Introduction

The outer membrane of *Neisseria meningitidis* contains a variety of proteins with the potential for inclusion in new meningococcal vaccines *(1)*. Studies on the vaccine potential of these proteins would be facilitated by the production of pure recombinant protein, free from other components of the *Neisseria* outer membrane. At present, the class 1 outer-membrane protein (OMP) is generally regarded as the most promising candidate. In this chapter, we describe four protocols involved in the preparation of recombinant class 1 OMP for vaccine development. This integrated set of methods can also be readily used to study the potential of other meningococcal OMP as vaccine candidates, and moreover, their utilities make them attractive for vaccine studies relating to many other human pathogens.

The class 1 OMP is encoded by the *porA* gene, a fragment of which was first cloned and expressed as a fusion protein with β-galactosidase in the bacteriophage vector λgt11 *(2)*. Subsequently, cloning of the entire *porA* gene *(3)* enabled the construction of a plasmid vector, designed to express constitutively the protein in the Gram-negative heterologous host *Escherichia coli (4)*. This method yielded a low level of expression of class 1 protein in the form of insoluble inclusion bodies that were able to induce antibodies that recognized denatured protein. However, these antibodies were nonbactericidal for meningococci, highlighting the need to present the protein in a native conformation. In an alternative strategy, Nurminen and colleagues *(5)* cloned and expressed the class 1 porin as a fusion protein with an 11 amino acid leader peptide in the Gram-positive organism *Bacillus subtilis*. Bactericidal antibodies were induced to this protein when complexed with exogenous LPS *(5)* and when incorpo-

From: *Methods in Molecular Medicine, vol. 66: Meningococcal Vaccines: Methods and Protocols*
Edited by: A. J. Pollard and M. C. J. Maiden © Humana Press Inc., Totowa, NJ

rated into the artificial membranes of liposomes *(6,7)*. In general, however, *E. coli* is the usual choice of host organism for cloning and expression of heterologous proteins, and Ward et al. *(8)* reported high-level expression of the class 1 protein in *E. coli* using the p-GEMEX-1 vector. Despite the fact that this expression system was not optimal, owing to the addition of a large 28kD leader peptide N-terminal to the mature class 1 OMP, purified fusion protein incorporated into liposomes was able to induce the production of subtype-specific bactericidal antibodies *(8)*.

In this chapter, our first protocol involves cloning of the target *porA* sequence into a QIAGEN QIA*express*™ plasmid *(9)*. The general approach is to extract DNA from *N. meningitidis*, and to amplify *porA* sequences by polymerase chain reaction (PCR) with specific primers. The primers used introduce restriction sites for cloning into a QIA*express*™ plasmid, with the upstream primer designed so that the N-terminal modification of the expressed protein is as small as possible and with the signal peptide removed. The *porA* gene fragment is cloned into a pQE-30 plasmid, which is a type IV pQE vector with a His_6 affinity tag at the 5′ end of the polylinker that functions as a high-affinity nickel-binding domain in the translated protein. In a previous study, we used the pRSET vector system (Invitrogen) to clone and express the *porA* gene in *E. coli* and demonstrated that the recombinant protein could be readily purified with nickel-nitrilotriacetic acid (Ni-NTA) metal-affinity chromatography *(10)*. However, despite high-level expression of recombinant protein, the pRSET vector-expression system introduced the His_6 tag within a 3.4kD leader sequence N-terminal to the class 1 protein. In contrast, the QIA*express*™ vector expresses a fusion protein in *E. coli* that comprises mature class 1 OMP with only 10 extra amino acids, including the His_6 tag, at the N-terminus. Furthermore, unlike both the p-GEMEX *(8)* and pRSET vectors *(10)* previously used to produce recombinant class 1 OMP, the QIA*express* vectors lack an additional amino acid region required to provide a protease cleavage site between the *porA* gene and the His_6 tag.

The second protocol involves expression of the *porA*-pQE-30 plasmid construct in a heterologous host, namely *E. coli*. The general approach is to prepare high-quality expression plasmids by inducing *E. coli* JM109 cells to competence for the uptake of ligated *porA*-pQE-30 vector constructs, and selecting the transformants by screening for antibiotic resistance. These plasmids are subsequently purified and used to transform the *E. coli* strains (M15 or SG13009) included with the QIA*express*™ system. Class 1 OMP expression is induced from transformed *E. coli* strain M15 with the addition of isopropyl-β-D-thiogalactoside (IPTG). The QIA*express*™ vectors use an IPTG-inducible T5 promoter with a choice of position and reading frame for the His_6 affinity tag. High levels of the *lac* repressor protein repress transcriptional regulation from the T5 promoter. The *E. coli* M15 strain contains a low-copy plasmid, pREP4, which constitutively expresses the *lac* repressor protein, and can be selected by resistance to the antibiotic kanamycin.

In our third protocol, the expressed recombinant protein is purified under denaturing conditions by affinity chromatography on the Ni-NTA matrix. The N-terminal His_6 tag on the class 1 OMP facilitates binding to Ni-NTA to a capacity of 5–10 mg protein/mL resin. The last protocol will describe the preparation of liposomes (artificial membranes) containing recombinant class 1 OMP. Liposomes are closed, concentric, phospholipid bilayers that have been used extensively by the pharmaceutical industry for targeted drug delivery to humans, and in trials of some human vaccines. The advantages of using liposomes for the preparation of class 1 OMP vaccines are that they are biodegradable, nontoxic and nonimmunogenic, and are capable of inducing both humoral and cell-mediated immunity with a large variety of antigens *(11)*. This immunoadjuvant activity, combined with the similarity of liposomes to biological membranes, provides a rationale for preparing human vaccines that present membrane proteins in a native conformation.

2. Materials

2.1. Bacterial Strains and Growth Conditions

N. meningitidis strain H44/76 (B:15: P1.7,16a) is stored in 1% (w/v) proteose-peptone and 8% (v/v) glycerol in water, under liquid nitrogen. *E. coli* strain JM109 and expression strains M15[pREP4] and SG13009[pREP4] are stored in Luria Bertani (LB) medium containing 10% (v/v) glycerol, under liquid nitrogen. GC agar is the medium of choice for growth of meningococci *(12)*, and LB agar for *E. coli*.

2.2. Polymerase Chain Reaction

1. Oligonucleotide primers:
   a. KAJ-105 (a 27-mer used as the upstream primer to introduce a *Bam*HI restriction site): 5′-GGCCGGATCCGATGTCAGCCTATACGG-3′
   b. KAJ-106 (a 25-mer used as the downstream primer to introduce a *Hind*III restriction site): 5′-AGCTATAAGCTTCACCGCCCCGATA-3′
   The primers are purchased as lyophilized pellets, which are resuspended in distilled, deionized water to prepare high-concentration stocks (1000 ng/mL). Lots (100 mL) are stored at –20°C. Working stocks (50 ng/mL) are prepared and dispensed in lots to minimize freeze/thaw cycles.
2. Bio-X-Act DNA polymerase (Bioline, cat. no. M12801B, supplied at 4 U/μL) and the proprietary 10X reaction buffer, lacking Mg^{2+}, supplied with the enzyme.

The enzyme is stored at –20°C in the buffer in which it is supplied. In use, the enzyme is kept on ice in an insulated benchtop cooler to protect the enzyme from temperature fluctuations.

3. 10X dNTP solution: 2 m*M* dATP, 2 m*M* dCTP, 2 m*M* dGTP, 2 m*M* dTTP in deionized water. We use dNTP set supplied by Promega (cat. no. 1240). The dNTPs are supplied at 100 m*M* each and these are combined into one solution. They are diluted 1:50 using deionized water to yield the solution containing 2 m*M* of each dNTP. This dNTP solution is dispensed into 100 μL aliquots and stored at –20°C. Multiple freeze-thaw cycles of the aliquots are to be avoided.

4. 50 m*M* MgCl$_2$. Supplied by Bioline with the polymerase.

5. Genomic DNA: *N. meningitidis* strain H44/76 is grown on GC agar plates overnight, and single colonies are picked and suspended in 10 μL distilled, deionized water in a sterile tube. To extract DNA, the bacteria are lysed with the addition of 10 μL 0.25 *M* KOH with boiling for 5 min. To adjust the pH for PCR, 10 μL of 0.5 *M* Tris-HCl, pH 7.5, buffer is then added. The lysed samples are then diluted to 300 μL with water, briefly centrifuged to remove any particulate material, and stored at –20°C. A negative control is also prepared from 10 μL deionized water treated similarly.

6. Tubes for carrying out the reaction (e.g., 0.2-mL thin-walled tubes from Genetic Research Instrumentation Ltd.).

2.3. Agarose Gel Electrophoresis of the PCR Product

1. 6X Loading buffer: 0.25% bromophenol blue, 0.25% xylene cyanol FF, 40% (w/v) sucrose in distilled, deionized water.

2. Agarose (Sigma, cat. no. A9539).

3. 1X TAE buffer: 40 m*M* Tris-acetate, 1 m*M* EDTA. A 50X stock is made up consisting of 24.2 g Tris-HCl, 10 mL 0.5 *M* EDTA, pH 8.0, and 5.71 mL glacial acetic acid/l.

4. Agarose gel: 1% agarose (w/v) in 1X TAE buffer.

5. 10 mg/mL ethidium bromide. This agent is a mutagen and should be handled in a contained area by personnel wearing suitable protective clothing. The chemical is stored at room temperature in the dark.

6. DNA molecular weight markers (Promega 1kb DNA ladder Cat. No. G5711).

2.4. Purification of PCR Product, Digested Vector and Expression Construct

1. Wizard PCR Preps DNA Purification System (Promega, cat. no. A7170).

2. Geneclean II kit. (Bio 101 Inc.).

3. QIAprep spin miniprep kit (Qiagen, cat. no. 27104).

2.5. Restriction Digestion of PCR Product and Expression Vector

1. *Bam*HI enzyme (New England Biolabs, cat. no. 136S, supplied at a concentration of 20 U/μL) with NEBuffer 1 (150 m*M* NaCl, 10 m*M* Tris-HCl, 10 m*M* MgCl$_2$, 1 m*M* dithiothreitol (DTT) (pH 7.9; supplemented with 100 μg/mL BSA).

2. *Hind*III enzyme (New England Biolabs, cat. no. 104S, supplied at a concentration of 20 U/µL) with NEBuffer 2 (50 mM NaCl, 10 mM Tris-HCl, 10 mM MgCl$_2$, 1 mM DTT, pH 7.9.

3. Calf alkaline phosphatase (New England Biolabs, cat no. 290S, supplied at a concentration of 10 U/µL).

2.6. Vector Ligation

The vector used for preparation of *porA* expression constructs is pQE-30 (Qiagen QIA*express*™ system). T4 DNA ligase (Promega, cat. no. M1801, supplied at 1–3 U/µL) and the 10X buffer (10X = 300 mM Tris-HCl, pH 7.8, 100 mM MgCl$_2$, 100 mM DTT, 10 mM ATP) supplied with the enzyme. The enzyme is stored frozen at –20°C. Similarly, the enzyme buffer is also stored at –20°C in small aliquots, in order to avoid freeze-thaw cycles, which decrease ATP activity.

2.7. Inducing Cells for Competence of Uptake of DNA and Transformation with Expression Construct

1. 25 mL LB medium (10 g/L bacto-tryptone, 5 g/L yeast extract, 10 g/L NaCl).
2. 100 mM MgCl$_2$ and 100 mM CaCl$_2$.

2.8. Screening of Expression Construct

1. STET buffer: 8% (w/v) sucrose, 5% (v/v) Triton X-100, 50 mM EDTA, 50 mM Tris-HCl, pH 8.0.
2. Alcohols (isopropanol and 80% ethanol).
3. Deionized water containing 20 µg/mL RNase A.
4. *Bam*HI and *Hind*III enzymes as described in **Subheading 2.5.1.** and **2.5.2.**

2.9. Transformation of Vector into Expression Hosts

1. *E. coli* strains M15[pREP4] and SG13009[pREP4].
2. Antibiotics (kanamycin and ampicillin at 25 µg/mL and 100 µg/mL final concentrations, respectively).
3. LB medium (10 g/L bacto-tryptone, 5 g/L yeast extract, 10 g/L NaCl).

2.10. Expression and Purification of Recombinant Class 1 Protein

1. Media: LB (**Subheading 2.1.**); 2 YT (16 g/L bacto-tryptone, 10 g/L yeast extract, 5 g/L NaCl); Super Broth (26 g/L bacto-tryptone, 15 g/L yeast extract, 5 g/L NaCl).
2. IPTG (Sigma).
3. Nickel-nitrilotriacetic acid (Ni-NTA) metal-affinity chromatography matrix (Qiagen).
4. Chromatography buffers: B. (8 M urea, 100 mM NaH$_2$PO$_4$, 10 mM Tris-HCl, pH 8.0 with 20 mM imidazole); C (8 M urea, 100 mM NaH$_2$PO$_4$, 10 mM Tris-HCl, pH 6.3 with 20 mM imidazole); D (8 M urea, 100 mM NaH$_2$PO$_4$, 10 mM Tris-HCl, pH6.3); E (8 M urea, 100 mM NaH$_2$PO$_4$, 10 mM Tris-HCl, pH 4.5).

Table 1
Preparation of PCR Master Mix

Reagent[a]	Volume (μL)	Final concentration
Distilled, deionized water	67.5	—
10X reaction buffer	15	1X
MgCl$_2$ (50 mM)	6	2 mM
dNTP solution (2 mM each)	15	200 μM each
Primer KAJ-105 (50 ng/μL)	15	250 ng/50 μL reaction
Primer KAJ-106 (50 ng/μL)	15	250 ng/50 μL reaction
Bio-X-Act (4 U/μL)	1.5	2 U/50 μL reaction

[a]The reagent volumes are sufficient for three reactions.

2.11. Liposomes

1. Purified recombinant class 1 proteins are stored lyophilized at –20°C with dessicant.
2. Reagents for lipid film: L-α-phosphatidylcholine (20 mg; Sigma) and Octyl-β-D-glucopyranoside (100 mg; Sigma).
3. Sephadex G50 (Pharmacia) and chromatography column (dimensions at least 1.5 × 30 cm).

3. Methods

3.1. Bacterial Strains and Growth Conditions

Grow *N. meningitidis* H44/76 on proteose-peptone (Difco) GC agar plates at 37°C for 18 h in an atmosphere of 5% (v/v) CO$_2$ *(12)*, and *E. coli* strains on Luria Bertani (LB) medium (Difco) agar plates and in LB liquid medium.

3.2. Polymerase Chain Reaction

Carry out PCR reactions with DNA from *N. meningitidis* H44/76 along with the negative (water) control.

1. Prepare a master mix as shown in **Table 1**, and dispense an aliquot (45 μL) into each reaction tube. Then, add the genomic DNA to the reaction tube for PCR. The tube receives 5 μL of DNA, bringing the final reaction volume to 50 μL.
2. Place the reaction tubes in a Perkin-Elmer 9600 thermal cycler or equivalent and subject to PCR with the following conditions: an initial denaturation at 96°C for 2 min, followed by 30 cycles each at 96°C for 40 s, 56°C for 40 s, and 72°C for 70 s.

3.3. Agarose Gel Electrophoresis of the PCR Product

1. Mix 5 μL aliquots of the PCR reactions with 1 μL of 6X loading buffer and load onto an agarose gel for electrophoresis. Load an additional lane with DNA molecular-weight markers.

2. Carry out electrophoresis at ~5 V/cm (measured as the distance between the electrodes) until the dyes in the loading buffer have separated 2–4 cm.
3. Stain the gel in electrophoresis buffer containing 0.5 µg/mL ethidium bromide for about 30 min. Then, rinse the gel in distilled water and visualize on an ultraviolet (UV) light box. A single band of ~1.2kb size is expected for the PCR product. There should be no corresponding band in the negative control lane.

3.4. Purification of the PCR Product

1. Clean the PCR products using a variety of commercially available kits. We use Wizard PCR preps from Promega, which effectively remove amplification primers and other components of the PCR reaction.
2. Following UV visualization of the PCR product, purify the remaining 45 µL of the reaction according to the manufacturer's instructions.
3. Elute the purified PCR product in 50 µL deionized water.

3.5. Restriction Digestion and Purification of PCR Product and Expression Vector

Digest the PCR product and the expression vector with the same restriction enzymes to facilitate cloning of the product into the vector.

1. Mix the 50 µL volume of eluted PCR product with 6 µL 10X *Bam*HI buffer, 0.6 µL 100 µg/mL BSA, 1.7 µL (34 U) *Bam*HI, and 1.7 µL (34 U) *Hind*III to make a final volume of 60 µL. Incubate in a water bath at 37°C for 3 h.
2. Five µg of the lyophilized pQE-30 vector is supplied. This can be used directly for the cloning experiments, or, if multiple experiments are to be done, it can be used to transform competent cells in order to purify greater quantities using standard midi-prep procedures.
   a. To use directly, dissolve the 5 µg of vector in 10 µL deionized water to make a 500 ng/µL solution.
   b. Add 4 µL (2 µg) aliquot of this vector to a solution containing 2 µL 10X *Bam*HI buffer, 2 µL 10 µg/mL BSA, 1 µL (20 U) *Bam*HI, 1 µL (20 U) *Hind*III, and 10 µL deionized water, in a final volume of 20 µL and incubate at 37°C for 3 h.
   c. Add 17.5 µL of deionized water, a further 2 µL 10X *Bam*HI buffer, and 0.5 µL (5 U) calf alkaline phosphatase to make a final volume of 40 µL, and incubate at 37°C for 1 h.
   d. Purify the digested PCR product as described in **Subheading 3.4.1.** using Promega Wizard PCR preps, and elute in 50 µL deionized water. The final concentration of DNA is 10–15 ng/µL, as estimated by comparison with standards on an agarose gel.
3. Run the digested vector on an agarose gel and stain with ethidium bromide as described in **Subheading 3.3.**
4. Locate the band representing the linearized vector, lacking the small polylinker excised by the restriction reactions, using a hand-held UV lamp.

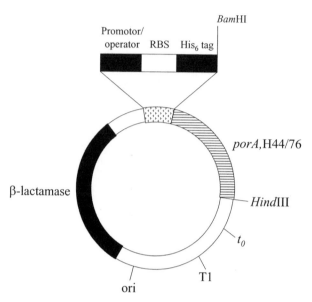

Fig. 1. H44/76 *porA* expression plasmid constructed from Qiagen QE-30 expression vector. RBS: Ribosomal binding site; t_o: Transcriptional terminator from phage λ; T1: Transcriptional terminator from the *rrnB* operon of *E. coli*; ori: ColE1 origin of replication

5. Cut out the band from the agarose using a clean razor blade and transfer it to a sterile 1.5-mL centrifuge tube, ensuring that the smallest cut possible is made while removing the entire band.

6. Elute the DNA from the agarose using a variety of commercially available extraction kits. We routinely use the Geneclean protocol, following the manufacturer's instructions whereby linearized vector is eluted in 20 µL deionized water at a final concentration of ~100 ng/µL.

3.6. Vector Ligation

1. Set up a ligation reaction for the H44/76 *porA* construct, consisting of the following: 1 µL linearized vector (~100 ng/µL), 5 µL (10–15 ng/µL) purified *porA* PCR product, 1 µL 10X ligase buffer, 2 µL deionized water, 1 µL T4 DNA ligase (1–3 U).

2. Set up a control reaction containing linearized vector but no insert DNA to check for background levels of incomplete cleavage or re-ligation of vector.

3. Incubate both ligation reactions in a water bath at 15°C overnight. An example of the H44/76 *porA* plasmid (pKAJ108) constructed from the pQE-30 vector is shown in **Fig. 1**.

3.7. Inducing Cells for Competence of Uptake of DNA and Transformation

1. Inoculate LB medium (25 mL in a 100 mL conical flask) with 1 mL of overnight culture of *E. coli* JM109 cells. Incubate the culture at 37°C with vigorous shaking (~250 rpm) until the A_{550} reaches 0.4–0.5.

2. Chill the culture on ice for 20 min, and decant 20 mL to an ice-cold sterile tube and centrifuge (1300g for 10 min at 4°C). Remove the supernatant solution and resuspend the cell pellet in 10 mL of ice-cold 0.1 M MgCl$_2$ and immediately centrifuge as above (1300g for 10 min at 4°C).
3. Remove the supernatant solution and resuspend the cells in 1 mL of ice-cold 0.1 M CaCl$_2$ and leave on ice for at least 1 h. This produces competent cells for use up to 24 h later.
4. Mix aliquots (150 μL) of competent JM109 cells with the ligation reactions described in **Subheading 3.6.** and leave on ice for 30 min. Mix occasionally by flicking the tubes.
5. Heat-shock the cells by placing in a water bath for 2 min at 42°C and then return them to ice for 30 min. Subsequently, plate out the cells (50 μL) onto LB agar containing 100 μg/mL ampicillin and incubate overnight at 37°C.
6. Following incubation, each agar plate containing bacteria transformed with the ligation mixture with the H44/76 *porA* insert should have ~200–500 colonies. The control plate should have few or no colonies.

3.8. Screening of Expression Construct

1. Plate out individual colonies from the transformed cell plates onto fresh LB-ampicillin plates; up to 12 colonies can be screened on each plate.
2. Incubate overnight at 37°C and transfer streaks of bacterial growth about 2 cm in length from the plates, using sterile toothpicks, to 0.6 mL micro-centrifuge tubes each containing 100 μL STET buffer. Add lysozyme (8 μL of a 10 mg/mL solution) to the bacterial suspensions and then incubate for 5 min at room temperature.
3. Place the suspensions in a boiling water bath for 40 s and then centrifuge (13,000g for 10 min). Transfer the supernatant solutions (usually 50–70 μL) to clean micro-centrifuge tubes and add equal volumes of isopropanol. Place the samples at –20°C for 1 h to precipitate the nucleic acids.
4. Centrifuge the samples (13,000g for 5 min), discard the supernatant solutions and add 100 μL of 80% (v/v) ethanol to each of the nucleic-acid pellets.
5. Briefly vortex-mix the tubes, centrifuge for 2 min at 13,000g and remove the ethanol with a micropipet.
6. Dry the pellets by vacuum or air and resuspend in 15 μL deionized water containing 20 μg/mL RNase A. This is a low-quality DNA preparation that is adequate for screening, and there is enough DNA present to allow for at least two restriction digestions.
7. Set up two restriction digests for each sample; one reaction is to linearize the vector in order to determine its size and the other to excise any insert to determine its identity.
   a. The first restriction digestion contains 7 μL DNA preparation, 1 μL of 10 μg/mL BSA, 1 μL 10X *Bam*HI buffer, and 1 μL (20 U) of *Bam*HI enzyme.
   b. The second restriction digestion contains 7 μL DNA preparation, 1 μL of 10 μg/mL BSA, 1 μL *Bam*HI buffer, 0.5 μL (10 U) of *Bam*HI and 0.5 μL (10 U) of *Hind*III enzyme.

8. Incubate the restriction digests at 37°C for 1 h and then run on an agarose gel. For strains with a plasmid containing the *porA* insert, the first restriction digest should have a single band at ~4.6kb; the second digest should show two bands corresponding to the vector at ~3.4kb and the insert at ~1.2kb.

9. For short-term storage, re-streak the strains identified as containing inserts onto LB-ampicillin agar plates. Make small-scale preparations of higher quality of these expression plasmids using a commercial miniprep kit. We recommend QIAprep™ spin miniprep kits from Qiagen.

3.9. Transformation of Vector into Expression Hosts

The Qiagen expression host cells, *E. coli* M15 [pREP4] and *E. coli* SG13009 [pREP4] are made competent and transformed with the H44/76 *porA* construct by the method explained for *E. coli* JM109 cells (*see* **Subheadings 3.6., 3.7.**), using 1 μL of miniprep plasmid DNA. The only difference is that the LB growth medium and plates contain kanamycin (25 μg/mL) to maintain selection for the pREP4 *lac* repressor plasmid present in these strains, in addition to ampicillin (100 μg/mL) for selection of the expression plasmids.

3.10. Expression and Purification of Recombinant Class 1 Protein

1. Prepare a starter culture by inoculating LB liquid medium (50 mL) containing ampicillin (100 μg/mL) and kanamycin (25 μg/mL), with a single colony of *E. coli* M15 [pREP4] transformed with the H44/76 *porA* expression plasmid, and incubate at 37°C for 18 h. Then, use a 20 mL volume of this starter culture to inoculate 500 mL of pre-warmed SuperBroth liquid medium (containing antibiotics) in a 2-L flask. Inoculate two flasks and incubate for 1 h at 37°C with agitation (250 rpm).

2. In order to induce expression, add a solution of 1 mM IPTG (5.25 mL of a 100 mM stock) to each flask and incubate the cultures for a further 3 h.

3. Harvest the cultures by centrifugation (8000g, for 1 h at 25°C), remove the supernatant solution, and store the pellets at –20°C overnight.

4. Resuspend the cell pellets in lysis Buffer B (5 mL per gram wet weight of cells), pool the pellets, and disrupt using 30-s bursts of sonication (MSE Soniprep 150), with cooling in an ice/water slurry for 90 s between bursts, until a cleared lysate is obtained.

5. Centrifuge the cell lysate (18,000g for 1 h at 25°C) and keep the supernatant on ice.

6. Prepare a Pharmacia column (0.5 × 15 cm) containing a bed volume of between 5–15 mL of the nickel-nitrilotriacetic acid (Ni-NTA) affinity-chromatography gel matrix (Qiagen). Wash the matrix with five column volumes of distilled, deionized water and equilibrate with five column volumes of Buffer B. Load the supernatant onto the matrix at a flow rate of 15 mL/h, collect the flow-through, and re-circulate.

7. Wash the matrix sequentially with five column volumes each of Buffer B and Buffer C, and then elute with Buffer D and Buffer E. Collect fractions of 6 mL

volume, and analyze by SDS-PAGE and Western blotting for the presence of class 1 protein. In general, the largest concentration of pure recombinant class 1 protein is eluted in Buffer E.

8. Precipitate the class 1 protein from these fractions with the addition of four volumes of ethanol at 4°C overnight, collect the pellet by centrifugation (3000g for 30 min), and wash twice with water to remove traces of urea.

9. Store the purified recombinant protein at –20°C with dessicant until use.

3.11. Production of Liposomes Containing Recombinant Class 1 Protein

1. Stock solution of recombinant protein.
   a. Prepare a stock solution (5 mg/mL) of lyophilized recombinant class 1 protein in 100 mM Tris-HCl buffer, pH 8.0, containing 2% SDS.
   b. Dilute this solution in 100 mM Tris-HCl buffer, pH 8.0, containing KCl (100 mM), octyl-β-D-glucopyranoside (2% w/v) and SDS (0.4% w/v) to give a final protein concentration of 1 mg/mL.
   c. Heat this protein solution at 100°C for 10 min for denaturation, then dilute to 5.0 mL with the addition of 100 mM Tris-HCl buffer, pH 8.0, containing octyl-β-D-glucopyranoside (2% w/v), and leave at room temperature for 3 h.

2. Lipid film.
   a. Dissolve *L*-α-phosphatidylcholine (20 mg) and octyl-β-D-glucopyranoside (100 mg) in 3 mL chloroform/methanol (2:1) and place in a 50 mL round-bottomed flask.
   b. Produce a lipid film by rotary evaporation (Buchi) under vacuum and with immersion in a water bath at 25°C.
   c. Dry the lipid film for 3 h under vacuum.

3. Small unilamellar liposomes (SUV) containing recombinant protein are prepared with size-exclusion chromatography (SEC) *(6,10)*.
   a. Add the recombinant protein solution (5 mL) to the lipid film and gently resuspend.
   b. Leave this mixture at room temperature for 1 h to induce the formation of multi-lamellar liposomes.
   c. Pass the suspension over a column of Sephadex G50 at a flow rate of 3.0 mL/ min and collect fractions (4.0 mL).
   d. Assay the fractions for the presence of lipid by turbidity, and for protein by SDS-PAGE.
   e. Pool turbid fractions containing both lipid and protein and store at –20°C until used.
   f. Analyse the liposomes by electron microscopy (EM) for small unilamellar vesicles, and with immuno-gold labeling for the presence of surface-exposed class 1 protein epitopes *(8)*. Generally, the yield of protein-liposomes is approx one-third of the initial protein concentration.

4. Notes

1. It is recommended that those unfamiliar with procedures for cloning and expressing recombinant proteins consult a practical manual such as *Current Protocols in Molecular Biology (13)*.

2. Lamps emitting long-wavelength UV light must be used to locate digested vectors on agarose gels, in order to minimize UV damage to the DNA.

3. During restriction digestion (**Subheading 3.5., step 2c**), dephosphorylation of the digested vector is necessary to prevent self-ligation and hence reduce the vector background during the later ligation stage.

4. In screening of the expression constructs, a higher proportion of strains containing an insert are found by picking the smallest colonies. Presumably the slower growth is owing to some constitutive expression of *porA* in these strains. We also sequence the plasmid inserts to check for PCR-induced errors, even though Bio-X-act is a proof-reading enzyme. Standard plasmid-sequencing protocols can be used, but descriptions of these are beyond the scope of this chapter.

5. Prior to large-scale growth of plasmid-expressing *E. coli*, initial expression trials are strongly recommended. In these experiments, inoculate 10 mL cultures of LB medium with 500 μL of overnight culture of cells containing the expression plasmid(s). Culture of bacteria and induction of plasmid expression are as described above (**Subheadings 3.1.–3.9.**). We have found that all our expression strains produce large quantities of recombinant protein, representing at least 80% total cell protein as estimated by SDS-PAGE. We also find *E. coli* M15 [pREP4] to be the better host strain.

6. A time-course experiment for the determination of plasmid expression from host cells grown in different media is also strongly recommended. We have tested LB, 2YT, and SuperBroth liquid media, and found that SuperBroth gave the maximum yields of expressed protein.

7. The QIA*express*™ system does not use phage induction of plasmid expression. If the recombinant protein of choice cannot be expressed maximally using the QIA*express*™ system, we suggest using a vector based on the T7 promoter, such as the pRSET expression system (Invitrogen).

8. Purification of the His_6 tagged recombinant protein is carried out under denaturing conditions, in that Buffers B, C, D, and E all contain 8 *M* urea. However, only Buffers B and C contain 20 m*M* imidazole, which reduces the nonspecific binding of background proteins and leads to greater purity in fewer chromatography steps.

9. The histidine residues in the His_6 tag have a pK_a of ~6.0 and will become protonated when the pH is reduced (pH 4.5–5.3). Under these conditions the His_6-tagged recombinant protein can no longer bind to Ni ions and will dissociate from the Ni-NTA matrix.

10. The Ni-NTA matrix can be regenerated for further use as described by the manufacturer. We have used it as least six times without any loss in binding efficiency.

11. Exposure of the Ni-NTA matrix to reducing agents (e.g. dithiothreitol) or chelating agents (e.g. EDTA) reduces the binding of His_6-tagged proteins. We recom-

mend that *E. coli* cells not be lysed with these reagents or ionic detergents such as SDS.

12. We have used the QIA*express*™ system to produce purified recombinant class 1 protein from four different meningococcal strains, with yields of approx 80–110 mg/L culture medium. We recommend that the purity of the final product be assessed using SDS-PAGE, and Western blotting with specific antibodies. The absence of contaminating LPS can be checked with low molecular-weight gels and silver staining or Limulus assay. Purity of our preparations is >99%.

13. The N-terminal leader sequence can be removed from the purified recombinant protein. Our attempts at removing N-terminal leader sequences, with the introduction of specific protease-cleavage sites between the mature class 1 protein and the leader polypeptide, have been unsuccessful *(8,10)*. The enzymes we used (Factor Xa and recombinant enterokinase) are nonspecific under the conditions used and cleave sites within the class 1 protein, despite the fact that the meningococcal porin does not contain defined cleavage sites recognized by these proteases. If necessary, we recommend chemical cleavage of the leader peptide, and in the case of the class 1 protein expressed in *B. subtilis* a methionine residue was introduced prior to the mature porin protein for CNBr cleavage *(7)*. This procedure produced mature protein with no leader sequence, but was dependent, however, on replacement of a methionine residue (Met^{144}) present in the porin to preclude internal cleavage.

14. We prepare SUV containing recombinant protein by dialysis-sonication *(8,10)* and size exclusion chromatography (SEC). Both methods yield similar liposomes with respect to vesicle size and immunogenicity *(10)*. However, we find the SEC method more facile and less time-consuming.

15. In order to separate the protein-containing liposomes from contaminating detergents, a chromatography column at least 30 cm in height must be used when preparing liposomes by SEC.

Acknowledgments

We are indebted to the National Meningitis Trust, Medical Research Council, World Health Organization, and the University of Southampton Strategic Development Fund for supporting this research.

References

1. Poolman, J. T., van der Ley, P. A., and Tommassen, J. (1995) Surface structures and secreted products of meningococci, in *Meningococcal Disease* (Cartwright, K. A. V., ed.), John Wiley and Sons, Chichester, UK, pp. 21–34.

2. Barlow, A. K., Heckels, J. E., and Clarke, I. N. (1987) Molecular cloning and expression of *Neisseria meningitidis* class 1 outer membrane protein in *Escherichia coli* K12. *Infect. Immun.* **55,** 2734–2740.

3. Barlow, A. K., Heckels, J. E., and Clarke, I. N. (1989) The class 1 outer membrane protein of *Neisseria meningitidis*: gene sequence and structural and immunological similarities to gonococcal porins. *Mol. Microbiol.* **3,** 131–139.

4. White, D. A., Barlow, A. K., Clarke, I. N., and Heckels, J. E. (1990) Stable expression of meningococcal class 1 protein in an antigenically reactive form in outer membranes of *Escherichia coli*. *Mol. Microbiol.* **4**, 769–776.

5. Nurminen, M., Butcher, S., Idanpaan-Heikkila, I., Wahlstrom, E., Muttilainen, S., Runeberg-Nyman, K., et al. (1992) The class 1 outer membrane protein of *Neisseria meningitidis* produced in *Bacillus subtilis* can give rise to protective immunity. *Mol. Microbiol.* **6**, 2499–2506.

6. Muttilainen, S., Idanpaan-Heikkila, I., Wahlstrom, E., Nurminen, M., Makela, P. H., and Sarvas, M. (1995) The *Neisseria meningitidis* outer membrane protein P1 produced in *Bacillus subtilis* and reconstituted into phospholipid vesicles elicits antibodies to native P1 epitopes. *Microb. Pathog.* **18**, 423–436.

7. Muttilainen, S., Butcher, S. J., Runeberg, K., Nurminen, M., Idanpaan-Heikkila, I., Wahlstrom, E., and Sarvas, M. (1995) Heterologous production of the P1 porin of *Neisseria meningitidis* in *Bacillus subtilis*: the effect of an N-terminal extension on the presentation of native-like epitopes. *Microb. Pathog.* **18**, 365–371.

8. Ward, S. J., Scopes, D. A., Christodoulides, M., Clarke, I. N., and Heckels, J. E. (1996) Expression of *Neisseria meningitidis* class 1 porin as a fusion protein in *Escherichia coli*: the influence of liposomes and adjuvants on the production of a bactericidal immune response. *Microb. Pathog.* **21**, 499–512.

9. QIAGEN (1997) The *QIAexpressionist*. A handbook for high-level expression and purification of 6xHis-tagged proteins.

10. Christodoulides, M., Brooks, J. L., Rattue, E., and Heckels, J. E. (1998) Immunisation with recombinant class 1 outer membrane protein from *Neisseria meningitidis*: influence of liposomes and adjuvants on antibody avidity, recognition of native protein and the induction of a bactericidal immune response against meningococci. *Microbiology* **144**, 3027–3037.

11. Gregoriadis, G. (1995) Liposomes as immunological adjuvants, in *The Theory and Practical Application of Adjuvants* (Stewart-Tull, D. E. S., ed.), John Wiley and Sons Ltd., Chichester, UK, pp. 145–169.

12. Tinsley, C. R. and Heckels, J. E. (1986) Variation in the expression of pili and outer membrane protein by *Neisseria meningitidis* during the course of meningococcal infection. *J. Gen. Microbiol.* **132**, 2483–2490.

13. Ausebel, F. M., Brent, R., Kingston, R. E., Moore, D. D, Sedman, J. G, Smith, J. A, and Struhl, K. (1995) *Current Protocols in Molecular Biology*, John Wiley and Sons, New York.

14

Identification of Peptides that Mimic *N. meningitidis* LOS Epitopes Via the Use of Combinatorial Phage-Display Libraries

Paul J. Brett, Ian M. Feavers, and Bambos M. Charalambous

1. Introduction

Although capsular polysaccharide-based vaccines are effective at reducing the incidence of meningococcal disease caused by serogroups A, C, Y, and W135 *(1–3)*, immunization against serogroup B disease using similar strategies has proven unsuccessful *(4,5)*. The primary reason for this is that the $\alpha 2,8$-linked *N*-acetylneuraminic acid homopolymer expressed by serogroup B strains is poorly immunogenic in humans *(6)*. Consequently, considerable effort has been devoted towards the development of alternative strategies for vaccination against serogroup B disease. Many of these newer strategies include the use of lipooligosaccharide (LOS) as a protective antigen *(7)*. One of the approaches that we are currently pursuing involves the use of synthetic oligopeptides to stimulate antibody responses that are cross-reactive with LOS antigens expressed by serogroup B *Neisseria meningitidis* strains. An integral part of these studies has been the application of combinatorial phage-display technology. Described here is an overview of the methods that we have utilized to identify peptide mimics of LOS epitopes.

Meningococcal LOS moieties are low molecular-weight glycolipids with a $M_r = 3000–7000$ as estimated by sodium dodecyl sulfate-polyacrylamide gel electrophoresis (SDS-PAGE) *(8)*. They consist of oligosaccharides linked to lipid A through 2-keto-3-deoxyoctulosonic acid (KDO) and are structurally very similar to rough lipopolysaccharides (LPS) expressed by mutant strains of *Escherichia coli* and *Salmonella typhimurium* *(9,10)*. To date, some 12 LOS immunotypes have been identified, the majority via the use of immunotype-

From: *Methods in Molecular Medicine, vol. 66: Meningococcal Vaccines: Methods and Protocols*
Edited by: A. J. Pollard and M. C. J. Maiden © Humana Press Inc., Totowa, NJ

specific monoclonal antibodies (MAbs; *11*). The immunotype-specific epitopes recognized by these MAbs usually reside in the core component of the LOS antigen as demonstrated by Western-immunoblot analysis *(12)*. A number of LOS immunotypes, including L2-5, L7, and L9, possess a lacto-*N*-neotetraose (LNnT: Galβ1-4GlcNAcβ1-3Galβ1-4Glc) motif linked to the Heptose I (HepI) residue of the core complex *(13,14)*. An important feature of the LNnT motif is its ability to function as a receptor for sialic acid residues. By sialylating the terminal Galβ residue of the LNnT motif, many *N. meningitidis* strains increase their serum-resistance capacity by downregulating the activation of alternative complement-pathway components. Strains that lack the ability to synthesize the LNnT motif, on the other hand, are far more sensitive towards the bactericidal effects of serum because they are incapable of capping their LOS molecules with sialic acid *(15,16)*. Interestingly, the paragloboside, I, and i antigens expressed by human erythrocytes, lymphocytes, polymorphonuclear leukocytes, and other granulocytes also contain LNnT motifs *(14)*.

Various studies have demonstrated that LOS antigens expressed by *N. meningitidis* strains are both virulence determinants and protective antigens *(15,17,18)*. It is not surprising, therefore, that many of the newer serogroup B meningococcal-vaccine candidates include whole or detoxified LOS moieties in an attempt to exploit their immunostimulatory potential. The most promising of these candidates include outer-membrane vesicles (OMVs) prepared from the detergent extracts of whole cells and de-lipidated LOS-protein carrier conjugates *(19–22)*. Although preliminary evidence suggests that these vaccine preparations are capable of eliciting desirable immune responses in both humans and animals, specific concerns regarding their safety and efficacy remain. To address these issues, we have begun to examine the feasibility of utilizing peptide mimics of LOS epitopes to vaccinate against serogroup B meningococcal disease. In terms of quality control, cost of production, and shelf life, this approach offers several advantages over present strategies. These include the ability to cheaply synthesize large quantities of highly purified, chemically defined immunogens that can be stored or transported without refrigeration. Additionally, the use of synthetic peptides to mimic LOS structures allows for undesirable epitopes, such as those associated with LNnT motifs, to be eliminated from vaccine preparations. By conjugating synthetic peptides to carrier proteins or immunostimulating complexes (ISCOM), T-cell dependent-type immune responses can also be raised with these antigens.

During the past decade, significant advances in the development of combinatorial peptide libraries have been achieved via the introduction of novel, coliphage-based peptide-expression systems. The advantage of bacteriophage-

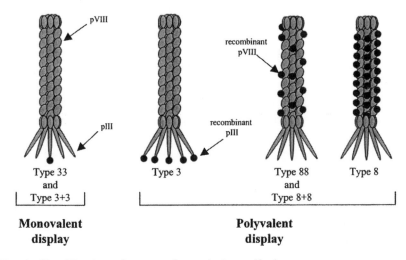

Fig. 1. Classification of commonly used phage-display systems.

display libraries over other peptide-display technologies is that the phenotype of a surface-displayed peptide is intimately linked to the genotype that encodes it. Furthermore, the power of using phage particles for display of diverse peptide libraries is that large numbers of variants can be quickly and easily assembled and screened. The most commonly employed vectors for phage display of peptides are variants or phagemid derivatives of filamentous *E. coli* bacteriophage (fd and M13). These consist of single-stranded, circular genomic DNA packaged into particles of about 65 Å in diameter and 1 μm in length *(23)*. Five structural proteins are required in the assembly of a mature virion *(24,25)*. Two of these antigens, pVIII and pIII, possess surface-exposed N-terminal domains that tolerate the insertion of foreign peptides. The major coat protein (pVIII) is represented by ~2800 copies per phage particle, whereas the minor protein (pIII), essential for the attachment of phage to F[+] *E. coli* strains, is present at 3–5 copies *(26)*. By genetically manipulating the genes encoding these proteins, both linear and conformationally constrained peptide motifs can be displayed on the surface of the phage particles.

Illustrated in **Fig. 1** are some of the systems commonly used to display foreign peptides on the surfaces of filamentous phage. A Type 3 system has a single recombinant gene-*III* encoding for all copies of pIII; the remaining genes are wild-type. Some large foreign peptides are not well-tolerated in Type 3 systems because they may disrupt the normal structure and/or function of pIII *(27)*. Type 33 vectors alleviate this problem by providing two gene-*III* alleles, one wild-type and one recombinant. Phage particles based on this approach display a mixture of pIII molecules, only some of which are fused to foreign peptides. Type 33 systems can tolerate foreign inserts more readily than Type 3 because recombinant pIII antigens need not be functional as long as they are incorporated into mature particles along with wild-type copies of the protein *(27)*. Type 3 + 3 vectors resemble Type 33 systems in having two gene-*III* alleles, however, the recombinant gene resides on a phagemid genome. When phagemid-harboring cells are superinfected with a helper phage, both helper and phagemid genomes are packaged into phage particles. Consequently, host cells secrete two types of particles, both of which possess a mixture of recombinant and wild-type pIII. Owing to the presence of antibiotic resistance markers on phagemid genomes, selective pressures can be imposed on F^+ strains to independently isolate phagemid particles from mixed populations. Type 8, 88, and 8 + 8 systems are the gene-*VIII* equivalents of those based on gene-*III* *(28)*. One of the distinct advantages of using pIII fusion libraries over pVIII systems is the ability to decrease potential chelate or avidity effects that might occur during the selection process. In general, it has been found that monovalent display systems are most useful for detecting high-affinity ligand/receptor interactions, whereas, polyvalent systems are best suited for identifying peptide motifs which have lower affinities for a target molecule *(29,30)*.

The general approach used to identify and characterize peptide mimics of carbohydrate antigens is outlined in **Fig. 2**. Basically, the wells of a polystyrene microtiter plate are coated with a purified target molecule in order to generate an activated solid support for biopanning. Phage libraries are then added to the wells of the plate and allowed to incubate for a fixed period of time in order to facilitate the interaction of the phage particles with the immobilized target molecules. Following the incubation, phage particles that have not been captured by the activated support are eliminated from the system by washing. During this stage, the stringency of the selection process can be adjusted to satisfy individual requirements by manipulating the ionic strength and/or detergent concentration of the wash buffers. The phage particles that remain in the wells after washing, owing to ligand/receptor interactions, are eluted from the system with a brief incubation in a low pH buffer. Rescued phage are then amplified using a suitable host strain and the process repeated 2–3 more times. Subsequent to the last round of biopanning, individual phage clones are isolated, amplified, and the nucleic acid from each purified and sequenced to facilitate the identification of peptide consensus motifs. At this point, it is important to confirm that individual phage clones bind only to the target molecule by panning each against a series of positive and negative controls or via enzyme-linked immunosorbent assay (ELISA) techniques. This precaution is

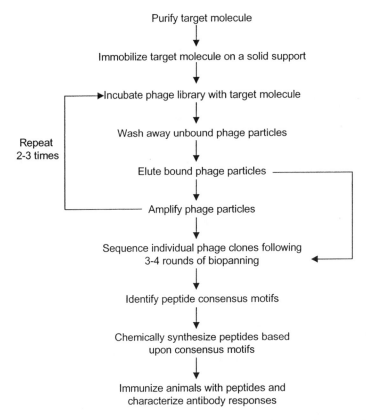

Fig. 2. A summary of the steps utilized to identify and characterize peptide mimics of carbohydrate antigens using phage-display libraries.

necessary because the isolation of "plastic binders" is a common occurrence when using polystyrene plates. Once it has been established that the peptide motifs associated with individual phage clones are carbohydrate mimics, they can be chemically synthesized and conjugated to carrier proteins to facilitate the evaluation of their immunogenic potential in animal models.

Described here are the materials and methods used to: 1) identify and 2) characterize peptide mimics of an L3,7,9 epitope following their selection from a conformationally constrained phage-display library (Ph.D.-C7C). The phage library was biopanned against the LOS specific 9-2-L379 MAb.

2. Materials

Unless otherwise stated, all chemicals were purchased from Sigma or BDH. Tryptone, yeast extract, and bacteriological agar were purchased from Oxoid,

Table 1
Monoclonal Antibodies in This Protocol

Hybridoma	MAb[a]	Specificity	Isotype	Reference
4BE12C1	9-2-L379	Immunotype L3,7,9	IgG_{2a}	*(11)*
MN14C11.6	MN14C11.6	Serosubtype P1.7	IgG_{2a}	*(31)*

[a]The source of the MAbs can be either ascites or hybridoma-culture supernatants.

the agarose from Sigma. The pH of all solutions was adjusted accordingly using 5 *M* NaOH or HCl.

2.1. Target Molecule Purification

1. Monoclonal antibodies (*see* **Table 1**).
2. HiTrap Protein G affinity columns: 1 or 5 mL (Pharmacia LKB Biotechnology).
3. Start Buffer: 20 m*M* sodium phosphate. Adjust pH to 7.0. Make fresh before use.
4. IgG Elution Buffer: 100 m*M* glycine-HCl. Adjust pH to 2.5. Make fresh before use.
5. Neutralizing Buffer: 1 *M* Tris-HCl. Adjust pH to 9.0. Make fresh before use.
6. Dialysis membranes: 10K MWCO Slide-A-Lyzer cassettes and 10K MWCO SnakeSkin dialysis tubing (Pierce Chemical Company).

2.2. Phage Titering and Biopanning

1. 96-well microtiter plates: Nunc-Immuno™ Plate MaxiSorp™ Surface (Nalge Nunc International).
2. Coating Buffer A: 100 m*M* NaHCO₃. Adjust pH to 8.6. Autoclave and store at room temperature.
3. Blocking Buffer A: Coating buffer A plus 5 mg/mL bovine serum albumin (BSA; Sigma). Adjust pH to 8.6. Filter-sterilize and store at 4°C.
4. Ph.D.-C7C Phage library: 2×10^{13} pfu/mL stored in TBS with 50% glycerol at –20°C (New England Biolabs). Complexity of the library is 3.7×10^9 transformants (*see* **Note 1**).
5. Tris-Buffered Saline (TBS): 50 m*M* Tris-HCl, 150 m*M* NaCl. Adjust pH to 7.5. Autoclave and store at room temperature.
6. TBST: TBS plus 0.1% or 0.5% (v/v) Tween 20. Adjust pH to 7.5. Make fresh before use.
7. Phage Elution Buffer: 200 m*M* glycine-HCl. Adjust pH to 2.2. Autoclave and store at room temperature.
8. Neutralization Buffer (*see* **Subheading 2.1.**, step 5).
9. Phage host strains: *E. coli* ER2537 (New England Biolabs; *see* **Note 2**).
10. 2X M9 salts: 12 g Na₂HPO₄, 6 g KH₂PO₄, 1 g NaCl, 2 g NH₄Cl, qs to 1000 mL with deionized water. Filter-sterilize and store at room temperature.

11. Minimal Medium Agar (MMA): 500 mL 2X M9 salts, 500 mL 3% agar, 20 mL 20% glucose, 2 mL 1 M MgSO$_4$, 0.1 mL 1 M CaCl$_2$, 1 mL thiamine (10 mg/mL). Filter-sterilize the glucose and thiamine. Autoclave the remainder separately, cool to 70°C, and combine all components. Pour plates and store at 4°C.
12. LB Broth: 10 g tryptone, 5 g yeast extract, 5 g NaCl, qs to 1000 mL with dH$_2$0. Autoclave and store at room temperature.
13. LB Agar: LB broth plus 1.5% agar bacteriological (agar no.1). Autoclave, cool to 70°C before pouring plates. Store at 4°C.
14. Overlay Agarose: 10 g tryptone, 5 g yeast extract, 5 g NaCl, 1 g MgCl$_2$•6H$_2$O, 7 g agarose, qs to 1000 mL with deionized water. Autoclave, dispense into 50 mL aliquots, and store at room temperature. Prior to use, melt in a microwave oven then equilibrate to 45°C in a water bath.
15. Falcon 14-mL polypropylene round bottom "snap-cap" tubes (Becton Dickinson Labware).
16. PEG/NaCl: 20% (w/v) polyethylene glycol (PEG)-8000, 2.5 M NaCl. Autoclave and store at room temperature.

2.3. Nucleic Acid Isolation and Sequencing

1. Phage host strains (*see* **Subheading 2.2., item 9**).
2. LB Broth (*see* **Subheading 2.2., item 12**).
3. Falcon 14-mL polypropylene round-bottom "snap-cap" tubes.
4. Wooden tooth-picks: Autoclave to sterilize.
5. PEG/NaCl (*see* **Subheading 2.2., item 16**).
6. TE Buffer (TE): 10 mM Tris-HCl, 1 mM EDTA. Adjust pH to 8.0. Autoclave and store at room temperature.
7. Iodide Buffer: TE, 1 M NaI. Adjust pH to 8.0. Make fresh before use.
8. Ethanol (EtOH): 70% and absolute.
9. Sequencing primers:
   a. –96 pIII primer: 5'-CCCTCATAGTTAGCGTAACG-3'
   b. –28 pIII primer: 5'- GTATGGGATTTTGCTAAACAAC-3'

2.4. ELISAs

1. 96-well microtiter plates: Nunc-Immuno Plate MaxiSorp Surface.
2. Coating Buffer B: 1.59 g Na$_2$CO$_3$, 2.93 g NaHCO$_3$. Adjust pH to 9.6 and qs to 1000 mL with deionized water. Autoclave and store at room temperature.
3. NeutrAvidin Solution: Coating Buffer B plus 5 µg/mL NeutrAvidin (Pierce Chemical Company). Make fresh before each use.
4. BSA conjugated L3,7,9 LOS (*see* **Note 3**).
5. Synthetic peptides (*see* **Table 2**).
6. Phosphate-buffered saline (PBS): 16 g NaCl, 0.4 g KCl, 2.88 g Na$_2$HPO$_4$, 0.48 g KH$_2$PO$_4$. Adjust pH to 7.2 and qs to 2000 mL with deionized water. Autoclave and store at room temperature. It may be useful to make a 10X stock during frequent use.

Table 2
Sequence of the Consensus Peptides Synthesized
for Determining Binding Affinities to the Biopanning
Monoclonal Antibody 9-2-L379

Peptide[a]	Peptide sequence
C10-bio	amino-ACSWLHQPYCGGGSK-biotin
C22-bio	amino-ACNTIGGYECGGGSK-biotin

[a]The peptides were synthesized using standard FMOC chemistry (MedProbe, Oslo, Norway). Peptides were oxidized under controlled conditions in order to facilitate intramolecular-disulphide bridge formation between the cysteine residues located at positions C^2 and C^{10}. The resulting cyclic peptides were purified by high-performance liquid chromatography (HPLC) and determined to be >95% pure by mass spectrophotometer analysis.

7. Blocking Buffer B: PBS plus 3% (w/v) skim milk powder plus 0.05% (v/v) Tween 20. Adjust pH to 7.2. Make fresh prior to use.
8. PBST: PBS plus 0.05% (v/v) Tween 20. Adjust pH to 7.2. Make fresh prior to use.
9. Primary antibodies: 9-2-L379 MAb or mouse immune serum. Working concentration of the MAb should be determined prior to use.
10. Secondary antibody: Goat anti-mouse IgG (H + L) HRP conjugate (Sigma). Working concentration should be optimized prior to use.
11. HRP color development reagent: TM Blue; soluble form (Intergen Co.).
12. Stop Solution: $1\,M\,H_2SO_4$.

2.5. Immunization Studies

1. Synthetic peptides (*see* **Table 3**).
2. Carrier protein: BSA (Sigma).
3. Glutaraldehyde: Grade 1, 25% Aqueous solution (Sigma).
4. PBS (*see* **Subheading 2.4., item 6**).
5. Quenching Buffer: PBS, $1\,M$ glycine. Adjust pH to 7.2. Make fresh before each use.
6. 10K MWCO Slide-A-Lyzer cassettes.
7. Freund's complete adjuvant (FCA) and Freund's incomplete adjuvant (FIA; Sigma).
8. Balb/c mice: 45, female, ~14 g.

3. Methods

3.1. Target Molecule Purification (see Note 4)

1. Dialyze the ascites or hybridoma-culture supernatant against 3 changes of Start Buffer (4 L each time). Volumes <10 mL are most easily handled using the Slide-

**Table 3
Sequence of the Consensus Peptides Synthesized
for Conjugation to Carrier Protein**

Peptide	Peptide sequence
C10-K	amino-ACSWLHQPYCGGGSKKK-amide
C22-K	amino-ACNTIGGYECGGGSKKK-amide

A-Lyzer cassettes, whereas SnakeSkin dialysis tubing is best for samples >10 mL.

2. Pre-equilibrate the Protein G column with at least 5 column volumes of Start Buffer. Load the sample onto the column and wash with 5 column volumes of Start Buffer. Elute the bound MAb with 1–3 column volumes of IgG Elution Buffer (*see* **Note 5**). Collect 1.0-mL fractions into 1.5-mL microfuge tubes that contain 100 µL of Neutralizing Buffer.

3. Assay fractions for protein content at 210 nm. Pool positive fractions, dialyze against 3 changes of Start Buffer (4 L each time).

4. Determine the protein concentration of the dialyzed sample, then aliquot and store at –20°C until required for use (*see* **Note 6**).

3.2. Phage Titering

1. Inoculate 20 mL of LB Broth in a 250-mL Erlenmeyer flask with *E. coli* ER2537 picked fresh from a MMA plate. Incubate at 37°C with vigorous shaking until mid-log phase (OD_{600} ~0.5).

2. Melt the Overlay Agarose, dispense 3-mL aliquots into snap-cap tubes (1 for each phage dilution) and incubate in a 45°C water bath until required. Warm LB plates (1 for each phage dilution) to 37°C prior to use.

3. Prepare 10-fold dilutions of the phage stock in LB Broth. An amplified phage stock is ~10^{12}–10^{13} pfu/mL. Dispense 200 µL of the mid-log phase culture into microfuge tubes (1 for each phage dilution) and add 10 µL of each phage dilution to each tube. Vortex and incubate at room temperature for 1–5 min.

4. Transfer the infected cells one at a time to culture tubes containing the Overlay Agarose, vortex then quickly pour onto a pre-warmed LB plate. Tilt the plate to facilitate even spreading. Allow the plates to cool then incubate inverted overnight at 37°C.

5. Count plates that have ~10^2 plaques and multiply by the appropriate dilution factor to obtain a titer for the phage stock.

3.3. Biopanning

1. Day 1: Add 100 µL aliquots of the target molecule (9-2-L379 MAb) diluted in Coating Buffer A (50 µg/mL) to the wells of a microtiter plate and incubate overnight at 4°C. Make sure the plate is covered or placed in a humidification chamber.

2. Inoculate 5 mL of LB Broth in a snap-cap tube with *E. coli* ER2537 picked fresh from a MMA plate. Incubate overnight at 37°C with vigorous shaking. This will serve as a starter culture.

3. Day 2: Inoculate 50 mL of LB Broth in a 250-mL Erlenmeyer flask with 100 µL of the starter culture. Incubate at 37°C with vigorous shaking until required for use (this will serve as an *E. coli* source for phage titering and amplification).

4. Wash the wells 3× with TBST. Add 200 µL per well of the Blocking Buffer A and incubate for 60 min at room temperature.

5. Wash the wells 5× with TBST. Add 100 µL of the phage library diluted in TBST (10^{12} pfu/mL) to a well and incubate for 60 minutes at room temperature.

6. Wash the well 10× with TBST. Add 100 µL of the Phage-Elution Buffer to the well and incubate for 10 min at room temperature to elute bound phage. Pipet each eluate into 1.5-mL microfuge tubes containing 15 µL of Neutralization Buffer.

7. Titre 5 µL of the eluate to determine the number pfu recovered during the selection step.

8. Mix the remainder of the eluate with 20 mL of the *E. coli* inoculated prior to the start of the biopanning (cells should be in early-log phase at this point) and incubate at 37°C with vigorous shaking for 4–5 h.

9. Transfer the culture to a centrifuge tube and spin at 8,000*g* for 10 min at 4°C. Transfer the supernatant to a fresh tube and spin again.

10. Remove the upper 80% of the supernatant to a fresh tube and add a 1/6 volume of PEG/NaCl. Precipitate overnight at 4°C.

11. Day 3: Spin the precipitated supernatant at 8,000*g* for 10 min at 4°C. Discard the supernatant leaving the pellet behind and briefly spin again. Remove any excess liquid with a pipet.

12. Solubilize the pellet in 1 mL of TBS and transfer to a microfuge tube. Spin in a microfuge at top speed for 5 min at 4°C.

13. Transfer the supernatant to a fresh microfuge tube and precipitate with a 1/6 volume of PEG/NaCl for 1 h on ice. Spin for 5 min at 4°C. Discard the supernatant and briefly spin again. Remove any excess liquid with a pipet.

14. Solubilize the pellet in 200 µL of TBS and spin for 5 min at 4°C. Transfer the clarified supernatant to a fresh microfuge tube. This is the amplified phage stock. Titer 5 µL the supernatant and store the remainder at 4°C.

15. Add 100 µL aliquots of the target molecule (9-2-L379 MAb) diluted in Coating Buffer A (50 µg/mL) to the wells of a microtiter plate and incubate overnight at 4°C. Make sure the plate is covered or placed in a humidification chamber.

16. Inoculate 5 mL of LB Broth in a snap-cap tube with *E. coli* ER2537 to serve as a starter culture. Incubate overnight at 37°C with vigorous shaking.

17. Day 4: Conduct a second round of biopanning by repeating **steps 2–10**. This time, however, use the amplified phage stock prepared from the first round rather than the initial library stock. Increase the concentration of the Tween 20 in the TBST to 0.5% (v/v) for the wash steps.

18. Day 5: Repeat **steps 11–16**.

19. Day 6: Conduct a third round of biopanning by repeating **steps 2–7**. This time, however, use the amplified phage stock prepared from the second round rather than the first round. Maintain the concentration of the Tween 20 in the TBST at 0.5% (v/v) for the wash steps. Once the third round eluate has been used for titering, it should be mixed 1:1 with 40% glycerol and stored at –20°C until required (*see* **Note 7**).

20. Inoculate 5 mL of LB Broth in a snap-cap tube with *E. coli* ER2537 picked fresh from a MMA plate. Incubate overnight at 37°C with vigorous shaking.

3.4. Nucleic Acid Isolation and Sequencing

1. Day 7: Dilute the overnight culture (started on Day 6) 1:100 in LB Broth and dispense 36 × 1 mL aliquots into snap-cap tubes and number appropriately. Using sterile wooden toothpicks, transfer individual phage plaques (from the plates used for titering the third round eluate) into each tube. Use plates that have no more than 100 plaques.

2. Incubate the tubes with vigorous shaking at 37°C for 5 h.

3. Transfer the cultures to microfuge tubes and spin at top speed in a microfuge for 30 s. Transfer 500 μL of the supernatants to fresh tubes, mix 1:1 with 40% glycerol, and store at –20°C. Transfer the remaining 500 μL of the supernatants to fresh tubes, add 200 μL of PEG/NaCl, mix by inversion, then precipitate for 10 min at room temperature.

4. Spin the PEG precipitates for 10 min and discard the supernatants. Briefly spin again and remove the remainder of the liquid with a pipet.

5. Solubilize the pellet thoroughly in 100 μL of Iodide Buffer and add 250 μL of absolute EtOH. Incubate at room temperature for 10 min. Spin for 10 min and discard the supernatants. Wash the pellets with 70% EtOH and dry under vacuum. Solubilize the pellets in 30 μL of TE Buffer.

6. Sequence the DNA samples using the –28 or –96 pIII primers (*see* **Note 8**).

7. Translate the sequence data and search for peptide consensus motifs (*see* **Note 9**).

3.5. Peptide ELISAs (see Note 10)

1. Add 100 μL per well of the NeutrAvidin Solution to the microtitre plates and incubate overnight at 4°C. Make sure that the plate is covered or placed inside a humidification chamber.

2. Wash the wells with PBST. Add 200 μL per well of the Blocking Buffer B and incubate for 30 min at 37°C.

3. Wash the wells with PBST. Add 100 μL per well of the C10-bio or C22-bio peptides diluted in PBS (2 μg/mL) and incubate for 30 min at 37°C.

4. Wash the wells with PBST. Add 100 μL per well of the 1° antibodies (9-2-L379 MAb or mouse immune serum) diluted in Blocking Buffer B and incubate for 60 min at 37°C.

5. Wash the wells with PBST. Add 100 μL aliquots of the 2° antibody appropriately diluted in Blocking Buffer B and incubate for 60 min at 37°C.

6. Wash the wells with PBST. Add 100 µL per well of the TM Blue and develop (5–10 min at room temperature). Terminate the reaction by adding 100 µL per well of the Stop Solution. Read endpoint at 450 nm.

3.6. Competitive Inhibition ELISAs (see Note 11)

1. Dilute the 9-2-L379 mAb in Blocking Buffer B so that the absorbance of the solution is 0.75–1.0 when reacted against L3,7,9 LOS by ELISA.
2. Incubate the diluted MAb overnight at 4°C with varying concentrations of the C10-bio and C22-bio peptides. Incubate samples without the peptides to serve as positive controls. It is also useful to incubate an irrelevant peptide with the diluted MAb to serve as a negative control.
3. Add 100 µL per well of the BSA-L3,7,9 LOS conjugate diluted in Coating Buffer B (30 µg/mL) to the microtiter plates and incubate overnight at 4°C. Make sure that the plate is covered or placed inside a humidification chamber.
4. Wash the wells with PBST. Add 200 µL per well of the Blocking Buffer B and incubate for 30 min at 37°C.
5. Wash the wells with PBST. Add 100 µL per well of the peptide inhibited samples and incubate for 60 min at 37°C.
6. Wash the wells with PBST. Add 100-µL aliquots of the 2° antibody appropriately diluted in Blocking Buffer B and incubate for 60 min at 37°C.
7. Wash the wells with PBST. Add 100 µL per well of the TM Blue and develop (10–20 min at room temperature). Terminate the reaction by adding 100 µL per well of the Stop Solution. Read endpoint at 450 nm.

3.7. Immunization with Peptide Conjugates (see Note 12)

1. Solubilize BSA in PBS (2 mg/mL) and add 5 mL to a 10-mL bottle. Stir solution vigorously with magnetic stirrer bar.
2. Add 50 µL of the glutaraldehyde solution and continue stirring for 1 h at room temperature.
3. Dialyse overnight in the cold room with at least 3 changes of PBS (4 L each time).
4. Solubilize the C10-K and C22-K peptides in PBS (5 mg/mL). Mix 2 mL of a peptide solution with 1 mL (~2 mg) of glutaraldehyde-activated BSA and stir vigorously for 1 h at room temperature.
5. Add 0.5 mL of the Quenching Buffer and continue to stir for an additional 1 h.
6. Dialyse overnight in the cold room with at least 3 changes of deionized water (4 L each time) to eliminate unconjuagted peptide.
7. Transfer the conjugate solutions (C10-BSA and C22-BSA) to suitable tubes and lyophilize.
8. Re-suspend conjugates in PBS.
9. Immunize 3 groups of 15 Balb/c mice with C10-BSA, C22-BSA, or BSA emulsified 50/50 with FCA (see Note 13). Immunize each mouse subcutaneously with 25 µg of immunogen in a volume no greater than 100 µL.

10. Boost the mice on days 14 and 28 using FIA as the emulsifying agent. Cull mice in groups of 5 on days 14, 28, and 42. Store serum samples at −70°C until required for use.

11. Titer the serum samples against purified L3,7,9 LOS using ELISA to demonstrate their cross-reactive capacity. Also, titer against biotinylated peptides to determine the magnitude of the response against the conjugates.

4. Notes

1. Although the Ph.D.-C7C phage-display library was useful for identifying peptide mimics an L3,7,9 LOS epitope, the library best-suited for use with alternative target molecules will need to be empirically defined. It has been our experience, however, that carbohydrate mimics are best obtained from conformationally constrained display libraries.

2. *E. coli* ER2537 is an excellent host strain for the propagation of filamentous phage owing to its rapid growth rate. Other *E. coli* stains that harbor the F-factor can be substituted for ER2537 if this strain is not available. If using *E. coli* ER2537 as the host strain, however, it is important to maintain it on MMA in order to prevent the loss of the F-factor. Because ER2537 is Δ(*lac-proAB*), it will not grow on MMA unless complemented by the *proAB locus* on the F-factor. Plates should be incubated at 37°C and then stored at 4°C wrapped in parafilm for up to 1 mo.

3. Because purified LOS binds very poorly to the wells of microtiter plates, titering of antibodies against this antigen using ELISA is often complicated by a low signal-to-background ratio. We have found that by conjugating the LOS to BSA this problem can be rectified. Basically, 1 mg of LOS and 2 mg of BSA are solubilized in 900 μL of 100 m*M* MES buffer, pH 5.0, and stirred at room temperature. Add 100 μL of an 1-Ethyl-3-(3-Dimethylaminopropyl) carbodiimide Hydrochloride solution (EDC: 10 mg/mL in deionized water) and stir for a further 2 h at room temperature. Following this, the conjugate can be stored at −20°C until required. The simplicity of this approach is that no purification step is required prior to the use of the conjugate as a coating antigen.

4. The method described here is specific for the purification of IgG isotypes. If different target molecules are to be used for biopanning, alternative purification strategies should obviously be implemented.

5. One or five mL pre-packed HiTrap Protein G affinity columns should be chosen for use depending on the quantity of the MAb to be purified. For loading sample volumes >10 mL, a peristaltic pump is recommended rather than a syringe.

6. Once the target molecule has been purified, it is important to analyze the sample by SDS-PAGE in order to detect the presence of contaminants. If present during biopanning, contaminating antigens might facilitate the selection of irrelevant phage clones.

7. The plates used for titering phage eluates following the third round of biopanning can be utilized as a plaque source for nucleic acid sequencing. The plates, how-

ever, should be incubated for no longer than 18 h if they are to be used for this purpose.

8. In our lab, we employ an automated sequencing approach using the ABI PRISM BigDye Terminator Cycle Sequencing Ready Reaction Kit and an ABI PRISM 377 Sequencer. The –96 pIII primer is best-suited for this. If manual sequencing is to be conducted, then the –28 pIII primer should be used.

9. Once peptide consensus motifs have been identified, individual phage clones should be "re-panned" against a series of controls to demonstrate their affinity for the target molecule. For our purposes, the positive control was the 9-2-L379 MAb, while the negative controls were the MN14C11.6 MAb and BSA. Because MN14C11.6 is the same antibody subclass as the 9-2-L379 MAb, the specificity of the phage clones for the target associated paratope only can be assessed. The BSA control is useful for eliminating the "plastic binders."

10. When peptide motifs have been confirmed as carbohydrate mimics, they should be chemically synthesized to facilitate immunization studies. It is often useful to biotinylate some of the peptide sample for immuno-assay purposes. Biotinylated peptides can be readily immobilized on ELISA plates that have been "activated" with avidin, streptavidin, or NeutrAvidin.

11. The competitive inhibition assay outlined here is based on that described by Van Dam et al. *(32)*. Using this approach, 50% inhibitory concentrations (IC_{50}) can be calculated using the formula: $I(\%) = \{[A(O)-A(X)/A(O)]\}100\%$ where I = inhibition coefficient, $A(O)$ = the absorbance of the positive control minus the background, and $A(X)$ = the absorbance of a MAb dilution (+ inhibitor) minus the background. Using the I values as the ordinate and the corresponding inhibitor concentrations (in the MAb dilution) as the abscissa, inhibition curves can be constructed and the IC_{50} derived from these.

12. Because the N-terminal amino group associated with the peptides is a critical feature of the epitope recognized by the target molecule, we could not block this group nor couple the peptides to BSA through this end. By adding multiple lysine (K) residues to the C-terminus of the peptide, we have biased the coupling orientation of the peptides to the BSA carrier.

13. Immunization with phage particles is a suitable alternative to the use of peptide conjugates. When using this approach, mice should be inoculated with 10^{10}–10^{12} pfu/100 µL emulsified in FCA/FIA.

References

1. Twumasi, P. A., Jr., Kumah, S., Leach, A., O'Dempsey, T. J., Ceesay, S. J., Todd, J., et al. (1995) A trial of a group A plus group C meningococcal polysaccharide-protein conjugate vaccine in African infants. *J. Infect. Dis.* **171**, 632–638.

2. Anderson, E. L., Bowers, T., Mink, C. M., Kennedy, D. J., Belshe, R. B., Harakeh, H., et al. (1994) Safety and immunogenicity of meningococcal A and C polysaccharide conjugate vaccine in adults. *Infect. Immun.* **62**, 3391–3395.

3. Lieberman, J. M., Chiu, S. S., Wong, V. K., Partridge, S., Chang, S.-J., Chiu, C.-Y., et al. (1996) Safety and immunogenicity of a serogroups A/C *Neisseria meningitidis* oligosaccharide-protein conjugate vaccine in young children. *JAMA* **275**, 1499–1503.

4. Wyle, F. A., Artenstein, M. S., Brandt, B. L., Tramont, E. C., Kasper, D. L., Altieri, P. L., et al. (1972) Immunologic response of man to group B meningococcal polysaccharide vaccines. *J. Infect. Dis.* **126**, 514–521.

5. Granoff, D. M., Bartoloni, A., Ricci, S., Gallo, E., Rosa, D., Ravenscroft, N., et al. (1998) Bactericidal monoclonal antibodies that define unique meningococcal B polysaccharide epitopes that do not cross-react with human polysialic acid. *J. Immunol.* **160**, 5028–5036.

6. Finne, J., Leinonen, M., and Makela, P. H. (1983) Antigenic similarities between brain components and bacteria causing meningitis; implications for vaccine development and pathogenesis. *Lancet* **ii**, 335–337.

7. Diaz Romero, J. and Outschoorn, I. M. (1994) Current status of meningococcal group B vaccine candidates: capsular or noncapsular? *Clin. Microbiol. Rev.* **7**, 559–575.

8. Schneider, H., Hale, T. L., Zollinger, W. D., Seid, R. C., Hammack, C. A., and Griffiss, J. M. (1984) Heterogeneity of molecular size and antigenic expression within lipooligosaccharides of individual strains of *Neisseria gonorrhoeae* and *Neisseria meningitidis. Infect. Immun.* **45(3)**, 544–549.

9. Jennings, H. J., Beurret, M., Gamian, A., and Michon, F. (1987) Structure and immunochemistry of meningococcal lipopolysaccharides. *Antonie van Leeuwenhoek* **53**, 519–522.

10. Jennings, H. J., Bhattacharjee, A. K., Kenne, L., Kenny, C. P., and Calver, G. (1980) The R-type lipopolysaccharides of *Neisseria meningitidis. Can. J. Biochem.* **58**, 128–136.

11. Scholten, R. J., Kuipers, B., Valkenburg, H. A., Dankert, J., Zollinger, W. D., and Poolman, J. T. (1994) Lipo-oligosaccharide immunotyping of *Neisseria meningitidis* by a whole-cell ELISA with monoclonal antibodies. *J. Med. Microbiol.* **41**, 236–243.

12. Tsai, C. M., Mocca, L. F., and Frasch, C. E. (1987) Immunotype epitopes of *Neisseria meningitidis* lipooligosaccharide types 1 through 8. *Infect. Immun.* **55**, 1652–1656.

13. Tsai, C. M. and Civin, C. I. (1991) Eight lipooligosaccharides of *Neisseria meningitidis* react with a monoclonal antibody which binds lacto-N-neotetraose (Gal beta 1-4GlcNAc beta 1-3Gal beta 1-4Glc). *Infect. Immun.* **59**, 3604–3609.

14. Mandrell, R. E., Griffiss, J. M., and Macher, B. A. (1988) Lipooligosaccharides (LOS) of *Neisseria gonorrhoeae* and *Neisseria meningitidis* have components that are immunochemically similar to precursors of human blood group antigens. *J. Exp. Med.* **168**, 107–126.

15. Kahler, C. M., Martin, L. E., Shih, G. C., Rahman, M. M., Carlson, R. W., and Stephens, D. S. (1998) The (α2-8)-linked polysialic acid capsule and

lipooligosaccharide structure both contribute to the ability of serogroup B *Neisseria meningitidis* to resist the bactericidal activity of normal human serum. *Infect. Immun.* **66,** 5939–5947.

16. Estabrook, M. M., Griffiss, J. M., and Jarvis, G. A. (1997) Sialylation of *Neisseria meningitidis* lipooligosaccharide inhibits serum bactericidal activity by masking lacto-N-neotetraose. *Infect. Immun.* **65,** 4436–4444.

17. Mackinnon, F. G., Borrow, R., Gorringe, A. R., Fox, A. J., Jones, D. M., and Robinson, A. (1993) Demonstration of lipooligosaccharide immunotype and capsule as virulence factors for *Neisseria meningitidis* using an infant mouse intranasal infection model. *Microb. Pathog.* **15,** 359–366.

18. Jones, D. M., Borrow, R., Fox, A. J., Gray, S., Cartwright, K. A., and Poolman, J. T. (1992) The lipooligosaccharide immunotype as a virulence determinant in *Neisseria meningitidis*. *Microb. Pathog.* **13,** 219–224.

19. Dalseg, R., Wedege, E., Holst, J., Haugen, I. L., Hoiby, E. A., and Haneberg, B. (1999) Outer membrane vesicles from group B meningococci are strongly immunogenic when given intranasally to mice. *Vaccine* **17,** 2336–2345.

20. Fischer, M., Carlone, G. M., Holst, J., Williams, D., Stephens, D. S., and Perkins, B. A. (1999) *Neisseria meningitidis* serogroup B outer membrane vesicle vaccine in adults with occupational risk for meningococcal disease. *Vaccine* **17,** 2377–2383.

21. Quakyi, E. K., Frasch, C. E., Buller, N., and Tsai, C. M. (1999) Immunization with meningococcal outer-membrane protein vesicles containing lipooligosaccharide protects mice against lethal experimental group B *Neisseria meningitidis* infection and septic shock. *J. Infect. Dis.* **180,** 747–754.

22. Verheul, A. F., Braat, A. K., Leenhouts, J. M., Hoogerhout, P., Poolman, J. T., Snippe, H., and Verhoef, J. (1991) Preparation, characterization, and immunogenicity of meningococcal immunotype L2 and L3,7,9 phosphoethanolamine group-containing oligosaccharide-protein conjugates. *Infect. Immun.* **59,** 843–851.

23. Glucksman, M. J., Bhattacharjee, S., and Makowski, L. (1992) Three-dimensional structure of a cloning vector. X-ray diffraction studies of filamentous bacteriophage M13 at 7 Å resolution. *J. Mol. Biol.* **226,** 455–470.

24. Rasched, I. and Oberer, E. (1986) Ff coliphages: structural and functional relationships. *Microbiol. Rev.* **50,** 401–427.

25. Russel, M. (1991) Filamentous phage assembly. *Mol. Microbiol.* **5,** 1607–1613.

26. Makowski, L. (1993) Structural constraints on the display of foreign peptides on filamentous bacteriophages. *Gene* **128,** 5–11.

27. Greenwood, J., Willis, A. E., and Perham, R. N. (1991) Multiple display of foreign peptides on a filamentous bacteriophage. Peptides from *Plasmodium falciparum* circumsporozoite protein as antigens. *J. Mol. Biol.* **220,** 821–827.

28. De Bolle, X., Laurent, T., Tibor, A., Godfroid, F., Weynants, V., Letesson, J. J., and Mertens, P. (1999) Antigenic properties of peptidic mimics for epitopes of the lipopolysaccharide from Brucella. *J. Mol. Biol.* **294,** 181–191.

29. Lowman, H. B. (1997) Bacteriophage display and discovery of peptide leads for drug development. *Ann. Rev. Biophys. Biomol. Struct.* **26,** 401–424.

30. Lowman, H. B., Bass, S. H., Simpson, N., and Wells, J. A. (1991) Selecting high-affinity binding proteins by monovalent phage display. *Biochemistry* **30,** 10,832–10,838.

31. Poolman, J. T., Kriz, Kuzemenska, P., Ashton, F., Bibb, W., Dankert, J., et al. (1995) Serotypes and subtypes of *Neisseria meningitidis*: results of an international study comparing sensitivities and specificities of monoclonal antibodies. *Clin. Diagn. Lab. Immunol.* **2,** 69–72.

32. Van Dam, G. J., Verheul, A. F., Zigterman, G. J., De Reuver, M. J., and Snippe, H. (1989) Estimation of the avidity of antibodies in polyclonal antisera against Streptococcus pneumoniae type 3 by inhibition ELISA. *Mol. Immunol.* **26,** 269–274.

15

Testing Meningococcal Vaccines for Mitogenicity and Superantigenicity

Alexei A. Delvig, John H. Robinson, and Lee Wetzler

1. Introduction

Proteins with intrinsic mitogenic properties are widely represented in prokaryotes, such as in different *Streptococcus* species *(1–3)*, *Candida albicans (4)*, and *Eikenella corrodens (5)*. Specifically, several bacterial porins of *Escherichia coli*, *Shigella dysenteriae*, *Salmonella typhimurium*, *Fusobacterium nucleatum*, and pathogenic *Neisseria* species have been shown to induce nonspecific proliferation of lymphocytes *(6–12)*.

As early as in 1983, heat-killed meningococci and outer-membrane fractions derived thereof were described to induce lipopolysaccharide (LPS)-independent proliferation of B cells *(13)*, which was recently attributed to the outer-membrane porins *(14)*. In the latter study, the authors purified two porins from *Neisseria gonorrhoeae* (Protein IA and Protein IB) and two porins from *N. meningitidis* (class I protein [PorA] and class 3 protein [PorB]) to show that all four Neisserial porins were mitogenic for B cells in vitro and enhanced the expression of MHC class II, CD86, and intercellular adhesion molecule-1 (ICAM-1) molecules on this lymphocyte subpopulation. Interestingly, purified Neisserial porins had minimal effect on intact T cells or T cells activated by CD3 or T-cell receptor (TCR) cross-linking. In view of the fact that meningococcal porins are important protective components of meningococcal serogroup B vaccines *(15)* and efficient carriers for other vaccines *(16)*, it is important that porins in the particular protein vaccine formulation do not cause polyclonal activation (mitogenesis) of lymphocytes. Indeed, the initial B-cell polyclonal activation caused by several pathogenic microorganisms has been shown to lead paradoxically to subsequent immunosuppression and susceptibility to

From: *Methods in Molecular Medicine, vol. 66: Meningococcal Vaccines: Methods and Protocols*
Edited by: A. J. Pollard and M. C. J. Maiden © Humana Press Inc., Totowa, NJ

infection *(17)*, which at least partially can be accounted for by the ability of some pathogens and their products to induce apoptosis in different cell types. Thus, gonococcal PorB porin has been shown to trigger apoptosis in epithelial cells and monocytes by inducing calcium flux from the extracellular space, activation of cysteine proteases of the caspase family (e.g., caspase-3) and the calcium-activated cysteine protease calpain in the cytosol of target cells *(18)*. These authors hypothesized that upon translocation of Neisserial porins into the host membranes and reduction in intracellular ATP concentration, porin pores would initiate triggering of the programmed cell-death sequence consisting of cell-membrane depolarization, calcium flux, and activation of caspases. Indeed, according to our unpublished observations, different formulations of outer-membrane vesicle (OMV) vaccines may acquire mitogenic properties for B and T cells leading to apoptosis of lymphocytes. Consequently, it is becoming increasingly important to screen all potential meningococcal vaccines for nonspecific immunomodulation, owing to the risk of adverse effects such mitogenicity may have on vaccinees. The question of whether the presence of the mitogenic activity, especially for antigen-presenting cells (APCs) (including B cells), as well as for T cells, is beneficial or detrimental is controversial. On one hand, the efficacy of a vaccine might depend on the mitogenic activity of its components (such as porins or LPS) to allow induction of a robust and long-lived protective immune response. This might especially be true if some of the components of the vaccine are T-cell independent antigens, like bacterial capsular polysaccharide. This is the basis for the successful development of conjugate vaccines using bacterial polysaccharide conjugated to Neisserial porins, including *Haemophilus (19)*, *Streptococcus (20,21)*, and, significantly for this chapter, *N. meningitidis (22,23)*. Moreover, the presence of mitogenic activity in meningococcal-vaccine candidates can have a specific adjuvant effect precluding the use of potentially toxic adjuvants like alum, monophosphoryl lipid A, or non-ionic block polymers. However, on the other hand it is also believed that nonspecific immune stimulation by mitogens potentially present in vaccines might have a detrimental systemic effect, seen occasionally with the administration of potent immune stimulators like LPS, cytokines, and so on. This chapter cannot address this issue in its entirety and only offers various methods to measure the mitogenic activity of potential meningococcal vaccines. However, it is likely that some nonspecific mitogenic activity will need to be present, as either an inherent part of the vaccine, or added by the addition of various adjuvants, to allow maximum efficacy of the vaccines.

Here we described several methods to test candidate vaccines for potential LPS-independent non-antigen specific polyclonal activation of murine B and

T lymphocytes in mouse systems in vitro. Mitogenic responses of murine lymphocytes are assayed using routine proliferation methods in unseparated lymphoid spleen cells obtained from naïve animals. This is followed by more advanced techniques using purified and cloned lymphocytes to evaluate the mechanisms of the mitogenic effects for B- and T-cell compartments that enable polyclonal activation and superantigenicity to be distinguished. Finally, flow-cytometry assays allowing detection of early stages of apoptosis occurring in mononuclear cells and lymphocyte subpopulations are described.

2. Materials
2.1. Strains of Mice

1. BALB/c ($H-2^d$) and BALB.K ($H-2^k$). The combination of these strains addresses whether the responses are not restricted to the particular H-2 haplotype ($H-2^d$ versus $H-2^k$).
2. BALB/c ($H-2^d$) and B10.D2 ($H-2^d$). This combination addresses whether the responses are dependent on non-MHC genes (BALB/c vs B10.D2, both $H-2^d$).
3. C3H/HeJ ($H-2^k$). This strain of mice has been shown to be LPS-hyporesponsive owing to three specific defects in the cytoplasmic portion of the LPS coreceptor-Toll Like Receptor 4 (TLR4) *(24–26)*. TLR4 is essential for transduction of a signal upon binding of LPS to its receptor CD14, which explains why mice with defective TLR4 (such as strains C3H/HeJ and B10SnCCR) respond extremely poorly to LPS. However, these strains of mice retain the ability to respond to other immune stimulators, such as tumor necrosis factor (TNF)-α, interferon (IFN)-γ, interleukin (IL)-1, and to the TLR-independent mitogens, such as ConA, phytohemagglutinin (PHA), lipopeptides, muramyldipeptide and, importantly, to Neisserial porin proteins.
4. C3H/HeOuJ. This strain is similar in all respects to strain C3H/HeJ, but has an intact TLR4 gene and therefore is characterized by the normal response to LPS.

2.2. Culture Media, Materials, and Equipment
2.2.1. Culture Media

1. The complete RPMI 1640 medium: RPMI 1640 (Sigma Chemical Co., supplied in 500-mL bottles, #R0883), 3.0 mM L-glutamine (Sigma, #G7513, supplied in 100-mL bottles), 0.05 mM 2-mercaptoethanol (2-ME, Sigma, #M7522, supplied in 100-mL bottles, 14.3 M stock) and 10% fetal bovine serum (v/v) (FBS, Sigma, #F7524, supplied in 500-mL bottles) (*see* **Note 1**). High concentration stock of 2-ME is prepared (0.0143 M in sterile deionized water) and stored at 2–8°C. The complete RPMI 1640 medium is used in proliferation assays.
2. RPMI with antibiotics (R10 + antibiotics medium): RPMI 1640 (BioWhittaker, #12-702F) pH 7.4, 10% fetal calf serum (FCS, HyClone Laboratories, Inc., Logan UT, #A-1111L, heat inactivate 56°C for 30 min, then store at –20°C in

50-mL aliquots; *see* **Note 1**), 50 μM 2-ME (JT Baker, Phillipsburg, NJ, #4049-00), 2 mM glutamine (BioWhittaker, #17-605E), 100 U/mL penicillin, and 100 μg/mL streptomycin (BioWhittaker, #17-602E).

3. Hanks' Balanced Salt Solution, Modified, (HBSS; Sigma, supplied in 500-mL bottles, #H8264).

4. Diluent for flow cytometry: HBSS supplemented with 2% FBS, 0.01 M HEPES buffer (Sigma, #H0887, stock 1.0 M, supplied in 100-mL bottles) and 0.1% Sodium Azide (NaN$_3$, Sigma, #S8032, stock 10.0% in sterile deionized water and stored at room temperature). Stored at 2–8°C.

5. Medium for B cell isolation: HBSS without Calcium chloride, Magnesium sulphate, and phenol red (Ca/Mg-free HBSS) (Sigma, #H6648) supplemented with 5 mM ethylenediaminetetraacetic acid (EDTA) (Sigma, #E6758) and 0.5% bovine serum albumin (BSA; fraction V, Sigma, #A4503). Stored at 2–8°C.

6. Phosphate-buffered saline (PBS; Dulbecco 'A', OXOID, #BR14a). Dissolve 1 tablet in 100 mL deionized water, autoclave at 115°C for 10 min.

7. Medium for lymphocyte staining: PBS containing 2% FCS. Prepare 500-mL aliquots, sterile-filter, and re-filter prior to each use. It must be filtered to remove particles.

8. MiniMACS separation buffer (PBS supplemented with 5 mM EDTA and 0.5% BSA). Stored at 2–8°C.

9. Stock solution of Penicillin (10,000 U/mL) and Streptomycin (10,000 μg/mL) (in PBS with 2% FCS) (BioWhittaker, #17-602E), use at a dilution of 1 : 100.

10. Proteose Peptone #3 (DIFCO, #0122-17-4) used for meningococcal media.

11. Neisseria liquid media: double-distilled water, 250 mL; Proteose Peptone, 15.0g (Difco #0122-17-4); K$_2$HPO$_4$, 4.0g; KH$_2$PO$_4$, 1.0 g; NaCL, 5.0 g; add ddH$_2$O to 1000 mL. Following autoclaving (115°C, 10 min), add Isovitalex Enrichment BBL 10 mL/L (1% solution, Fisher #B11876).

2.2.2. Antibodies, Conjugates, and Complement

All reagents are stored at 2–8°C. Each lot of MAb has its optimal concentration to use in flow cytometry. This should be determined experimentally. Most MAb will stain well at 10 μg/mL.

1. Anti-mouse CD3 ε chain FITC-labeled MAb (clone 145-2C11; PharMingen, #01084D, 0.5 mg) (an alternative supplier: Caltag, #RM3401-3).

2. Anti-mouse CD4 (rat IgG2b, TIB 207, clone GK1.5, ATCC).

3. Anti-mouse CD4 FITC-labeled MAb (Caltag, #RM2501-3).

4. Anti-mouse CD8 (rat IgG2b, TIB 211, clone 3.155, ATCC).

5. Anti-mouse CD8 FITC-labeled MAb (Caltag, #RM2201-3).

6. Anti-mouse CD11b/Mac1 FITC-labeled MAb (macrophage-specific) (Caltag, #RM2801).

7. Anti-mouse CD16/CD32 MAb (Fc Block®, clone 2.4G2 specific for FcγIII/II Receptor, PharMingen, #01241D, 0.5 mg).

8. Anti-mouse CD19 PE-labeled MAb (clone 1D3, PharMingen, #09655B, 0.2 mg, pre-dilute 1 : 30).
9. Anti-mouse CD45R/B220 FITC-labeled MAb (B cell-specific) (clone RA3-6B2, PharMingen, #01124D, 0.5 mg).
10. Anti-mouse CD45/B220 PE-labeled MAb (B cell-specific) (Caltag, San Diego, CA, #RM2604-3).
11. Anti-mouse CD80/B7-1 FITC-labeled MAb (PharMingen, #09604D).
12. Anti-mouse CD86/B7-2 FITC-labeled MAb (Pharmingen, #09274D).
13. Anti-mouse CD90.2/Thy1.2 FITC-labeled MAb (T cell-specific) (PharMingen, #01004D).
14. Anti-FITC MicroBeads (Miltenyi Biotec, #487-01, supplied in 2.0-mL vials). Magnetic beads for magnetic isolation of B cells.
15. Anti-mouse $\alpha\beta$TCR PE-labeled MAb (PharMingen, #01305A, 1.0 mg, pre-dilute 1 : 500).
16. Isotype control antibodies:
    a. rat IgG2bκ fluorescein isothiocyonate (FITC)-labeled (PharMingen, #11034C, 0.25 mg).
    b. rat IgG2aκ PE-labeled (PharMingen, #11025A, 0.1 mg).
17. Mouse TCR Vβ Screening Panel (PharMingen, #0143KK). This kit contains 15 prediluted FITC-conjugated MAb against: TCR Vβ2; Vβ3; Vβ4; Vβ5.1,5.2; Vβ6; Vβ7; Vβ8.1,8.2; Vβ8.3; Vβ9; Vβ10[b]; Vβ11; Vβ12; Vβ13; Vβ14; and Vβ17[a]. The kit is sufficient to perform 50 tests.
18. Anti-mouse Thy1.2 (T cell-specific)(mouse IgM), TIB 188, clone HO.13.4, American Type Culture Collection (ATCC, Rockville, MD).
19. Anti-mouse MHC class II, I-A^k (used for labeling cells from C3H/HeJ and C3H/OuJ mice) (IgG2b, TIB 93, clone 10.2.16, ATCC).
20. Anti-mouse class MHC II, I-A^d (used for labeling cells from BALB/c and B10.D2 mice) (IgG2b, TIB 120, clone M5/114.15.2, ATCC).
21. Anti-murine MHC class II, I-A^d FITC-labeled MAb (PharMingen #06034D).
22. Guinea Pig Complement (Cappel, Westchester, PA, #55854).

2.2.3. Materials

1. 7-Amino-actinomycin D (Via-Probe™, PharMingen, #34321X, 100 tests). Stored at 2–8°C.
2. 96-well tissue-culture plates (Costar Scientific, Corning, NY, Fisher, Inc., #3595).
3. Annexin V FITC-labeled (PharMingen, #65874X, 100 tests). Stored at 2–8°C.
4. CM Sepharose CL-6B (Sigma, #CCL-6B-100).
5. DEAE Sepahrose CL-6B (Sigma, #DCL-6B-100).
6. Ficoll 400 (Sigma, #F-4375).
7. Hypaque (Sigma, #S-4506).
8. Lymphoprep™ (Nycomed, #221395) is used for separation of lymphocytes by density centrifugation. Stored at 2–8°C.

9. MiniMACS Separation Columns (type MS, Miltenyi Biotec Inc., #422-01). One column is used for separation of 10^7 lymphocytes.
10. Nylon wool (for depletion of B cells) (Robbins Scientific Corporation, #1078-02-0).
11. Propidium iodide (PI) Staining Solution (PharMingen, #66211E).
12. Recombinant mouse IL-2 (Cambridge BioScience, #CMI-038).
13. Sephacryl S-300 (Sigma, #S-300-HR).
14. TiterMax Adjuvant (Sigma, #H4397, supplied in 0.5-mL vials) is used for footpad immunizations of mice. Stored at 2–8°C (*see* **Note 2**).
15. Tritiated thymidine (Amersham, #TRA310, specific activity 2.0 Ci/mmol). High-concentration stock is prepared (14.8 µCi/mL in complete RPMI 1640 medium). An alternative supplier: New England Nuclear (Boston, MA #NET-027). Stored at 2–8°C.
16. Tubes for flow cytometry (polystyrene tubes, size 12 × 75 mm, Elkay Eireann, #000-2052-001).
17. Type A/E Glass-fiber filter (Gelman Sciences, #p/n 61638, size 20.3 × 25.4 cm). Cut the filters to the size of a 96-well plate 8.0 × 12.5 cm).
18. Zwittergent 3-14 (Calbiochem, #693017).

2.2.4. Equipment

1. Cell harvester, such as Packard Micromate 196 (Packard, Canberra Packard, Berks, U.K).
2. Beta counter, such as Packard Matrix 9600 (Packard Instrument Company, Meridan, CT).
3. MiniMACS Separation Unit (High-energy permanent magnet, Miltenyi Biotec, #421.02).
4. MACS MultiStand (holds up to 4 MiniMACS Separation Units, Miltenyi Biotec, #423-03).
5. Flow cytometer, such as Becton Dickinson FACScan® (Becton Dickinson, Mount View, CA).
6. CellQuest™ Analysis and Acquisition Software (Becton Dickinson on Macintosh G4 computer).
7. Scintillation counter (Tracor Analytic Delta300, Searle Analytic, Inc.).

2.3. Test Vaccines and Control Antigens

2.3.1. Test Vaccines

The methods described in this chapter were set up to test protein-related LPS-independent mitogenicity of noncapsular meningococcal vaccines, such that any vaccine of this type can be used.

2.3.2. Control Antigens

1. Concanavalin A from *Canavalia ensiformis* type IV-S (ConA, Sigma, #C5275) is a lectin with mitogenic properties for T cells. High-concentration stock of ConA is prepared (1.0 mg/mL, sterile deionized water) and stored at –20°C.

2. LPS (*E. coli*, serotype 0111:B4, Sigma, #L4130) is a potent B-cell mitogen. Stock solution of LPS is prepared (1.0 mg/mL) and stored at –20°C. Meningococcal LPS can also be used.
3. Ovalbumin (OVA) (Albumin, Chicken Egg, grade VII, Sigma, #A7641) is used as a control protein antigen to distinguish antigen-specific from antigen nonspecific responses in activated lymphocytes.
4. Staphylococcal enterotoxin B from *S. aureus* (SEB, Sigma, #S4881) is a potent superantigen specific for murine TCR Vβ8 T cells, as shown previously (*27*).
5. Pure Neisserial porins and proteosomes (*see* **Note 3** for details of the purification procedure).

3. Methods

Testing vaccines for mitogenicity and superantigenicity consists of several separate procedures:

1. Testing antigen-nonspecific (mitogenic) proliferative responses in naïve mice.
2. Testing antigen-specific vs antigen-nonspecific (mitogenic) proliferative responses in activated mononuclear cells.
3. Testing mitogenicity for purified naïve B and T lymphocytes.
4. Testing the effect of the test vaccines on B-cell activation.
5. Testing mitogenicity for ConA-activated T lymphocytes.
6. Testing for superantigenicity for naïve T lymphocytes.
7. Testing for apoptosis of mononuclear cells.

The procedures described in **Subheadings 3.1.** and **3.2.** are essential for establishing whether or not the particular test vaccine is mitogenic. Should the test vaccine be found mitogenic, all other tests are to be performed to assess the particular subpopulation of lymphocytes affected (**Subheadings 3.3., 3.4.,** and **3.5.**), to check superantigenicity for T lymphocytes (**Subheading 3.6.**), and to determine whether mitogenic activation leads to apoptosis of mononuclear cells and particular lymphocyte subpopulations (**Subheading 3.7.**).

3.1. Testing Antigen-Nonspecific (Mitogenic) Proliferative Responses in Naïve Mice

The experimental protocol described in **Subheadings 3.1.** and **3.2.** were adjusted for measuring antigen nonspecific proliferative responses occurring within first 1–2 d in the mouse system. The lack of mitogenicity is established if no lymphocyte proliferation is observed to the test vaccine: 1) in naïve mice (*see* **Subheading 3.1.**), and 2) after foot-pad immunization with OVA (*see* **Subheading 3.2.**). Mitogenic responses are characterized by the vigorous proliferation of lymphocytes to the test vaccine: 1) in naïve mice, and 2) in mice immunized with OVA (**Fig. 1 A, B,** respectively). Note that the antigen-specific responses develop later in the mouse system, such that responses to OVA in OVA-immunized mice (**Fig. 1B**) are still relatively low.

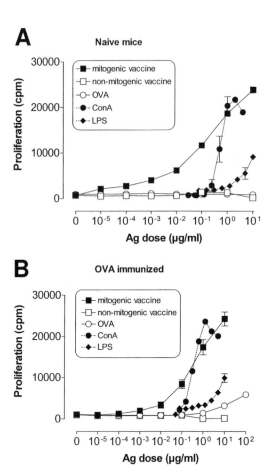

Fig. 1. Dose-response curves representing proliferation of lymphocytes from BALB/c mice in response to a mitogenic vaccine (closed squares), nonmitogenic vaccine (open squares), OVA (open circles), Con A (closed circles), or LPS (diamonds) (*see* **Note 4**). (**A**) Proliferative responses in spleen cells from naïve mice. (**B**) Proliferative responses in PLN cells from OVA-immunized mice. Error bars denote SD of the mean. The mitogenic meningococcal vaccine was deoxycholate-extracted outer-membrane vesicle (OMV) vaccine from the PorB-deficient strain 44-76/HIII5 *(42)* grown in a synthetic medium with high aeration (60%). The nonmitogenic meningococcal vaccine was prepared under GMP conditions for human vaccines from strain 44/76 (ET-5 complex; B:15:P1.7,16:P5.5,C:L3,7) grown in Frantz medium with lower aeration. This particular strain was used for production of the Norwegian OMV vaccine *(44)*.

1. Obtain spleen cells from naïve mice (*see* **Subheading 2.1.**) and add them to the round-bottomed 96-well microtiter plates (at 3×10^5/well) to test mitogenic activity of test vaccines for naïve lymphocytes.
2. Prepare a 10-fold dilution series of test vaccine or OVA (100 µg/mL starting concentration), and a twofold dilution series of ConA or LPS (starting concentration 10 µg/mL) in sterile, round-bottomed, 96-well microtiter plates in triplicates (*see* **Note 4**). Use the wells containing complete RPMI 1640 medium alone as a negative control.
3. Incubate plates for 24 h at 37°C in a humidified CO_2 incubator, pulse triplicate cultures overnight with 0.3 µCi/well of [^{3}H]-thymidine (20 µL of concentrated stock 14.8 µCi/mL) and harvest on Type A/E glass-fiber filters using a cell harvester. Measure the amount of radioactivity in each well using a beta counter.

3.2. Testing Antigen-Specific vs Antigen-Nonspecific (Mitogenic) Proliferative Responses in Activated Mononuclear Cells

1. Immunize mice (BALB/c, BALB.K, B10.D2, and C3H/HeJ; 2 animals each) in foot pads with 10 µg of the test vaccine, or the irrelevant antigen OVA emulsified in TiterMax adjuvant according to the manufacturer's instructions (*see* **Note 2**).
2. Seven days later, get the popliteal lymph nodes (PLN) cells and distribute them in sterile round-bottomed 96-well microtiter plates (at 2×10^5/well). Prepare a 10-fold dilution series of the test vaccine or OVA (100 µg/mL starting concentration) (*see* **Note 4**), and a twofold dilution series of ConA or LPS (10 µg/mL starting concentration) in the control wells in triplicates.
3. After 24 h incubation, pulse triplicate cultures overnight with 0.3 µCi of [^{3}H]-thymidine (20 µL of concentrated stock 14.8 µCi/mL) and harvest, as described in **Subheading 3.1., step 3**.

3.3. Testing Mitogenicity for Purified Naïve B and T Lymphocytes

This method assays mitogenic properties of test vaccines with respect to naïve B and T lymphocytes. The method involves magnetic separation of B lymphocytes, which also provides a sample of enriched T lymphocytes. The procedure described yields approx $1-2 \times 10^7$ positively selected 97–99% pure B lymphocytes (B220$^+$ by flow cytometry), as well as $3-5 \times 10^6$ negatively-selected 75% pure T lymphocytes (CD3$^+$ by flow cytometry). For separation of B and T lymphocytes, we modified the method described elsewhere *(28)*. Murine B and T cells can be also obtained from single-cell suspensions of splenocytes *(29)* (*see* **Note 5**).

Figure 2 shows that both fractions of lymphocytes showed typical patterns of proliferative responses either to the B-cell mitogen LPS or to the T-cell mitogen Con A. A strong mitogenic effect with respect to purified B cells, as well as to enriched T-cell populations, was characteristic for the mitogenic

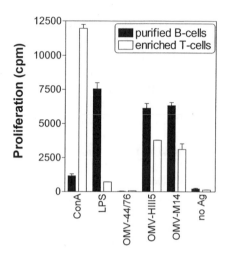

Fig. 2. Proliferation of different lymphocyte subsets to different mitogenic stimuli in vitro. Responses of purified B cells (filled bars) and enriched T cells (empty bars) fractions obtained by magnetic beads from spleens of naïve BALB/c mice. OMV-M14 was extracted from the PorA-deficient strain *(42)*. Other details as in the legend to **Fig. 1**.

OMV vaccine. The purity of B cells used also suggests that the mitogenic OMV vaccine could directly stimulate B cells. In contrast, no mitogenic responses were detected when the nonmitogenic OMV vaccine was tested. Typical results using purified gonococcal Por are displayed in **Fig. 3**. Note that Por-induced proliferation of HeJ B cells, while both Por or LPS induces proliferation of HeOuJ B cells. Neither Por or LPS induces T-cell proliferation.

1. Use spleen cells from 4 naïve BALB/c mice for isolation of B lymphocytes. Place spleen cells in glass flasks and allow them to adhere for 90 min at 37°C in a humidified CO_2 incubator.
2. Discard adherent cells (dendritic cells and macrophages), collect the remaining cells (B and T lymphocytes), and wash them in medium for B-cell isolation. Add anti-CD45R/B220 FITC-labeled MAb (diluted 1 : 250) to the cell suspension and incubate for 30 min at 4°C. Add 1.0 mL MiniMACS buffer and collect cells by centrifugation (200g, 5 min).
3. Add 80 µL MiniMACS buffer and 20 µL anti-FITC MicroBeads to the cells, and incubate cells for 15 min at 4°C. Add 1.9 mL MiniMACS buffer is added, and proceed with the magnetic isolation procedure, as described in **Subheading 2.2.4.–3.3.5.**
4. Place two MiniMACS Separation Columns on the MiniMACS Separation Unit attached to the MACS MultiStand. Wash the Separation columns twice with 0.5 mL MiniMACS buffer, and label the cell suspension with anti-FITC MicroBeads from

C3H/HeJ (LPS Non-responsive)

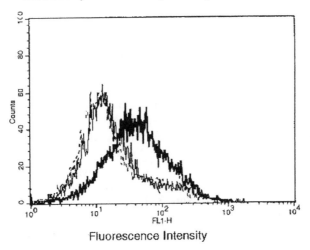

Fluorescence Intensity

C3H/HeOuJ (LPS Responsive)

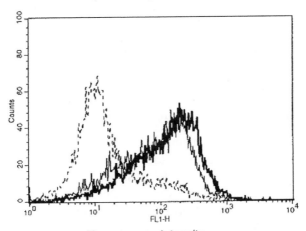

Fluorescence Intensity

Fig. 3. Purified B lymphocytes from either the LPS nonresponsive murine strain C3H/HeJ and from the LPS responsive strain C3H/HeOuJ at a concentration of 5×10^6 per mL were incubated with purified Neisserial LPS (10 µg/mL, 3 nM), Protein IB (PIB)(10 µg/mL, 0.3 nM) or medium alone for 48 h. The surface expression of B7-2 (CD86) was then determined by labeling with anti-B7-2-FITC conjugate and subsequent analysis by flow cytometry. Ten thousand cells were analyzed per sample. Media incubated B lymphocytes, dashed line; LPS incubated B lymphocytes, thin solid line; PIB incubated B lymphocytes, thick solid line. The data displayed is from one typical experiment, experiments were performed three times. Adapted with permission from **ref. *14***.

step 2, and add cells in two 0.5-mL portions to each column. Wash the columns 3 times with 0.5 mL MiniMACS buffer to remove unbound cells (according to our experience, this fraction of negatively-selected cells contains about 75% $\alpha\beta T$ cells).

5. Remove MiniMACS Separation Columns from the MiniMACS Separation Unit, and wash the columns twice with 0.5 mL MiniMACS buffer to elute B lymphocytes. Collect the positively selected cells by centrifugation (200g, 5 min) and resuspend B cells in complete RPMI 1640 medium.

6. To test the mitogenic effect of the test vaccine selectively on B and/or T cells, place positively and negatively selected cell populations from spleen in round-bottomed, 96-well microtiter plates (at 2×10^5/well) and mix them with the complete RPMI 1640 medium (or R10 + antibiotics medium, (negative control), or with the following antigens: 10 µg/mL test vaccines or 10 µg/mL (0.3 nM) porin proteins or proteosomes *see* **Note 3**, 10 µg/mL (approx 3 nM) LPS, 5 µg/mL Con A, 10 µg/mL OVA (*see* **Note 4**). Purified B lymphocytes could be also incubated with dextran (20 µg/mL) (Sigma), which has been previously shown to induce activation markers, including the costimulatory molecules B7-1 or B7-2, on the surface of B lymphocytes *(30)*.

7. After 48 h incubation, pulse triplicate cultures with tritiated thymidine as described in **Subheading 3.1., step 3**. Alternatively, pulse the cells with 1 µCi ^{3}H-thymidine (10 µL of a 100 µCi/mL solution) per well. After an additional 18 h incubation, harvest the wells onto filter paper discs and quantitate the ^{3}H -thymidine incorporation on a beta scintillation counter (such as in **Subheading 2.2.4., item 7**), as a measure of porin- or LPS-induced proliferation.

3.4. Testing the Effect of the Test Vaccines on B-Cell Activation

Potential vaccine antigens, membrane fragments, and purified porin proteins are tested for the ability to induce B-cell activation, i.e., induction of MHC class II molecules and CD80/CD86 expression. The expression of B-lymphocyte surface antigens that can be altered upon activation is studied by flow cytometry of single-cell suspension using a flow cytometer (such as in **Subheading 2.2.4., item 5**) and software (such as CellQuest™). To demonstrate that the stimulatory ability of the test vaccine or the porin protein is *not* LPS-dependent, B cells from the hyporesponsive murine strain, C3H/HeJ are used. To further support his hypothesis, B cells from these mice and from LPS-responsive mice C3H/HeOuJ can be incubated with LPS at a concentration between 0.01 and 10 µg/mL. B cells from C3H/HeJ mice should only respond to Por, whereas C3H/OuJ B cells should respond to both LPS and Por.

1. Incubate B lymphocytes (5×10^6/mL) in R10 + antibiotics medium with Por/ proteosomes at a concentration of 10 µg/mL, for 48 h in a humidified, 5% CO_2 incubator at 37°C in 96-well, sterile tissue-culture plates. Use wells incubated with dext-

ran (20 µg/mL) as a positive control, and wells containing R10 + antibiotics medium alone as a negative control. Harvest the B cells and separate life cells from dead cells and debris by density-gradient centrifugation with Ficoll-Hypaque. Test cell viability by trypan blue exclusion.

2. Collect the cells by centrifugation (400g, 10 min), and resuspend in R10 + antibiotics medium or medium for lymphocyte staining at a density of 10^5–10^7 cells per mL. To reduce the nonspecific labeling, block Fcγ receptors by Fc Block (20 µL of 1 : 50 dilution per tube in diluent for flow cytometry) and incubate cells for 30 min at 4–8°C in the dark.

3. Place cells on ice and add 25–50 µL of the cell suspension into a 12 × 75 mm polystyrene tube. Add MAb to each tube (to be tested anti-CD80, anti-CD86, anti-MHC class II, anti-CD45). A convenient amount is 1 µL of a 250 µg/mL solution (ending up with a 5–10 µg/mL dilution). Incubate on ice for 30 min.

4. While the cells are incubating, if a second Ab is needed (e.g., the FITC or PE conjugate), take medium for lymphocyte staining, sterile-filter prior to each use) and add the second reagent (e.g., FITC goat anti-mouse IgG at 1 : 100–500). Spin this antibody solution in an Eppendorf tube at 10,000g, 2 min to remove aggregates.

5. Wash cells with the first MAb with 2 mL per tube of the same medium. Decant tube, break up pellet by tapping the side of the tube, and add 50 µL of the second antibody solution per tube. Incubate on ice for 30 min, then wash with PBS/FCS, 2 mL per tube.

6. Resuspend the pellet in 400–500 µL of PBS/FCS. If so desired, add 1 µg/mL of propidium iodide per tube to stain the nuclei of dead cells. This will show up on the FL-2 channel and therefore can be used only when FITC is used.

3.5. Testing Mitogenicity for ConA-activated T Lymphocytes

This method characterizes mitogenic properties of the test vaccine for activated T lymphocytes. ConA-activated T cells from spleen are used as a source of polyclonal T cells. **Figure 4** demonstrates proliferation of a BALB/c ConA-activated T-cell line in response to a mitogenic and nonmitogenic test vaccine. Clearly, ConA or the mitogenic test vaccine induced vigorous proliferation of T cells, whereas the nonmitogenic test vaccine did not induce proliferation.

1. Develop polyclonal ConA-activated T-cell lines from mice (*see* **Subheading 2.1.**) by stimulating spleen cells with ConA (5.0 µg/mL) for 3 d followed by separation of live cells by density centrifugation (Lymphoprep™) and cultivation in the presence of 1.0 ng/mL recombinant mouse IL-2 for 4 d. Replace half of the medium with the fresh medium and incubate cells for a further 7 d.

2. Add T-cell lines to wells of round-bottomed, 96-well microtiter plates (at 2 × 10^4/well), mix them with irradiated (30 Gy) syngeneic spleen cells (at 7.5 × 10^5/well) and complete RPMI 1640 medium (negative control) or the following antigens:

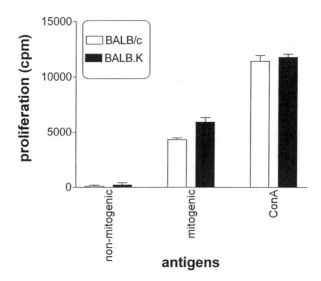

Fig. 4. Proliferative responses of ConA-stimulated BALB/c T cell line to mitogenic and nonmitogenic test vaccines in vitro using isogeneic (open bars), or allogeneic (black bars, BALB.K) spleen cells. Other details as in the legend to **Fig. 1**.

    10 µg/mL test vaccines, 10 µg/mL LPS, 5 µg/mL Con A, 10 µg/mL OVA (*see* **Note 4**).

3. T-cell lines can be used to test whether the mitogenic effect of the test vaccine is MHC class II restricted. To this end, add ConA-activated T cells (2×10^4/well) in flat-bottomed, 96-well microtiter plates and mix them with irradiated syngeneic or allogeneic spleen cells (at 7.5×10^5/well) in the presence of complete RPMI 1640 medium (negative control) or the following antigens: 10 µg/mL test vaccines (*see* **Note 4**), 10 µg/mL LPS, 5 µg/mL Con A, 10 µg/mL OVA, or the antigen that the clone is specific for.

4. After 24 h incubation, add tritiated thymidine to the triplicate cultures and incubate overnight as described in **Subheading 3.1., step 3**.

3.6. Testing for Superantigenicity for Naïve T Lymphocytes

    Several bacterial or viral proteins have been described to interact with the Vβ domain of the TCR from a number of different Vβ families and with MHC class II molecules on the surface of APCs, resulting in polyclonal activation of large fractions (5–20%) of T lymphocytes *(31)*. For example, staphylococcal enterotoxin B (SEB) predominantly activates T cells expressing the Vβ8 TCR family, such that the percentage of Vβ8 TCR T cells rise from about 30% to more than 50% of the CD3+ T cells *(27)*, providing a positive control for superantigenicity. In contrast, ConA stimulated T cells express a full range of TCR Vβ chains, and

Table 1
**The Distribution of Different T-Cell Receptor Vβ Chains in BALB/c
Spleen T Cells Induced by Porin-Deficient OMV Vaccines**[a]

TCR Vβ chain distribution	In uncultured spleen cells	In spleen cells stimulated with:		
		ConA	SEB	Mitogenic vaccine
Vβ2	6.4	8.1	6.8	9.0
Vβ3	3.6	0	1.3	8.9
Vβ4	9.1	8.2	5.3	11.3
Vβ5.1/5.2	0.8	0.5	0.5	1.2
Vβ6	10.0	11.8	7.6	10.5
Vβ7	3.4	3.8	6.4	3.4
Vβ8.1/8.2	22.5	23.6	31.9	21.6
Vβ8.3	8.7	10.7	19.2	11.2
Vβ9	1.1	1.1	1.2	1.5
Vβ10b	5.3	6.3	4.2	9.2
Vβ11	1.4	1.7	1.6	7.8
Vβ12	0	0	0	0.7
Vβ13	3.0	2.8	4.3	4.2
Vβ14	10.0	7.2	5.8	11.3
Vβ17a	0.4	0.2	0.7	1.4

[a]Typical values reflecting the distribution of Vβ TCR chains in activated T cells are presented as percentages of Vβ+ T cells from the total population of CD3+ T cells. Values for the nonmitogenic vaccine were similar to those observed for the uncultured spleen.

provide a control for nonsuperantigenicity. **Table 1** shows the typical distribution of Vβ TCR chains in mitogen/superantigen-activated T cells.

1. Separate mononuclear cells from spleen cells of naïve BALB/c mice by density centrifugation. Incubate cells with complete RPMI 1640 medium (negative control), the test vaccine (10.0 μg/mL) (*see* **Note 4**), or control antigens: SEB (1 μg/mL, 10^{-6} *M*), Con A (5.0 μg/mL) or LPS (10.0 μg/mL) for 48 h.
2. Distribute mononuclear cells into flow cytometry tubes (3–5 × 10^5 cells per), collect cells by centrifugation (400*g*, 5 min), and wash them in diluent for flow cytometry (*see* **Subheading 2.2.1., item 4**).
3. To reduce the nonspecific labeling, block Fcγ receptors by adding Fc Block (20 μL of 1:50 dilution per tube in HBSS for flow cytometry). Incubate cells for 30 min at 4–8°C in the dark.
4. Label all mitogen/superantigen-activated CD3+ T cells with anti-mouse CD3 ε chain (20 μL of the pre-diluted 1:25 stock) and incubate the cell suspension for 30 min at 4–8°C. Use the diluent for flow cytometry for dilution of MAb.

5. Label different TCR Vβ chains in T lymphocytes individually with mouse TCR Vβ FITC-labeled MAb (10 μL of each MAb, listed in **Subheading 2.2.2., item 17**). Incubate cells for 30 min at 4–8°C, and wash them using the diluent for flow cytometry. Add the same diluent (1.0 mL per tube) before flow cytometry.

6. Analyze the distribution of different TCR Vβ chains on T lymphocytes using a flow cytometer (such as FACScan® Becton Dickinson) with the following typical instrument settings:
   a. Voltage, SSC-299, FL1-682, FL2-690, FL3-150;
   b. Compensation, FL1 1% of FL2, FL2 25% of FL1;
   c. Threshold, FSC-120.
      For each sample 10,000 events are collected. Mononuclear cells are gated on forward vs side scatter.

3.7. Testing for Apoptosis of Mononuclear Cells

Apoptosis is programmed cell death characterized by a series of morphological alterations associated with cell death, including cell shrinkage, plasma- and nuclear-membrane blebbing, organelle relocalization and chromatin condensation *(32)*. In apoptosing cells, the membrane phospholipid phosphatidylserine (PS) is translocated to the outer leaflet of the plasma membrane and is ligated by the macrophage CD36-PS receptor complex, which is a component of multiple recognition systems used by macrophages to phagocytose apoptotic lymphocytes *(33)*. Annexin V is a phospholipid-binding protein, which binds to PS with high affinity in the presence of calcium, thus lending itself as a powerful tool for detecting cells entering apoptosis at an earlier stage, preceding the nuclear changes *(34)*. In addition to apoptosis, PS is expressed also during necrosis, such that a nucleic acid dye ViaProbe™ can be used to exclude nonviable cells during flow-cytometry analysis. The advantage of the ViaProbe dye is that its fluorescence is detected in the far red range of the spectrum (650 nm), which opens the possibility to use ViaProbe in combination with PE-labeled MAb in three-color analysis. Therefore, apoptosis can be studied in the total leukocyte population, as well as in CD19+ (B cells) and TCRαβ+ (T cells) subpopulations. Thus, labeling with ViaProbe plus Annexin V-FITC in combination with anti-CD19 MAb (*see* **Subheading 2.2.2., item 8.**) for the three-color labeling to test for apoptosis in B lymphocytes, or in combination with anti-TCRαβ PE-labeled MAb to test for apoptosis in T lymphocytes (*see* **Note 6**).

Figure 5 demonstrates that a mitogenic test vaccine doubled the percentage of mononuclear cells that undergo apoptosis, similar to the effect of ConA. In contrast, LPS and a nonmitogenic vaccine did not enhance the percentage of apoptosing leukocytes.

1. Separate mononuclear cells from spleen cells of naïve BALB/c mice by density centrifugation. Incubate the cells with complete RPMI 1640 medium (negative

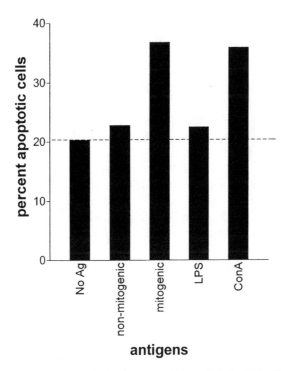

antigens

Fig. 5. Percentage of apoptotic leukocytes (Annexin V$^+$, PI$^-$) after 18-h culture in the absence of antigen, or in the presence of the test vaccines (10.0 µg/mL), LPS (10 µg/mL), or ConA (5 µg/mL). Leukocytes were gated on forward vs side scatter. Other details as in the legend to **Fig. 1**.

    control), with the test vaccine (10.0 µg/mL) (*see* **Note 4**), LPS (10 µg/mL), or ConA (5 µg/mL) for 18 h.

2. Distribute the cells into the flow cytometry tubes ($3-5 \times 10^5$ cells per tube), collect them by centrifugation (400g, 5 min), and wash in diluent for flow cytometry.
3. Block Fcγ receptors by Fc Block, as described in **Subheading 3.4., step 2**.
4. Add Annexin V FITC-labeled (10 µL) to label apoptotic/necrotic cells. At this stage, add also anti-CD19 PE-labeled MAb (20 µL of 1 : 60 pre-diluted stock), or anti-TCRαβ PE-labeled MAb (20 µL of 1 : 500 pre-diluted stock) for labeling B or T lymphocytes, respectively. Incubate cells for 30 min at 4–8°C.
5. Add ViaProbe (10 µL per test, 5×10^5 cells) to distinguish apoptotic vs necrotic cells, and incubate cells are for 10 min at 4–8°C before the assay.
6. After washing in diluent for flow cytometry, collecte cells by centrifugation (400g, 5 min), resuspend them in the same medium (1.0 mL) and analyze by flow cytometry.
7. Use the following controls for the single-color protocol:
   a. isotype control—rat IgG2a/IgG2b (PE/FITC) (20 µL of 1 : 400 pre-diluted stock, *see* **Subheading 2.2.2., item 16**);

b. Annexin V; and

c. ViaProbe.

Use the following controls for the two-color protocol:

a. Annexin V plus ViaProbe (in addition to adjusting instrument settings, this combination also allows to measure percentage of apoptosing leukocytes);

b. CD19 PE-labeled MAb plus ViaProbe (for FL2 and FL3 compensation);

c. anti-TCRαβ PE-labeled MAb plus ViaProbe (for FL2 and FL3 compensation);

d. Annexin V plus CD19 PE-labeled MAb plus ViaProbe (for FL1 and FL2 compensation); and

e. Annexin V plus anti-TCRαβ PE-labeled MAb (for FL1 and FL2 compensation).

8. Analyze apoptosis in mononuclear cells using a flow cytometer with the following typical instrument settings for the three-color labeling protocol:

a. Voltage, SSC-297, FL1-650, FL2-750, FL3-800;

b. Compensation, FL1 0.2% of FL2, FL2 86% of FL1, FL2 0% of FL3, and FL3 12.4% of FL2;

c. Threshold, FSC-60.

For each sample collect 10,000 events. Gate mononuclear cells on forward vs side scatter (*see* **Note 6**).

4. Notes

1. Different lots of FBS/FCS can have distinct effects on B-cell proliferation and activation, especially if B cells are obtained from LPS-sensitive mice, like C3H/HeOuJ mice, because of minor LPS contamination and the presence of other serum proteins. It is recommended that the vendor is contacted to obtain small samples of each batch they have and make up separate lots of media with each sera batch. Then each lot of media containing the different batches of sera should be tested for their ability to induce B-cell proliferation by itself. Only those batches of sera that induces the least amount of baseline proliferation should be used.

2. We have used also TiterMax Gold Adjuvant (Sigma, cat. No. T2684, 1.0 mL), which appears to be equally effective.

3. Neisserial porins are the major outer membrane component and can be isolated from organisms utilizing a method originally developed by Blake and Gotschlich *(35)* with subsequent modifications *(36,37)*. Gonococcal porin (Por or Protein I in older nomenclature, two types, PIA or PIB of one allele) can be isolated from strains that lack the reduction-modifiable protein (Rmp or Protein III in older nomenclature) *(38)*. Meningococci contain two porins in two different alleles, PorA (class1 protein in older nomenclature) or PorB (class 2 or 3 protein in older nomenclature). They also contain a reduction-modifiable protein (RmpM) termed class 4 protein in older nomenclature). Strains have been genetically modified to allow purification of either PorA or PorB without contamination by the other porin of by RmpM *(39–42)*. This method will discuss the purification of PorB from a meningococcal strain lack both RmpM and PorA. Similarly, this method can be used to purify meningococcal PorA from strains lacking PorB and RmpM.

The reason for isolating these proteins from strains lacking Rmp and other porins is to improve the purity of the subsequent porin preparation.

Grow 6–12 L of meningococci in Neisseria liquid media (as in **Subheading 2.2.1., item 11**) containing isovitalex (BBL). Obtain pellets of organisms and resuspend bacteria in an equal volume of 1 M NaAcetate, pH 4.0, with 1 mM 2-dimercaptopropanol. Then add 6 volumes of 5% Zwittergent 3-14 (Z3-14) (as in **Subheading 2.2.3., item 18**) in 0.5 M CaCl$_2$, and then after 1 h stirring, add ethanol to a concentration of 20% (v/v) to precipitate DNA and nuclear and cellular fragments. After centrifugation at 17,000g, precipitate the protein present in the supernatant (mainly containing Por) by the addition of ethanol to a concentration of 80% (v/v). After an overnight incubation at 4°C, obtain crude Por by centrifugation, resuspend Por in 50 mM Tris, pH 8.0, with 10 mM EDTA and 5% Z3-14 and clarify the preparation by a subsequent centrifugation at 12,000g. Clear the subsequent solution of major contaminants by passage over two ion exchange columns (DEAE followed by CM sepaharose in tandem). Precipitate the protein present in the flow-through once more by the addition of ethanol to a concentration of 80% (v/v), and resuspend the subsequent precipitate in as small a volume as possible of 50 mM Tris, pH 8.0, with 10 mM EDTA and 5% Z3-14. Clarify this solution again as previously, and place it on a molecular sieve column (Sephacryl S-300). Collect 10-mL fractions and analyze the fractions containing the porin by gel electrophoresis.

Proteosomes, pure protein micelles, are prepared from purified Por in order to remove detergent, which can be potentially cytotoxic with respect to immune cells. To this end, precipitate the chromatographically purified Por by the addition of ethanol to a concentration of 70% (v/v). Wash the precipitate once with 70% ethanol and then resuspend it in a solution containing the dialyzable detergent 10% D-octyl glucoside (w/v) (Sigma) in 10 mM HEPES, pH 7.2, to a concentration of 1 mg Por per mL. Dialyze this solution against 10 mM phosphate buffer, pH 8.0, with multiple changes of the dialyzing buffer to remove any remaining detergent. An oily-appearing precipitate is obtained consisting of pure protein. Determine the protein concentration by any standard assay (e.g., Coommassie blue, Pierce BCA assay, etc.). Using this procedure to purify Por and form them into proteosomes allows for minimal LPS contamination, less than 0.01% as demonstrated by Limulus Lysate Assays or silver staining of gels.

4. A different concentrations range of the test vaccine may prove to be more appropriate for testing. The concentrations given reflect our experience with meningococcal membrane-vesicle vaccine extracted from the PorB-deficient strain 44-76/HIII5 and from the PorA-deficient strain 44/76/M14 *(42)*.

5. First, deplete single-cell suspensions of spleens of red blood cells by treatment with 0.85% NH$_4$Cl in PBS *(29)*. To obtain pure B lymphocytes, resuspend spleen cells at 10^6/mL in R10 + antibiotics medium, and incubate them with anti-T cell MAbs (anti-Thy 1.2, anti-CD4, and anti-CD8) diluted 1:3 to 1:4 (the optimum concentration should be tested beforehand) for 45 m in a humidified, 5% CO$_2$ incubator at 37°C,

and wash in R10 + antibiotics medium. Add the complement at a dilution of 1 : 10 for 30 min to remove T cells. Remove adherent cells by passing the cell suspension via a G10 Sephadex column, and remove dead cells and debris by density centrifugation over Ficoll-Hypaque *(29).* Obtain T helper cells (CD4 positive) by enrichment over a nylon wool column and subsequent complement lysis using anti-class II MHC (anti-I-A^k/I-A^d) and anti-CD8 MAbs, with guinea pig complement as above. Test the purity of the preparations by flow cytometry *(43)* using antibodies against cell markers listed in **Subheading 2.2.2.**

6. Alternatively, if only a two-color labeling protocol is available, the DNA intercalating dye PI can be used to distinguish the total population of apoptotic leukocytes (Annexin V$^+$, PI$^-$) from necrotic cells (Annexin V$^+$, PI$^-$). The typical flow cytometer settings for the two-color labeling protocol are:
   a. Voltage, SSC-297, FL1-750, FL2-750, FL3-800;
   b. Compensation, FL1 0.6% of FL2, FL2 29.8% of FL1, FL2 9.1% of FL3, and FL3 7.8% of FL2;
   c. Threshold, FSC-60.

   For each sample 10,000 events are collected. Leukocytes are gated on the forward vs side scatter.

References

1. Ferreira, P., Brás, A., Tavares, D., Vilanova, M., Ribeiro, A., Videira, A. and Arala-Chaves, M. P. (1997) Purification, and biochemical and biological characterization of an immunosuppressive and lymphocyte mitogenic protein secreted by *Streptococcus sobrinus*. *Int. Immunol.* **9,** 1735–1743.
2. Arala-Chaves, M. P., Ribeiro, A. S., Santarem, M. M., and Coutinho, A. (1986) Strong mitogenic effect for murine B lymphocytes of an immunosuppressor substance released by *Streptococcus intermedius*. *Infect. Immun.* **54,** 543–548.
3. Santarem, M. M., Porto, M. T., Ferreira, P., Soares, R., and Arala-Chaves, M. P. (1987) Semi-purification of an immunosuppressor substance secreted by *Streptococcus mutans* that plays a role in the protection of the bacteria in the host. *Scand. J. Immunol.* **26,** 755–761.
4. Tavares, D., Salvador, A., Ferreira, P., and Arala-Chaves, M. P. (1993) Immunological activities of a *Candida albicans* protein which plays an important role in the survival of the microorganism in the host. *Infect. Immun.* **61,** 1881–1888.
5. Proqulske, A., Mishell, R., Trummel, C., and Holt, S. C. (1984) Biological activities of Eikenella corrodens outer membrane and lipopolysaccharide. *Infect. Immun.* **43,** 178–182.
6. Roy, S. and Biswas, T. (1996) Murine splenocyte proliferation by porin of *Shigella dysenteriae* type 1 and inhibition of bacterial invasion of HeLa cell by anti-porin antibody. *FEMS Microbiol. Lett.* **141,** 25–29.
7. Vordermeier, H.-M. and Bessler, W. G. (1987) Polyclonal activation of murine B lymphocytes in vitro by *Salmonella typhimurium* porins. *Immunobiology* **175,** 245–251.

8. Vordermeier, H.-M., Drexler, H., and Bessler, W. G. (1987) Polyclonal activation of human peripheral blood lymphocytes by bacterial porins and defined porin fragments. *Immunol. Lett.* **15**, 121–126.

9. Otsuka, J. (1986) Immunobiological activity of 41K protein (porin) derived from the cell envelope of *Fusobacterium nucleatum*. *Nippon Shishubyo Gakkai Kaishi* **28**, 445–467.

10. Minetti, C. A. S. A., Tai, J. Y., Blake, M. S., Pullen, J. K., Liang, S. M., and Remeta, D. P. (1997) Structural and functional characterization of a recombinant PorB class 2 protein from *Neisseria meningitidis*. Conformational stability and porin activity. *J. Biol. Chem.* **272**, 10,710–10,720.

11. Liu, M. A., Friedman, A., Oliff, A. I., Tai, J., Martinez, D., Deck, R. R., et al. (1992) A vaccine carrier derived from *Neisseria meningitidis* with mitogenic activity for lymphocytes. *Proc. Natl. Acad. Sci. USA* **89**, 4633–4637.

12. Ulmer, J. B., Burke, C. J., Shi, C., Friedman, A., Donnelly, J. J., and Liu, M. A. (1992) Pore formation and mitogenicity in blood cells by the class 2 protein of *Neisseria meningitidis*. *J. Biol. Chem.* **267**, 19,266–19,271.

13. Melancon, J., Murgita, R. A., and DeVoe, I. W. (1983) Activation of murine B lymphocytes by *Neisseria meningitidis* and isolated meningococcal surface antigens. *Infect. Immun.* **42**, 471–479.

14. Wetzler, L. M., Ho, Y., and Reiser, H. (1996) Neisserial porins induce B lymphocytes to express costimulatory B7-2 molecules and to proliferate. *J. Exp. Med.* **183**, 1151–1159.

15. Poolman, J. T. (1995) Development of a meningococcal vaccine. *Infect. Agents Dis.* **4**, 13–28.

16. Fusco, P. C., Michon, F., Laude-Sharp, M., Minetti, C. A. S. A., Huang, C.-H., Heron, I., and Blake, M. S. (1998) Preclinical studies on a recombinant group B meningococcal porin as a carrier for a novel *Haemophilus influenzae* type b conjugate vaccine. *Vaccine* **16**, 1842–1849.

17. Arala-Chaves, M. P. (1992) Is prophylactic immunostimulation of the host against pathogenic microbial antigens an adequate strategy of immunoprotection? *Scand. J. Immunol.* **35**, 495–500.

18. Müller, A., Günther, D., Düx, F., Naumann, M., Meyer, T. F., and Rudel, T. (1999) Neisserial porin (PorB) causes rapid calcium influx in target cells and induces apoptosis by the activation of cysteine proteases. *EMBO J.* **18**, 339–352.

19. Donnelly, J. J., Deck, R. R., and Liu, M. A. (1990) Immunogenicity of *Haemophilus influenzae* polysaccharide: *Neisseria meningitidis* outer membrane protein complex conjugate vaccine. *J. Immunol.* **145**, 3071–3079.

20. Giebink, G. S., Koskela, M., Vella, P. P., Harris, M., and Le, C. T. (1993) Pneumococcal capsular polysaccharide-meningococcal outer membrane protein complex conjugate vaccines: immunogenicity and efficacy in experimental pneumococcal otitis media. *J. Infect. Dis.* **167**, 347–355.

21. Paradiso, P. R. and Lindbberg, A. A. (1996) Glycoconjugate vaccines: future combinations. *Dev. Biol. Stand.* **87**, 269–275.

22. Mackinnon, F. G., Ho, Y., Blake, M. S., Michon, F., Chandraker, A., Sayegh, M. H., and Wetzler, L. M. (1999) The role of B/T costimulatory signals in the immunopotentiating activity of Neisserial porin. *J. Infect. Dis.* **180,** 755–761.

23. Fusco, P. C., Michon, F., Tai, J. Y., and Blake, M. S. (1998) Preclinical evaluation of a novel group B meningococcal conjugate vaccine that elicits bactericidal activity in both mice and nonhuman primates. *J. Infect. Dis.* **175,** 364–372.

24. Poltorak, A., He, X., Smirnova, I., Liu, M. Y., Huffel, C. V., Du, X., et al. (1998) Defective LPS signaling in C3H/HeJ and C57BL/10ScCr mice: mutations in Tlr4 gene. *Science* **282,** 2085–2088.

25. Takeuchi, O., Hoshino, K., Kawai, T., Sanjo, H., Takada, H., Ogawa, T., et al. (1999) Differential roles of TLR2 and TLR4 in recognition of gram-negative and gram-positive bacterial cell wall components. *Immunity* **11,** 443–451.

26. Poltorak, A., Smirnova, I., He, X., Liu, M. Y., van Huffel, C., McNally, O., et al. (1999) Genetic and physical mapping of the Lps locus: identification of the toll-4 receptor as a candidate gene in the critical region. *Blood Cells Mol. Dis.* **25,** 78.

27. Robinson, J. H., Pyle, G., and Kehoe, M. A. (1992) Influence of major histocompatibility complex haplotype on the mitogenic response of T cells to staphylococcal enterotoxin B. *Infect. Immun.* **59,** 3667–3672.

28. Kleijmeer, M. J., Ossevoort, M. A., van Veen, C. J. H., van Hellemond, J. J., Neefjes, J. J., Kast, W. M., et al. (1995) MHC class II compartments and the kinetics of antigen presentation in activated mouse spleen dendritic cells. *J.Immunol.* **154,** 5715–5724.

29. Kruisbeek, A. M. (1994) In vitro assays for lymphocyte function, in *Current Protocols in Immunology* (Coligan, J. E., Kruisbeek, A. M., Margulies, D. H., Shevach, E. M., and Strober, W., eds.), John Wiley and Sons, Inc., New York, pp. 3.0.1–3.19.7.

30. Calvin, F., Freeman, G. J., Razi-Wolf, Z., Hall, W. Jr., Benacerraf, B., Nadler, L., and Reiser, H. (1992) Murine B7 antigen provides a sufficient costimulatory signal for antigen-specific and MHC-restricted T cell activation. *J. Immunol.* **149,** 3802–3808.

31. Li, H., Llera, A., Malchiodi, E. L., and Mariuzza, R. A. (1999) The structural basis of T cell activation by superantigens. *Ann. Rev. Immunol.* **17,** 435–466.

32. McConkey, D. J., Zhivotovsky, B., and Orrenius, S. (1996) Apoptosis: molecular mechanisms and biological implications. *Mol. Aspects Med.* **17,** 1–110.

33. FadoK, V. A., Warner, M. L., Bratton, D. L., and Henson, P. M. (1998) CD36 is required for phagocytosis of apoptotic cells by human macrophages that use either a phosphatidylserine receptor or the vitronectin receptor (α v β 3). *J. Immunol.* **161,** 6250–6257.

34. Vermes, I., Haanen, C., Steffens-Nakken, H., and Reutelingsperger, C. (1995) A novel assay for apoptosis. Flow cytometric detection of phosphatidylserine expression on early apoptotic cells using fluorescein labelled Annexin V. *J. Immunol. Methods* **184,** 39–51.

35. Blake, M. S. and Gotschlich, E. C. (1982) Purification and partial characterization of the major outer membrane protein of *Neisseria gonorrhoea. Infect. Immun.* **36,** 277–283.

36. Lytton, E. J. and Blake, M. S. (1986) Isolation and partial characterization of the reduction-modifiable protein of *Neisseria gonorrhoea*. *J. Exp. Med.* **164,** 1749–1759.

37. Wetzler, L. M., Blake, M. S., and Gotschlich, E. C. (1988) Characterization and specificity of antibodies to protein I of *Neisseria gonorrhoeae* produced by injection with various protein I-adjuvant preparations. *J. Exp. Med.* **168,** 1883–1897.

38. Wetzler, L. M., Gotschlich, E. C., Blake, M. S., and Koomey, J. M. (1989) The construction and characterization of *Neisseria gonorrhoeae* lacking protein III in its outer membrane. *J. Exp. Med.* **169,** 2199–2209.

39. Guttormsen, H.-K., Wetzler, L. M., and Solberg, C. O. (1994) Humoral immune response to class 1 outer membrane protein during the course of meningococcal disease. *Infect. Immun.* **62,** 1437–1443.

40. Guttormsen, H.-K., Wetzler, L. M., and Næss, A. (1993) Humoral immune response to the class 3 outer membrane protein during the course of meningococcal disease. *Infect. Immun.* **61,** 4734–4742.

41. Klugman, K. P., Gotschlich, E. C., and Blake, M. S. (1989) Sequence of the structural gene (*rmpM*) for the class 4 outer membrane protein of *Neisseria meningitidis*, homology of the protein to gonococcal protein III and *Escherichia coli* OmpA, and construction of meningococcal strains that lack class 4 protein. *Infect. Immun.* **57,** 2066–2071.

42. Tommassen, J., Vermeij, P., Struyve, M., Benz, R., and Poolman, J. T. (1990) Isolation of *Neisseria meningitidis* mutants deficient in class 1 (PorA) and class 3 (PorB) outer membrane proteins. *Infect. Immun.* **58,** 1355–1359.

43. Otten, G., Yokohoma, Y. M., and Holmes, K. L. (1994) Immunofluorescence and cell sorting, in *Current Protocols in Immunology* (Coligan, J. E., Kruisbeek, A. M., Margulies, D. H., Shevach, E. M., and Strober, W., eds.), John Wiley and Sons, Inc., New York, pp. 5.0.1–5.8.8.

44. Bjune, G., Høiby, E. A., Grønnesby, J. K., Arnesen, O., Fredriksen, J. H., Halstensen, A., et al. (1991) Effect of outer membrane vesicle vaccine against group B meningococcal disease in Norway. *Lancet* **338,** 1093–1096.

16

Early Experiences with Nasal Vaccines against Meningococcal Disease

Johan Holst and Bjørn Haneberg

1. Introduction

In common with most infectious agents, meningococci invade mucosal membranes before causing disease *(1)*. An attractive vaccine strategy is therefore to induce immunological responses at the mucosal surfaces, with the possibility of blocking microbial invasion, as well as to induce systemic immunity with the capacity of inactivating the microbes.

The current parenteral vaccines against group B meningococcal disease have important shortcomings *(2)*, e.g., a high degree of strain- and serosubtype-specific immune responses in infants, and side effects presumably caused by lipopolysaccharide (LPS). There is thus reason for exploring alternative strategies for vaccination.

1.2. Mucosal Vaccines

Vaccines given directly onto mucosal surfaces are meant to mimic the natural pathways of invading microorganisms. In this manner, the possibility is exploited that such mucosal vaccines might stimulate the mucosal immune system that is characterized mainly by the secretion of dimeric or polymeric immunoglobulin A (IgA) *(3)*. As opposed to injectable vaccines, mucosal vaccines are in fact more likely to induce local and secretory immune responses, capable of acting as a barrier to further invasion by specific pathogens *(4,5)*. It has also been shown that these vaccines can induce systemic immunity, e.g., functional, bactericidal antibodies at the same level as the vaccines given by injections *(6,7)*. In addition to being more practical in use, they have thus the

From: *Methods in Molecular Medicine, vol. 66: Meningococcal Vaccines: Methods and Protocols*
Edited by: A. J. Pollard and M. C. J. Maiden © Humana Press Inc., Totowa, NJ

potential of inducing immune responses of better functional quality than have the corresponding injectable vaccines.

The administration of vaccines consisting of attenuated live microbes onto mucosal surfaces, where the "wild" microbes would have its habitat, is so close to mimicking the natural infection as is possible. The success of the live oral polio vaccine shows that such vaccines can be highly effective. It has recently also been proposed to use live attenuated *Neisseria* strains in vaccines against meningococcal disease *(8)*. However, the use of live attenuated microbes is connected with some inherent risks, although small, of creating serious infection *(9–11)*. In cases of immune deficiencies, the risk of vaccine induced diseases may be even greater *(12)*.

An alternative strategy, that might be better and more applicable, is to develop mucosal vaccines that do not replicate or cause any infection. So far, an oral vaccine against cholera consisting of killed *Vibrio cholera*, plus the B-subunit of cholera toxin (CT) as a mucosal adjuvant (*see* **Subheading 1.3.**) is the only representative on the market of a nonreplicating mucosal vaccine *(13)*. However, there is both a theoretical basis and clinical evidence for the belief that this type of vaccines might be useful in other instances, e.g., against meningococcal disease *(3,6)*.

1.3. Mucosal Adjuvants

The mucosal surfaces are designed to be nonreactive and to tolerate the exposure to foreign nonliving material, such as in ingested food. Soluble proteins, which otherwise are immunogenic, may even induce a state of immunological tolerance to further exposure after first being given orally *(14)*. In order to create immune responses with the intent of protecting against infectious diseases, this tendency to tolerance induction should therefore be specifically abrogated by mucosal adjuvants *(15)*. In several respects, mucosal adjuvants might differ from conventional immunological adjuvants used together with vaccines for injection *(16)*.

Cholera toxin and the heat-labile toxin (LT) of *Escherichia coli* are known as the most powerful mucosal adjuvants. However, both are too toxic to be used in humans *(17)*, but there are promising results for making nontoxic mutants *(18,19)*. Although their nontoxic B-subunits, CTB or LTB, possess some adjuvant activity on the mucosa, the observation that CTB may induce a state of T-cell tolerance *(20)* have negative impact on the prospects for their use as mucosal adjuvants for vaccines against infectious diseases.

From studies in animals, it became apparent that whole heat- or formaldehyde-inactivated bacteria, and outer membrane vesicles (OMVs) from group B *Neisseria meningitidis*, may act as mucosal vaccines, even without the use of additional adjuvants *(21–24)*. This was most pronounced when such bacteria-derived particles were given intranasally, and not into the intestines via the rectal route. A possible explanation might be that they all represents airway pathogens, i.e., *Neisseria meningitidis*, *Streptococcus pneumoniae*, group B streptococcus, and *Bordetella pertussis*. The effect on antibody responses to a nasal whole-cell *B. pertussis* vaccine was even less when CT was added, than without *(24)*. It appeared, thus, that these particles possessed some kind of self-adjuvanticity.

Studies in humans have confirmed that meningococcal OMVs alone can actually function as a nasal vaccine *(6,7,25,26)*. An adjuvant effect of the meningococcal OMVs and whole heat-killed *N. meningitidis*, as well as formaldehyde-inactivated *B. pertussis*, was further substantiated by increased mucosal and systemic antibody responses to a killed whole virus influenza vaccine given intranasally *(27,28)*.

1.4. Formulations of Nasal Vaccines

In the few studies in humans done so far *(6,7,26)* rather straightforward formulations have been used. For group B meningococci they have been either the same OMVs as used in parenteral vaccines *(6)*, or the 'native vesicles' (i.e., not exposed to detergent treatment and with high LPS content) as used by Drabick et al. (*7* and *see* **Note 1**). Moreover, Berstad et al. used simple suspensions of killed whole-cell *B. pertussis* in saline. No other extra adjuvant or any special pharmaceutical exipients were added to the formulations. Some groups however, have studied the properties of CTB and others propose to use LT mutants as well *(29)*.

The doses of nasal vaccines have been substantially higher than for those of parenteral formulations, i.e., mostly 10-fold more antigen per dose than for injectable formulations (*6,7* and **Note 2**). The rationale has been that the waste and spillage will be much greater when presented as nasal drops or spray *(31–33)*.

Various issues regarding formulation and other pharmaceutical-chemical properties for nasal vaccines need further study. There is reason to believe that particle concentration, as well as size and charge, may influence uptake by immunocompetent structures and cells. Also, the effects of increasing the viscosity or use of extra bioadhesives have so far not been fully investigated.

1.5. Characterization and Quality Control of Nasal Vaccines

For manufacture and quality control of OMV vaccines for nasal use, nearly all the issues given for parenteral OMV vaccines apply (*see* **Chapter 7**).

The manufacturing conditions for the nasal OMV-vaccine used in the clinical trial in Norway *(6)* were the same as for the parenteral vaccine because this latter vaccine was already available. International regulatory bodies have not formally acknowledged the manufacturing conditions and specifications for nasal vaccines. There is precedence, however, for the view that aseptic quality during manufacture and demand for sterility of the end product might be less stringent for nasal vaccines than for traditional formulations (*34,35*). Nevertheless, monitoring of the microbial quality of the manufacturing environment, determination of the bioburden, and other measures for assuring that no harmful contamination had occurred should be performed.

The vesicular or particulate nature for the active ingredient might be the most important of the vaccine characteristics. For quality control of parenteral formulations, electron microscopy (EM) has traditionally been used (*36,37* and **Chapter 7** in this volume). The use of low-angle laser scattering or laser diffraction, as for other colloidal or particulate drug formulations in the pharmaceutical industry (*38*), might be of value for characterization and stability study purposes. New methods, like "Sedimentation Field-Flow Fractionation" (SedFFF), might also be valuable (*39*). In addition, measurements of zeta potentials for OMVs in the nasal-vaccine formulation might be important for development of an optimal formulation (*40*).

1.6. Administration of Nasal Vaccines

In mice, up to 30 µL of the liquid vaccine formulation would be easily inhaled after being applied as small drops on the nares, with the animals held in a supine position and head down to prevent the vaccine from flowing into the mouth. Intranasal administration in this way was easier to perform when the animals had received a general anaesthetic (propofol; Diprivan) intravenously (*see* **Note 3**). However, both serum and saliva antibodies were induced whether or not the animals had been put to sleep during immunization (B. Haneberg, unpublished results). It also appeared that the immunogenic effect of a particulate vaccine derived from *S. pneumoniae* was far better when given intranasally than by the oral and gastric routes, even with regard to induction of intestinal mucosal antibodies (*22*).

In humans, a meningococcal OMV vaccine might be given either as nasal spray, with the vaccinee sitting, or as drops with the vaccinee lying on a couch and head tilted backwards (**Fig. 1**). Strong as well as weak immune responses were seen with both ways of administering the vaccine (*6*). There was thus no evidence that the vaccine had to reach the bronchial airways to be effective (*see* **Note 4**).

1.7. Immunization Schedules

From previous experiments in animals, it seemed that nasal vaccines had to be given repeatedly in order to induce sizable antibody responses (*41*). A recent

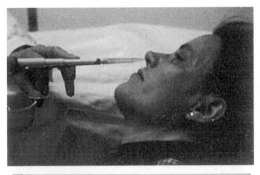

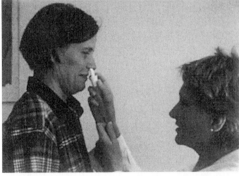

Fig. 1. Vaccine given intranasally as drops, with the head tilted backwards (top), and as nasal spray (bottom).

study with a meningococcal OMV vaccine showed that antibody responses in both serum and secretions was better with four small intranasal doses given 1 wk apart, than with one dose equivalent to the sum of the four *(42)*. It also appeared from studies with intervals varying from 1 h to several weeks that this effect was owing to induction of immunological memory, and not to the vaccine having resided longer at the mucosal surface. Two of the larger doses given 2 mo apart seemed sufficient for induction of ample antibody responses in both serum and saliva *(42)*. For practical reasons, therefore, nonreplicating mucosal vaccines may be administered at intervals largely as for injections.

As opposed to serum antibodies, which reflect production over time, antibodies measured in secretions at one time represent some that are produced shortly before *(3)*. In order to attain high concentrations of antibodies in secretions, therefore, nonliving mucosal vaccines might be given shortly before the suspected exposure of a pathogen. Available data with a meningococcal OMV-vaccine indicate that repeated intranasal administration does not have any ill effects such as induction of tolerance *(42)*.

1.8. Sampling Techniques

Studies in animals have shown that secretions may be easily collected by absorbent material and later extracted for analyses of antibodies *(43)*. It is also likely that antibodies in mucus collected by such material applied directly onto mucosal surfaces will mainly represent those that have been secreted locally at that mucosal area or segment, and not some from adjacent or remote areas *(44)*. In mice, ample amounts of IgA-containing saliva can be obtained from the drooling mouth with small absorbent "wicks" within minutes after they have been given pilocarpine by injections as a stimulus for secretion. Because the concentrations of IgA antibodies in saliva seem to mirror those in lung secretions, the collection of samples representing airway secretions may be limited to saliva, and the number of experimental animals can thus be reduced *(22* and **Note 6**).

In humans, saliva can be collected for antibody analyses with similar absorbent devices, but without the need for a pharmacological stimulus of secretion *(6)*. Recently, it has also been shown that antibodies in air-dried saliva can be preserved for months without refrigeration *(45)*. In addition, it appears that small but measurable amounts of IgG antibodies derived from serum or underlying tissues can be found in saliva *(45)*. The collection and storage of saliva can thus be made under very simple conditions, and the saliva samples may even substitute for blood in the analyses of systemic antibodies.

For analyses of IgA antibodies in nasal secretions of human volunteers, it was sufficient to collect some drops flowing out at the nares after spraying the nasal cavities with plain saline solution from a standard metered nasal spray device *(6*, **Subheading 3.4.**, and **Note 6**). This simple sampling technique was also painless and without risk, and showed that the most pronounced secretory antibody response to nasal vaccines occurred at the site of vaccination, i.e., of the nasal and not the oral mucosa *(6,26)*.

Because the concentrations of IgA-antibodies in secretions may vary owing to fluctuations in secretory flow or degree of dilution during extractions, they should be related to the corresponding secretion of total IgA *(43)*. In mice that can be exposed to more standardized sampling conditions, however, such corrections of antibody concentrations do not seem to be necessary *(21)*.

1.9. Analyses of Immune Responses

Vaccine-specific antibodies in both secretions and serum can be analyzed by enzyme-linked immunosorbent assay (ELISA) and further characterized by immunoblotting techniques *(6,21)*. Studies in both animals and human volunteers have shown that intranasal immunizations will induce antibodies against a more limited range of antigens than with an injectable vaccine *(6)*. The quan-

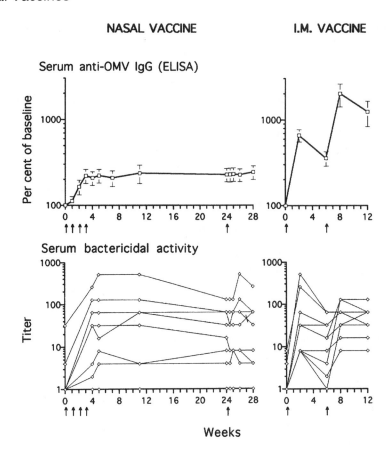

Fig. 2. Serum antibodies to meningococcal OMVs, measured by ELISA, and serum bactericidal activity against the vaccine strain of meningococci, after immunizations (marked by arrows) of 11 volunteers with a nasal OMV vaccine (no additional adjuvant), and of 10 volunteers with an intramuscular (I.M.) OMV vaccine adsorbed to Al-hydroxide. The ELISA antibodies are given as mean increments from baseline values ± standard errors (upper panels), and the bactericidal activities as individual titers (lower panels). Adapted with permission from **ref.** *(6)*.

tity of antibodies in serum after a nasal meningococcal OMV-vaccine, without additional adjuvant, was also less than after intramuscular vaccinations with the same type of vaccine plus aluminum hydroxide as adjuvant (**Fig. 2**). The bactericidal activity or the proportion of functional antibodies that had been induced, however, was surprisingly strong *(6)*. Except in some vaccinees who did not respond to the nasal vaccine, this bactericidal activity was equal to that attained with the intramuscular vaccine. It seems, therefore, that the antibodies induced by the nasal vaccine were of very high quality *(6,7)*. To judge the effect of new nasal vaccines, it is thus of importance that the functional ability of the antibodies is taken into account.

In addition to both systemic and local mucosal antibody response, the nasal meningococcal OMV-vaccine induced T-cell responses measured as antigen-specific in vitro proliferation of peripheral blood mononuclear cells *(25)*. Similar vaccine-specific T-cell responses were seen after a nasal vaccine against whooping cough *(46)*. It appears from these observations that the vaccines had a "balanced" immune response that seemed to involve both Th1- and Th2-cells. Nonreplicating nasal vaccines based on particles derived from bacteria may thus fulfill the criteria for vaccines to be used in the future, at least for vaccines against diseases caused by airway pathogens.

1.10. Areas for Further Exploration

The early experiences with nasal vaccines against meningococcal disease hold high promise, i.e., nonreplicating nasal vaccines appear to be a realistic alternative. A prerequisite for success in this area, however, will be to use immunological assays for measuring functional immune responses. Ideally, such assays should also correlate to protection against disease. It seems that the test for bactericidal activity in serum fulfils these criteria for the group B meningococcal vaccine developed at National Institute of Public Health (NIPH), Oslo *(47,48)*.

Still, there is need for dose-response studies and testing of various regimens to establish how nasal vaccines best should be given. A primary vaccination series consisting of four intranasal immunizations at weekly interval *(6)* is not practical on a larger scale unless the vaccine can be self-administered. Preliminary studies indicate that intranasal immunization schedules can in fact be simplified (B. Haneberg, unpublished results). Also, the use of parenteral immunization in combination with nasal vaccines might be considered *(42)*. Moreover, the usefulness of nasal vaccines in individuals with allergic rhinitis and infants with frequent upper-respiratory infections should be explored.

More work will be required to test for immunogenicity of other meningococcal antigens than OMVs, e.g., capsular polysaccharides from group A and C, and the respective protein conjugates.

OMVs have proved to function very well both as a nasal vaccine per se *(6)*, and as a mucosal adjuvant for nasal influenza vaccine *(27)*. As mentioned, no problems have been discovered in mice with respect to self-immunogenicity owing to repetitive intranasal immunizations. There is reason to believe, however, that strong immunogenic properties of mucosal adjuvants might in some instances be disadvantageous *(49)*. There is thus need for mucosal adjuvants that are not themselves immunogenic.

2. Materials

2.1. Vaccines

1. The intramuscular vaccine used for control contained OMVs from the group B meningococcal strain 44/76 (15:P1.7,16) adsorbed onto aluminum hydroxide *(36)*. The OMVs were prepared by extraction of bacteria with 0.5% deoxycholate in 0.1 M Tris-HCl, pH 8.6, containing 10 mM ethylene-diaminetetraacetic acid (EDTA), and purified by differential centrifugation. Each intramuscular dose of 0.5 mL consisted of 25 µg OMVs, measured as protein.
2. The nasal vaccine formulation was made from the original pool of OMVs used in the intramuscular vaccine, but without aluminum hydroxide. Each nasal dose of 0.5 mL consisted of 250 µg OMVs, measured as protein. *See* **Note 1** regarding the background and logic for choice of vaccine material.

2.2. Animals

1. Female Balb/C mice, obtained from Bomholtgård Breeding and Research Centre, Ry, Denmark, were used from the age of 8–10 wk.

2.3. Absorbent Materials

1. For collection of saliva from mice, use absorbent cylindrical wicks (2 × 25 mm) consisting of synthetic fibers and cellulose (Polyfiltronics Group Inc., Rockland, MA) after a single intraperitoneal injection of 0.1 mg pilocarpine-HCl (Sigma Chemical Co., St. Louis, MO) in 100 µL of PBS.
2. Collection of secretions from humans can be done by using the same wicks and/ or similar material in form of the "MucoSafe" system *(45)*.

2.4. Protease Inhibitors

1. If necessary, the following protease inhibitors may be added to the phosphate-buffered saline (PBS) buffer during extraction of immunoglobulins: 0.2 mM 4-(2-aminoethyl)-benzenesulfonylfluoride (AEBSF) (Boehringer Mannheim GmbH, Mannheim, Germany), 1 µg/mL Aprotinin (Sigma), 10 µM Leupeptin (Sigma), and 3.25 µM Bestatin (Sigma).

2.5. Additional Buffers

1. Buffer for use during homogenization: PBS, pH 7.2, with 3% sucrose.
2. 0.1 M phosphate-citrate buffer, pH 5.0, for the peroxidase reaction used in ELISA.

2.6. Additional Materials

1. For vaccine administration by spray: Minigrip metered spray device (Apodan, Copenhagen, Denmark).
2. For ELISA determination: Nunc-Immuno Plates, MaxiSorp F96 (A/S Nunc, Roskilde, Denmark).

3. For blocking unspecific binding in ELISA: 5% nonfat dry milk (Oxoid, Hampshire, UK), in PBS, pH 7.2.
4. Second antibody in ELISA: peroxidase-conjugated goat antibodies (Sigma).
5. Substrate for the peroxidase reaction: *o*-phenyldiaminehydrocloride (OPD; Sigma).
6. Readout of optical densities (ODs): Titertek Multiscan Plus MK II (Labsystems, Finland).
7. For detection of class-specific antibody binding: peroxidase-conjugated goat anti-mouse IgG or IgA. (DAKO A/S, Glostrup, Denmark).
8. For anesthesia of mice: propofol (Diprivan, AstraZeneca, Mölndal, Sweden).

3. Methods
3.1. Preparation of OMVs

1. Grow a suitable *N. meningitidis* strain until early stationary phase and extract OMVs by 0.1 *M* Tris-HCl, pH 8.6, 10 m*M* EDTA and 0.5% deoxycholate.
2. Purify by sequential centrifugation steps at 20,000*g* for 30 min, followed by ultra-centrifugation at 125,000*g* for 2 h.
3. Homogenize the pelleted OMVs in PBS, pH 7.2, with 3% sucrose. *See* also Chapter 7.

3.2. Immunization Procedure for Animals

1. Immunize groups of 10 mice intranasally, e.g., four times at weekly intervals with 250 µg OMVs (as protein) in volumes of 30 µL PBS.
2. For nasal immunizations: hold the animals in a supine position, fully awake with head down, while drops of the vaccine suspension is applied to the nares.
3. If general anesthesia is required, use propofol (*see* **Note 3**).

3.3. Immunization of Humans

1. The nasal vaccine might be given four times at weekly intervals (*6* and **Note 5**).
2. Administer the vaccine as nasal drops or spray (*see* **Note 4**).
3. If drops are used, administer by a regular pipet, 0.25 mL (125 µg protein) to each nostril, with the head of the vaccinees tilted backwards from a supine position to create a near vertical pathway to the upper nasal cavity. Keep the vaccinees in that position for 1 min after delivery.
4. If spray is used, administer as repeated douches by Minigrip metered spray device (Apodan) to total pre-measured volumes of 0.25 mL vaccine into each nostril with the vaccinees seated.
5. The parenteral vaccine for eventual comparison can be given twice in the deltoid muscle at a 6-wk-interval and a third immunization 6–10 mo after the second dose (*47*).

3.4. Collection of Samples

1. Obtain sera, separated from freshly drawn whole blood, oral secretions, and nasal fluid before immunizations, and at intervals starting 1 wk after the last dose (*6*).

2. Collect oral secretions (called saliva) by absorbent material placed between the lower gum and buccal mucosa at each side.

3. Collect nasal fluid by similar material at each nostril after spraying the nasal cavities with approx 0.4 mL luke-warm PBS, pH 7.2, using Minigrip metered spray devices.

4. Place the absorbent with saliva or nasal fluid into 1.5-mL microcentrifuge tubes, and record the combined weights of the wicks and tubes. The weights of the captured secretions can then be calculated (*see* **Note 6**).

5. Store all samples at –20°C until used.

3.5. Extraction of Immunoglobulins from Absorbent Material

1. Extract proteins by addition of 500 μL PBS with the protease inhibitors (*see* **Subheading 2.**).

2. After vortexing for 1 min, make a small hole into the bottom of each tube.

3. Place the tube containing the absorbent into another tube measuring 1.2 × 8 cm, and collect the extracts into the outer tube by centrifugation at approx 2,000*g* for 5 min at 4°C.

4. Store the extracts at –20°C until analyzed.

3.6. Quantitation of Antibodies and Immunoglobulins

1. Determine levels of IgA, IgG, and IgM antibodies to OMVs, and total IgA, IgG, and IgM concentrations by ELISA, using Nunc-Immuno Plates, MaxiSorp F96 (A/S Nunc).

2. Coat the plates for specific antibody assays by incubation with OMVs, 4 μg per mL in Tris-HCl buffer, pH 8.6, at 4°C for 1 wk. Block for nonspecific protein-binding sites with PBS, pH 7.2, containing 5% nonfat dry milk (Oxoid).

3. Transfer serum samples and mucosal extracts to the plates and serially dilute twofold in the blocking solution.

4. After 2 h incubation at 37°C, wash the plates five times with 0.05% Tween 20 in PBS and incubate 90 min with peroxidase-conjugated goat antibodies (Sigma) directed against mouse IgG or IgA (both 1 in 1,000) in blocking buffer.

5. After washing, detect bound antibodies with OPD (Sigma) (0.4 mg/ml) in 0.1 *M* phosphate-citrate buffer, pH 5.0, and read ODs at 492 nm.

6. Use a sample of saliva from one donor with high-titered IgA antibodies to OMVs, as reference standard for specific IgA antibodies in secretions. Likevise, use sera from donors with high-titered antibodies as reference standards for IgG antibodies in serum and secretions.

7. Express antibody titers as arbitrary units relative to the standard serum, and correct for the weights of the original samples and dilutions made.

8. Relate antibodies in secretions to total immunoglobulins of the same isotype.

3.7. Immunoblotting Analysis of the Antibody Responses

1. Separate antigens in OMV by sodium dodecyl sulfate-polyacrylamide gel electrophoresis (SDS-PAGE) on 7 × 8 cm 12% acrylamide gels and electroblot to nitrocellulose filters.

2. After electrotransfer and blocking, cut each blot into strips of 2.5 mm, corresponding to approx 1.8 μg protein per strip before transfer.
3. Incubate the strips overnight with 1:200 dilutions of sera and 1:25 of saliva.
4. Test all sera and extracts for antibody binding in the presence and absence of Empigen BB to increase renaturation of blotted antigens *(50)*.
5. Detect class-specific binding of antibodies by incubation for 2 h with a 1:1,000 dilution of peroxidase-conjugated goat anti-mouse IgG or IgA. (DAKO A/S).
6. Score the specific antibody binding visually *(50)*.
7. Use guide strips on each blot, incubated with specific monoclonal antibodies (MAbs) against the major outer-membrane proteins (OMPs) and other relevant components *(50)*.

3.8. Serum Bactericidal Assay (SBA)

1. For quantitation of functional immune responses, perform SBA in duplicate with an agar overlay method on microtiter plates in the presence of 25% human complement and bacterial inoculum of approx 100 colony-forming units (CFUs) per well with the *N. meningitidis* strain relevant for testing *(6,47,51)*.
2. Assay each serum by twofold serial dilutions.
3. Give the bactericidal titers as the highest serum dilutions that reduce the number of CFUs by more than 50%.

3.9. Statistical Analysis

1. Determine differences of significance between groups of animals/vaccinees, or values obtained at various times within groups, by the Mann-Whitney *U*-test and the Wilcoxon signed rank test, respectively *(6)*.

4. Notes

1. At NIPH we intended to study some of the basic differences and similarities between immune responses following parenteral and intranasal immunizations. The reason for starting with a formulation of OMV was that we in fact had the same material in hand, because it had previously been used in a large efficacy trial in Norway *(52)*. Also, we had already established an efficacy estimate with two doses of the parenteral vaccine, and a test for serum bactericidal activity as a surrogate marker for protection *(47,48)*.
2. The nasal-vaccine formulation was used in 10-times higher concentration, in terms of protein, than the corresponding formulation for parenteral use. This was done on a rather arbitrary basis, and no full dose-response study had been done for nasal immunization in humans. In mice, one-tenth the human dose is normally used, i.e., 2.5 μg OMV for subcutaneous and 25 μg for intranasal use. On the other hand, the nasal formulation did not contain any Al-hydroxide adjuvant, as did the parenteral vaccine (both for mice and man). The group lead by W. D. Zollinger, using native OMV, found that 8–10 times the parenteral dose

was required intranasally in mice to elicit equivalent bactericidal-antibody responses *(53)*.

3. The use of anesthetics during administration of nasal vaccine to mice will ease the handling of the animals and is probably important for delivering accurate doses. In our hands, with use of intravenous anesthetics, a higher dose of antigen might reach the lungs and higher systemic antibody responses will be seen, whereas no difference was observed on the secretory immune responses (B. Haneberg, unpublished results).

4. In humans, we have administered the vaccine as nasal drops by a metered pipet, or as spray with a metered spray device *(6)*. No striking differences on the immune responses have been observed among the few individuals who have been tested. For a more user-friendly nasal vaccine, that might be self-administered, a spray device will certainly be preferred. However, the logic behind the use of drops is that we then could have better control of the amount given, and the desired mucosal area of contact. With use of inhaled vaccines, studies in mice indicate that inflammatory reactions of the lungs should be taken into account *(53,54)*.

5. From the present clinical experiences with nasal vaccines, it is evident that more work is needed for finding the optimal and practical immunization schedule, (*see* **Subheading 1.7.**).

6. Special devices have been designed ("MucoSafe") for sampling of saliva from humans. In mice, the secretion of saliva has to be stimulated by intraperitoneal injection of 0.1 mg pilocarpine *(43)*. Care should be taken, however, to avoid that the mice might suffer from severe dyspnea during salivation.

7. Values that can be expected regarding net weights of captured saliva and nasal fluids in humans are: 74–310 mg (mean 248 mg) and 147–306 mg (mean 257 mg), respectively *(6)*.

References

1. Griffiss, J. M. (1995) Mechanisms of host immunity, in *Meningococcal Disease* (Cartwright, K. A. V., ed.), John Wiley and Sons, Chichester, UK, pp. 35–70.
2. Ala'Aldeen, D. A. A., and Griffiths, E. (1995) Vaccines against meningococcal disease, in *Molecular and Clinical Aspects of Bacterial Vaccine Development* (Ala'Aldeen, D. A. A. and Hormaeche, C. E., eds.) John Wiley and Sons, Chichester, UK, pp. 1–39.
3. Brandtzaeg, P., Farstad, I. N., Johansen, F.-E., Morton, H. C., Norderhagen, I. N., and Yamanaka, T. (1999) The B-cell system of human mucosae and exocrine glands. *Immunol. Rev.* **171,** 45–87.
4. McGhee, J. R., Mestecky, J., Dertzbaugh, M. T., Eldridge, J. H., Hirasawa, M., and Kiyono, H. (1992) The mucosal immune system: from fundamental concepts to vaccine development. *Vaccine* **10,** 75–88.
5. Walker, R. I. (1994) New strategies for using mucosal vaccination to achieve more effective immunization. *Vaccine* **12,** 387–400.

6. Haneberg, B., Dalseg, R., Wedege, E., Høiby, E. A., Haugen, I. L., Oftung, F., et al. (1998) Intranasal administration of a meningococcal outer membrane vesicle vaccine induces persistent local mucosal antibodies and serum antibodies with strong bactericidal activity in humans. *Infect. Immun.* **66**, 1334–1341.

7. Drabick, J. J., Brandt, B. L., Moran, E. E., Saunders, N. B., Shoemaker, D. R., and Zollinger, W. D. (2000) Safety and immunogenicity testing of an intranasal group B meningococcal native outer membrane vesicle vaccine in healthy volunteers. *Vaccine* **18**, 160–172.

8. Tang, C., Moxon, R., and Levine, M. M. (1999) For discussion: live attenuated vaccines for group B meningococcus. *Vaccine* **17**, 114–117.

9. American Academy of Pediatrics, Committee on Infectious Diseases (1999) Prevention of poliomyelitis: recommendations for use of only inactivated poliovirus vaccine for routine immunization. *Pediatrics* **104**, 1404–1406.

10. Bitnun, A., Shannon, P., Durward. A., Rota, P. A., Bellini, W. J., Graham, C., et al. (1999) Measles inclusion-body encephalitis caused by the vaccine strain of measles virus. *Clin. Infect. Dis.* **29**, 855–861.

11. Centers for Disease Control and Prevention (1999) Intussuspection among recipients of rotavirus vaccine: United States, 1998–1999. *MMWR Morb. Mortal. Wkly. Rep.* **48**, 577–581.

12. Talbot, E. A., Perkins, M. D., Silva, S. F. M., and Frothingham, R. (1997) Disseminated Bacille Calmette-Guérin disease after vaccination: case report and review. *Clin. Infect. Dis.* **24**, 1139–1146.

13. van Loon, F. P. L., Clemens, J. D., Chakraborty, J., Rao, M. R., Kay, B. A., Sack, D. A., et al. (1996) Field trial of inactivated oral cholera vaccines in Bangladesh: results from 5 years follow-up. *Vaccine* **14**, 162–166.

14. Richman, L. K., Chiller, J. M., Brown, W. R., Hanson, D. G., and Vaz, N. M. (1978) Enterically induced immunologic tolerance. I. Induction of suppressor T lymphocytes by intragastric administration of soluble proteins. *J. Immunol.* **121**, 2429–2434.

15. Ogra, P. L. (1996) Mucosal immunoprophylaxis: an introductory overview, in *Mucosal Vaccines* (Kiyono, H., Ogra, P. L., and McGhee, J. R., eds.), Academic Press, San Diego, CA, pp. 3–14.

16. Levine, M. M. and Dougan, G. (1998) Optimism over vaccines administered via mucosal surfaces. *Lancet* **351**, 1375–1376.

17. Holmgren, J., Lycke, N., and Czerkinsky, C. (1993) Cholera toxin and cholera B subunit as oral-mucosal adjuvant and antigen vector systems. *Vaccine* **11**, 1179–1184.

18. Agren, L., Lowenadler, B., and Lycke, N. (1998) A novel concept in mucosal adjuvanticity: the CTA1-DD adjuvant is a B cell-targeted fusion protein that incorporates the enzymatically active cholera toxin A1 subunit. *Immunol. Cell. Biol.* **76**, 280–287.

19. Douce, G., Giannelli, V., Pizza, M., Lewis, D., Everest, P., Rappuoli, R., and Dougan, G. (1999) Genetically detoxified mutants of heat-labile toxin from *Escherichia coli* are able to act as oral adjuvants. *Infect. Immun.* **67**, 4400–4406.

20. Sun, J.-B., Rask, C., Olsson, T., Holmgren, J., and Czerkinsky, C. (1996) Treatment of experimental autoimmune encephalomyelitis by feeding myelin basic protein conjugated to cholera toxin B subunit. *Proc. Natl. Acad. Sci. USA* **93**, 7196–7201.

21. Dalseg, R., Wedege, E., Holst, J., Haugen, I. L., Høiby, E. A., and Haneberg, B. (1999) Outer membrane vesicles from group B meningococci are strongly immunogenic when given intranasally to mice. *Vaccine* **17**, 2336–2345.

22. Hvalbye, B. K. R., Aaberge, I. S., Løvik, M., and Haneberg, B. (1999) Intranasal immunization with heat-inactivated *Streptococcus pneumoniae* protects mice against systemic pneumococcal infection. *Infect. Immun.* **67**, 4320–4325.

23. Hordnes, K., Tynning, T., Brown, T. A., Haneberg, B., and Jonsson, R. (1997) Nasal immunization with group B streptococci can induce high levels of specific IgA antibodies in cervicovaginal secretions of mice. *Vaccine* **15**, 1244–1251.

24. Berstad, A. K. H., Holst, J., Møgster, B., Haugen, I. L., and Haneberg, B. (1997) A nasal whole-cell pertussis vaccine can induce strong systemic and mucosal antibody responses which are not enhanced by cholera toxin. *Vaccine* **15**, 1473–1478.

25. Oftung, F., Næss, L. M., Wetzler, L. M., Korsvold, G. E., Aase, A., Høiby, E. A., et al. (1999) Antigen-specific T-cell responses in humans after intranasal immunization with a meningococcal serogroup B outer membrane vesicle vaccine. *Infect. Immun.* **67**, 921–927.

26. Berstad, A. K. H., Holst, J., Frøholm, L. O., Haugen, I. L., Wedege, E., Oftung, F., and Haneberg, B. (2000) A nasal whole-cell pertussis vaccine induces specific systemic and cross-reactive mucosal antibody responses in human volunteers. *J. Med. Microbiol.* **49**, 157–163.

27. Dalseg, R., Holst, J., Tangen, T., Stabbetorp, G., Simonsen, P., Jantzen, E., et al. (1996) Outer membrane vesicles from group B meningococci can act as mucosal adjuvant for influenza virus antigens, in *Vaccine 96; Molecular Approaches to the Control of Infectious Diseases* (Brown, E., Norrby, E., Burton, D., and Mekalanos, J., eds.), Cold Spring Harbor Laboratory Press, Cold Spring Harbor, NY, pp. 177–182.

28. Berstad, A. K. H., Andersen, S. R., Dalseg, R., Drømtorp, S., Holst, J., Namork, E., et al. (2000) Inactivated meningococci and pertussis bacteria are immunogenic and act as mucosal adjuvants for a nasal inactivated influenza virus vaccine. *Vaccine* **18**, 1910–1919.

29. Bergquist, C., Johansson, E.-L., Lagergård, T., Holmgren, J., and Rudin A. (1997) Intranasal vaccination of humans with recombinant cholera toxin B subunit induces systemic and local antibody responses in the upper respiratory tract and vagina. *Infect. Immun.* **65**, 2676–2684.

30. Del Giudice, G. and Rappuoli, R. (1999) Genetically derived toxoids for use as vaccines and adjuvants. *Vaccine* **17**, S44–S52.

31. Quraishi, M. S., Jones, N. S., and Mason, J. D. T. (1997) The nasal delivery of drugs. *Clin. Otolaryngol.* **22**, 289–301.

32. Lale, A. M., Mason, J. D. T., and Jones, N. S. (1998) Mucociliary transport and its assessment: a review. *Clin. Otolaryngol.* **23**, 388–396.

33. Winther, B. and Innes, D.J. (1994) The human adenoid. A morphologic study. *Arch. Otolaryngol. Head. Neck. Surg.* **120**, 144–149.
34. Anonymous (1997) Nasal preparations. *Ph. Eur.* 3rd Ed. (Council of Europe, Strasbourgh Cedex) pp. 1763–1765.
35. Anonymous (1997) Parenteral preparations. *Ph. Eur.* 3rd Ed. (Council of Europe, Strasbourgh Cedex) pp. 1765–1767.
36. Holst Fredriksen, J., Rosenqvist, E., Wedege, E., Bryn, K., Bjune, G., Frøholm, L. O., et al. (1991) Production, characterization, and control of Men B-vaccine "Folkehelsa": an outer membrane vesicle vaccine against group B meningococcal disease. *NIPH Ann.* **14**, 67–79.
37. Claassen, I., Meylis, J., van der Ley, P., Peeters, C., Brons, H., Robert, J., et al. (1996) Production, characterization and control of a *Neisseria meningitidis* hexavalent class 1 outer membrane protein containing vesicle vaccine. *Vaccine* **14**, 1001–1008.
38. Hammon, S. and Egelberg, P. (1999) Particle size and shape measurement by automated microscopy. *Eur. Pharm. Rev.* **4**, 16–20.
39. Anger, S., Caldwell, K., Niehus, H., and Müller, R. H. (1999) High resolution size determination of 20 nm colloidal gold particles by SedFFF. *Pharm. Res.* **16**, 1743–1747.
40. Woodle, M. C., Collins, L. R., Sponsler, E., Kossovsky, N., Papahadjopoulos, D., and Martin, F. J. (1992) Sterically stabilized liposomes. *Biophys. J.* **61**, 902–910.
41. Haneberg, B., Huynh, P., Nordsaeter, T., Haugen, I. L., Holst, J., and Aaberge, I. S. (1999) Intranasal immunization can generate better antibody responses when the antigen is given repeatedly in small doses. *Immunol. Lett.* **69**, 177.
42. Bakke, H., Haugen, I. L., Lie, K., Korsvold, G. E., Holst, J., Aaberge, I. S., et al. (1999) A bacterial outer membrane vesicle vaccine given intranasally can induce immunological memory with strong booster responses. *Immunol. Lett.* **69**, 178.
43. Haneberg, B., Kendall, D., Amerongen, H. M., Apter, F. M., Kraenhbuhl, J.-P., and Neutra, M. R. (1994) Induction of specific immunoglobulin A in the small intestine, colon-rectum, and vagina measured by a new method for collection of secretions from local mucosal surfaces. *Infect. Immun.* **62**, 15–23.
44. Haneberg, B., Kendall, D., Apter, F. M., and Neutra, M. R. (1997) Distribution of monoclonal antibodies in intestinal and urogenital secretions of mice bearing hybridoma 'backpack' tumours. *Scand. J. Immunol.* **45**, 151–159.
45. Vetvik, H., Grewal, H. M. S., Haugen, I. L., Åhrén, C., and Haneberg, B. (1998) Mucosal antibodies can be measured in air-dried samples of saliva and feces. *J. Immunol. Meth.* **215**, 163–172.
46. Berstad, A. K. H., Oftung, F., Korsvold, G. E., Haugen, I. L., Frøholm, L. O., Holst, J., and Haneberg B. (2000) Induction of antigen-specific T cell responses in humans after intranasal immunization with a whole-cell pertussis vaccine. *Vaccine* **18**, 2323–2330.
47. Perkins, B. A., Jonsdottir, K., Briem, H., Griffiths, E., Plikaytis, B. D., Høiby, E. A., et al. (1998) Immunogenicity of two efficacious outer membrane protein-

based serogroup B meningococcal vaccines among young adults in Iceland. *J. Infect. Dis.* **177,** 683–691.

48. Fuglesang, J.E., Høiby, E. A., Holst, J., Rosenqvist, E., and Nøkleby H. (1998) Increased and longer-lasting immune responses to the Norwegian meningococcal group B OMV vaccine in teenagers with a three-dose compared to a two-dose regimen, in *Eleventh International Pathogenic Neisseria Conference* (Nassif, X., Quentin-Millet, M.-J., and Taha, M.-K., eds.), Editions EDK, Paris, France, p. 174.

49. Bergquist, C., Lagergård, T., and Holmgren, J. (1997) Anticarrier immunity suppresses the antibody response to polysaccharide antigens after intranasal immunization with the polysaccharide-protein conjugate. *Infect. Immun.* **65,** 1579–1583.

50. Wedege, E., Bryn, K., and Frøholm, L. O. (1998) Restoration of antibody binding to blotted meningococcal outer membrane proteins using various detergents. *J. Immunol. Methods* **113,** 51–59.

51. Høiby, E. A., Rosenqvist, E., Frøholm, L. O., Bjune, G., Feiring, B., Nøkleby, H., and Rønnild, E. (1991) Bactericidal antibodies after vaccination with the Norwegian meningococcal serogroup B outer membrane vesicle vaccine: a brief survey. *NIPH Ann.* **14,** 147–156.

52. Bjune, G., Høiby, E. A., Grønnesby, J. K., Arnesen, O., Holst Fredriksen, J., Halstensen, A., et al. (1991) Effect of an outer membrane vesicle vaccine against serogroup B meningococcal disease in Norway. *Lancet* **338,** 1093–1096.

53. Saunders, N. B., Shoemaker, D. R., Moran, E. E., Larsen, T., and Zollinger, W. D. (1999) Immunogenicity of intranasally administered meningococcal native outer membrane vesicles in mice. *Infect. Immun.* **67,** 113–119.

54. Simecka, J. W., Jackson, R. J., Kiyono, H., and McGhee, J. R. (2000) Mucosally induced immunoglobulin E-associated inflammation in the respiratory tract. *Infect. Immun.* **68,** 672–679.

17

Animal Models for Meningococcal Disease

Andrew R. Gorringe, Karen M. Reddin, Pierre Voet, and Jan T. Poolman

1. Introduction

There are many in vitro systems for the study of meningococcal pathogenesis, but it is only in animal models of infection that the interactions of the bacteria with whole tissues and the humoral and cellular immune systems can be assessed. Animal-infection models are also of great importance for the assessment of the protective efficacy of existing and candidate vaccines. However, the relevance of these animal models to human disease and how well protection assessed in them corresponds to protection against human disease, must always be considered. Animal models for pathogenic *Neisseria* have been previously reviewed *(1)*.

As humans are the only natural hosts for *Neisseria meningitidis*, it has proved difficult to establish animal-infection models. Early attempts using monkeys *(2)*, rabbits *(3)*, and guinea pigs *(4)* proved unsuccessful. Different routes of inoculation of animals (intranasal [IN], intraperitoneal [IP] or intrathecal), were used in attempts to develop models that simulate the different phases or forms of meningococcal disease, i.e., colonization of the nasopharynx, invasion, bacteraemia, and/or meningitis. Intracranial injection of meningococci in rabbits produced clinical symptoms of meningitis *(3)*. However, it was shown that this was caused by the toxic effects of large numbers of bacteria, as a killed suspension of meningococci produced the same effect. Similar observations were found using guinea pigs *(4)*. A guinea-pig subcutaneous-chamber model has been used to study the immune response following infection *(5)* in which relatively low numbers of meningococci were required to infect the chambers and bacteria could be recovered for 6–8 d after infection.

From: *Methods in Molecular Medicine, vol. 66: Meningococcal Vaccines: Methods and Protocols*
Edited by: A. J. Pollard and M. C. J. Maiden © Humana Press Inc., Totowa, NJ

Large amounts of serum could be obtained for investigations but the infection did not progress to a disseminated infection.

Chick embryos have been used to differentiate the virulence of strains (6,7). However, the chick embryo lacks an active complement system, limiting its usefulness for studying meningococcal infection.

The model for meningococcal disease that has been most used is a mouse model first developed by Miller (8). This involved IP injection of meningococci suspended in hog gastric mucin into adult mice and was effective for differentiating the virulence of meningococcal strains (9). The minimum fatal dose for virulent strains was as low as 10 organisms, and from 100 to several thousands for avirulent strains. The addition of mucin to the inoculum was essential to produce a lethal infection. This IP challenge model was used by Branham and Pittman (10) for evaluation of anti-meningococcal serum. However, this model was difficult to standardize because the role of mucin was poorly understood. Also, because mucin is a poorly defined mixture of components, variability occurred in its capacity to augment infection. It is now understood that the mucin was providing an exogenous iron source for the infecting bacterial strain; this was required as the meningococcus has iron-acquisition systems that are specific for human iron proteins, particularly transferrin (11).

The important role of iron sources for establishing IP meningococcal infections in mice was demonstrated in a series of studies by Holbein; who monitored levels of bacteraemia and mortality in infected animals (12–15) and showed that iron dextran effectively augmented infection in a dose-dependent manner (12). Furthermore, iron-saturated human transferrin was also shown to be effective for enhancing meningococcal infection (13). Holbein also showed differential virulence between case and carrier isolates using this model (14). The role of iron supplements in the mouse IP challenge model was more recently studied by Schryvers and Gonzalez (16). Comparison of transferrins and lactoferrins from different species demonstrated that deaths of the mice only occurred when human forms of these proteins were used.

The susceptibility of different strains of mouse has also been investigated with inbred lines found to be more susceptible to IP meningococcal infection than outbred ones (17). Mouse strains with a range of phenotypes were also studied (18) and it was found that the lipopolysaccharide (LPS) locus, which influences a range of cellular responses to endotoxin, influenced the level of bacteraemia following IP infection.

The mouse IP challenge model has been useful for differentiation of virulence of meningococcal strains, including the effect of knockout mutants (19) and also in vaccine development for both active protection (20–22) and passive protection (22,23).

IP challenge of infant rats has also been developed as a model of meningo-coccal disease *(25–27)*. Compared with the mouse model, the advantages of using infant rats are that an additional iron source may not be required, lower inocula are required to produce disease, and the development of both bacter-aemia and meningitis can be determined by sampling of blood and cerebrospi-nal fluid. However, the use of infant animals does not allow the assessment of protection following active immunisation. Other disadvantages are that not all wild-type strains are virulent in this model and it is often necessary to increase the virulence of strains by animal passage. In addition, the duration of bacteraemia is short and mortality is low. However, this model has been used to demonstrate passive protection with antibodies against a number of menin-gococcal components *(24,26)* and has been adapted to evaluate human sera for protective immunity to group B meningococci *(27)*.

Although the IP models described have been shown to be effective for assessing virulence, immune protection, and the role of iron in infection, they do not incorpo-rate the pharyngeal-carriage phase that precedes bacteraemia and meningitis in humans. IN infection of mice, rats, and guinea pigs was performed by Salit *(28,29)*. The most successful infection was obtained with infant mice, with 40% of 2–5-d-old mice becoming bacteraemic by 48–72 h after inoculation with virulent meningococci. IN infection of infant mice was also investigated by Mackinnon et al. *(30)* and lipooligosaccharide (LOS) immunotype and capsule were found to be important factors for development of bacteraemia *(31)*. However, it was shown that the infection progressed from nasal colonisation to a lung infection followed by bacteraemia, rather than directly from the nasopharynx to bacteraemia as in humans. Iron supplements and high-inoculum doses were also required. In addi-tion, although this model was used reproducibly for some time in our laboratory, results were difficult to reproduce following a change in the source of the mouse strain (unpublished results).

Animal models for meningococcal disease do provide much valuable infor-mation for studies of pathogenesis and vaccine development. However, all the available models have some shortcomings in providing a model of human men-ingococcal disease. Methods for the most useful, reproducible, and widely used models of IP infection in mice and infant rats are provided.

2. Materials

2.1. Animals

1. NIH or Balb/c mice (Harlan) are used at 6–8 wk of age at the beginning of the immunization schedule.
2. Pregnant, pathogen-free Sprague Dawley rats are obtained from Iffa Credo (Lyon, France), and groups of 5–7-d-old pups used. Pups are randomly distributed in

litters in order to decrease variability between litters. Other rat species can also be used, such as albino Wistar rats *(27)*.

2.2. Active Protection in Mice

2.2.1. Preparation of the Subunit Vaccine

1. Freund's adjuvant: Complete and incomplete Freund's adjuvants are purchased from Sigma and stored in the original containers at 4°C until required. The adjuvant should be mixed immediately prior to use with the diluted antigen solution (*see* **Note 1**).
2. Aluminium adjuvants: Aluminium hydroxide and aluminium phosphate (Alhydrogel and Adju-Phos, respectively) are purchased from Superfos Biosector (Frederikssund, Denmark) as 2% sterile solutions. These are diluted and used as described in **Note 1**.

2.2.2. Preparation of the Whole-Cell Vaccine

1. Stock cultures: *N. meningitidis* strains are stored as lots (100–500 µL) at –70°C in Mueller-Hinton Broth (Oxoid) containing 30% (v/v) glycerol.
2. Blood agar plates: The seed stocks are thawed and subcultured onto two plates (*see* **Note 2**). One is used to produce a lawn of bacterial growth, which is used to inoculate 100 mL of MHB in flasks. The other plate is inoculated and streaked for single colonies to check the purity of the seed stock.
3. Mueller Hinton broth and agar (Oxoid).
4. Ethylenediamine-Di (o-Hydroxy-Phenylacetic acid) (EDDHA, Sigma) is prepared by dissolving 60 mg EDDHA in 0.36 M NaOH (7.2 mL 2 M NaOH + 20 mL distilled water), adjusting to pH 7.0, making up to 40 mL and sterilizing by filtration. This results in a stock solution of 1.5 mg/mL, which is diluted to give a final concentration of 5 µg/mL in the growth medium.

2.2.3. Immunizations

For Freund's adjuvant, glass syringes with Luer-lock fittings are used. The syringes are filled through a 21GA1/2-gauge needle, which is then replaced with a 25GA5/8-gauge needle for injecting. Aluminium adjuvants are administered using plastic syringes with 25GA5/8-gauge needles. Immunizations are given according to the requirements of the UK Home Office Animals (Scientific Procedures) Acts, 1986, or other equivalent national legislation.

2.2.4. Passive Protection

Monoclonal antibody (MAb) is normally obtained as tissue-culture fluid or ascitic fluid and is used either neat and/or diluted depending on the design of the experiment. Sera are raised by immunization using the appropriate animal model and the immunization schedule detailed in **Subheading 3.** The sera are diluted to the appropriate concentration prior to use.

3. Methods

All procedures involving animals were conducted according to the requirements of the UK Home Office Animals (Scientific Procedures) Acts, 1986, or other equivalent national legislation.

3.1. Active Protection in Mice

3.1.1. Preparation of Subunit Vaccines

Prepare the vaccine by diluting the antigen(s) to 100 μg/mL in sterile phosphate-buffered saline (PBS), and then diluting in the adjuvant (*see* **Note 1**) to give a solution of 50 μg/mL.

3.1.2. Preparation of Whole Cell Vaccine

1. To prepare the killed whole cell vaccine, grow the *N. meningitidis* strain on blood agar with overnight incubation at 37°C, 5% CO_2.
2. The following day, sub-culture the strain onto MH agar with or without EDDHA, depending on whether iron restriction is required, and incubate as above.
3. On day 3, scrape the growth from the plates using a sterile loop and resuspend in PBS containing 0.1% (w/v) thiomersal, 0.1% (v/v) formaldehyde. Adjust the optical density (OD) of this suspension to 0.05 at 600 nm using the same buffer. Leave the suspension at 4°C overnight and then check for sterility the next day by plating a loopful of the suspension onto blood agar.
4. Once sterility has been confirmed, dialyze the suspension overnight against PBS to remove the thiomersal and formaldehyde.
5. Prepare the vaccine by adding aluminium hydroxide to a concentration of 4 mg/mL (*see* **Note 1**).

3.1.3. Immunizations

1. Immunize NIH mice (Harlan) with the required dose of antigen in the appropriate adjuvant. Typical adjuvants include Freund's, aluminium hydroxide, and aluminium phosphate (*see* **Note 1**), and typically use a dose of 10 μg protein per mouse per dose. Administer the vaccines as sub-cutaneous injections, with each mouse receiving 0.1 mL at each of two sites sub-cutaneously (total = 0.2 mL, 10 μg antigen per dose).
2. Give animals three doses of vaccine on day 1, 21, and 28 prior to challenge with *N. meningitidis* on day 35. Where Freund's adjuvant is used, complete adjuvant is used to prepare the vaccine for the first dose and incomplete adjuvant for subsequent doses *(21)*.

3.1.4. Preparation of Challenge Inoculum

1. Store meningococcal strains at −70°C in Mueller Hinton Broth (MHB) containing 30% (v/v) glycerol (*see* **Note 2**).
2. Thaw the required strain and spread onto blood agar to produce a lawn of growth.
3. Incubate the agar plate(s) overnight at 37°C, in air with 5% CO_2.

4. Scrape the growth from the plate(s) into 100 mL MHB, with or without iron restriction as required by the protection experiment. Incubate flask(s) at 37°C with shaking for 4 h.

5. After 4 h, prepare a 1 : 10 dilution of the culture and measure the absorbance at 600 nm. Using this absorbance measurement, the amount of culture needed to give the required challenge dose (see **Note 3**) is calculated and mixed with the appropriate amount of iron source (see **Note 4**). An A_{600nm} of 0.1 is equivalent to 2×10^8 meningococci. Thus the inoculum is prepared using the formula:

$$\text{Total inoculum required (mL)} \times \frac{0.01}{A_{600nm} \text{ of } 1:10 \text{ dilution}} = \text{mL of neat culture required}$$

This volume will give 2×10^8 cfu/mL in the final challenge inoculum. Inject each mouse with 0.5 mL of the challenge inoculum IP therefore, each mouse receives 10^8 cfu. The number of viable bacteria in the inoculum is then determined by serial dilution and plating on MH agar.

6. Monitor the mice every 2–3 h after challenge over a 4-d period and signs of sickness, such as ruffled fur, eyes shut, or immobility, are recorded. Mice may exhibit one or more of these symptoms and must be humanely killed before the severity limit of the experiment is exceeded (Home Office Animals [Scientific Procedures] Act 1986).

3.2. Passive Protection in Mice

3.2.1. Immunizations

Administer 50 µL antibody solution or serum by IP injection to NIH mice 2 h before challenge and 2 h and 5 h after challenge. The antibody may be polyclonal antibody (PAb) or MAb, sera or purified immunoglobulins, depending on the design of the experiment. Purified antibody can be used neat or diluted. However, it is advisable to dilute sera before immunizing. PBS or the growth medium used to prepare the challenge inoculum can be used as the diluent.

3.2.2. Preparation of Challenge Inoculum

The challenge inoculum is prepared as described in **Subheading 2.2.4.**

3.3. Intraperitoneal Infection in Infant Rats

3.3.1. Preparation of the Challenge Inoculum for IP Challenge of Infant Rats

1. Plate 100 µL of the rat passaged (2×) H44/76 strain (see **Note 5**) on Mueller-Hinton (MH) agar with 1% (v/v) Polyvitex (Biomérieux, France) and 1% (v/v) heat inactivated horse serum (Sigma, H1138).

2. After overnight incubation at 37°C in air with 5% CO_2, bacteria are resuspended into Tryptic Soy Broth (TSB) medium containing 30 µM EDDHA and incubated

at 37°C using an orbital shaker until an OD of 0.4 is reached. The 0.4 OD corresponds to approx 10^9 CFU/mL in the mid-log phase.

3. Dilute the culture 10X in PBS buffer to a concentration of 10^8 bacteria/mL and prepare the several dilutions to be used for the challenge.
4. Challenge the pups with 100 μL of each dilution via the IP route. A challenge dose of 10^7 bacteria is routinely used in our laboratory, but 10^6 and 10^5 doses can also be used *(27)*.
5. Determine the exact number of viable bacteria in the challenge dose by plating the different prepared dilutions.

3.3.2. Passive Protection

1. Heat-inactivate the antibodies for 40 min at 56°C before use to destroy complement.
2. Passively immunize 4 groups of 8 pups with different concentrations/dilutions of the antibodies to be tested for protective efficacy.
3. Inject antibodies (100 μL) IP, from 24 h to 1 h before the bacterial challenge *(27)*.
4. Include appropriate controls (*see* **Note 6**).

3.3.3. Bacterial Challenge

1. Inject 10^4–10^7 cfu/pup (100–500 μL are generally used).
2. The selected dose depends on the virulence of the strain used. In our hands, a challenge dose of 10^7 bacteria from strain H44/76 is used (*see* **Note 7**).
3. Collect blood samples (250 μL) 3 h after the challenge (*see* **Note 8**) by cardiac puncture under anaesthesia and transfer into an EDTA anticoagulant tube containing 2.25 mL of TSB. This corresponds to the 1/10 dilution.

   Prepare further dilutions using TSB medium and plate 20 μL of each dilution on MH agar and colonies counted after an incubation period of 24 h. Do not use negative and confluent cultures to calculate the mean. (For calculation and analysis of results, *see* **Note 9**).
4. Collect cerebrospinal fluid (CSF) as follows *(25)*: hold the unanaesthetized rat in an immobile position with the head flexed forward. Locate the suboccipital region by palpation and enter the cisterna magna by puncture of the skin with a sterile 30-gauge needle. CSF flows into the hub of the needle and can be easily visualized with appropriately positioned lighting. Collect approx 15–20 μL of the CSF before withdrawal of the needle. Transfer the CSF into a micropipet and plate 10 μL in serial dilutions for enumeration.

4. Notes

1. Freund's complete and incomplete adjuvants: an equal volume is added to the 100 μg/mL antigen solution and this is homogenized to produce an emulsion. Aluminium adjuvants: the commercially available 2% solutions of aluminium phosphate or aluminium hydroxide are diluted 1:2.5 (v/v). An equal volume of this is then mixed with the 100 μg/mL antigen solution and mixed by rolling for

Table 1
Preparation of Challenge Inoculum

		Challenge dose		
		10^5	10^6	10^7
Vol. of culture	Neat	0.373 μL	3.73 μL	37.3 μL
	1 : 10 dilution	3.73 μL	37.3 μL	373 μL
Vol. of diluent (MHB)	Using a 1 : 10 dilution of the culture	4996.3 μL	4962.7 μL	4627 μL
Vol. of hTf 40 mg/mL in PBS		5 mL	5 mL	5 mL
Total volume		10 mL	10 mL	10 mL

If A600nm of a 4 h culture is 0.268 then using the formula, the volume of neat culture required for 10 mL of inoculum = 0.373 mL. So the challenge inoculum is prepared as follows for challenge doses of 10^5, 10^6, 10^7.

2 h at room temperature to allow the antigen to adsorb onto the adjuvant. This results in 4 mg/mL aluminium adjuvant in the final vaccine dose (*32*).

2. All *N. meningitidis* cultures and challenge inocula are prepared under ACDP category 2+ containment conditions. Challenge inocula are transported to the animal facilities in sealed containers. The challenge procedure is carried out on a down-draft table and a positive- or negative-pressure protective respirator is worn. To monitor the mice after challenge, a face mask with a 0.2-μm filter is worn.

3. The challenge dose used in an experiment depends on the virulence of the *N. meningitidis* strain used. This can be determined by a preliminary virulence titration using the methods described above in unimmunized mice. Typically, a range of three challenge doses are given to determine the virulence of a strain. The appropriate challenge doses are then used in the protection experiment, a typical challenge experiment would use 2–3 challenge doses.

   An example experiment using human transferrin (hTf) as the exogenous iron source is outlined in **Table 1**.

4. The exogenous iron source can be either human transferrin or iron dextran. Ten mg of iron-saturated human transferrin is given IP with the challenge dose and a further 10 mg per mouse is administered 24 h later. For iron dextran, 2 mg iron per mouse is given IP with the challenge dose and a further 2 mg is given 24 h later. Human transferrin is the preferred iron source as it requires a lower amount of iron to augment infection in the mouse model but is more costly.

5. *N. meningitidis* serogroup B strain H44/76 is the virulent strain commonly used in this model, but any other virulent strain may also be used (*27*). Strain H44/76 was originally isolated in 1976 in Norway (*33*).

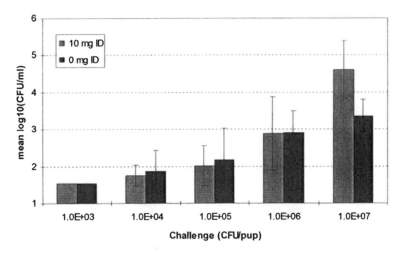

Fig. 1. Effect of several challenge doses and of iron dextran (ID) on bacteraemia.

6. Negative controls (buffer or medium without specific antibodies) and positive controls should be included in each experiment. Positive controls could be the protective monoclonal anti-PorA antibody (95/720, obtained from NIBSC, Potters Bar, UK) or anti-whole cell antibodies obtained from immunized Balb/C mice.

7. Determination of the optimal challenge dose, and effect of iron dextran in infant rats. Bacterial dose is of a great importance. Thus we have tested 10^4, 10^5, 10^6, and 10^7 cfu/mL of the rat-passaged H44/76 strain. Results indicated that, in our conditions, 10^7 cfu/pup from strain H44/76 appeared to be the optimal challenge dose (**Fig. 1**). We evaluated also the consequences in the model of 10 mg of iron dextran given 30 min before the challenge. Results we obtained indicated that higher bacteraemia was obtained with iron dextran at 10^7 challenge dose, compared to the control group.

8. Timing for blood collection. In a preliminary experiment, several timings have been evaluated in order to determine the best schedule for IP challenge of infant rats. Blood was taken 3, 6, or 18 h after the challenge and bacterial counts (not shown) indicated that rats eliminated group B meningococci quickly between 6 and 18 h after the challenge. In a second experiment, bacteraemia was evaluated 1, 2, and 3 h after the challenge, and 3 h appeared to be the optimal timing. At that time, all pups developed detectable bacteraemia (**Fig. 2**). The animals were challenged with 10^7 CFU H44/76 strain. The difference observed between the highest level of bacteraemia and the level obtained after passive transfer of the positive control, i.e., an anti-PorA MAb, is nearly a 2-log10 difference, which is highly significant (Anova 1 Tukey-HSD test).

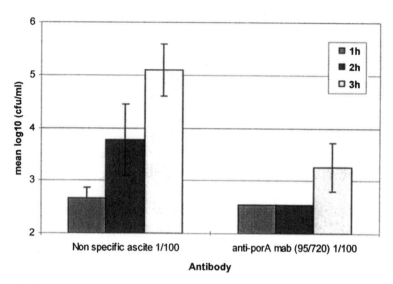

Fig. 2. Bacteraemia in infant rats 1, 2, or 3 h after challenge with 10^7 H44/76 bacteria.

9. For each animal, weighted means are calculated as follows:

$$\text{Weighted mean} = \frac{\text{(Sum of the CFU obtained at the different dilutions tested)}}{\text{(Sum of the corresponding initial blood volumes for plating*)}}$$

*, for the different dilutions tested.

As an example, 20 μL of the 1/10 dilution is equivalent of 2 μL of blood (0.002 mL). Twenty μL of the 1/100 dilution is equivalent to 0.0002 mL, etc.. Then, the sum is 0.0022 if colonies are counted only from these two dilutions. See also the example calculation in **Table 2**.

Geometric means of CFU obtained for each group are then transformed to logarithmic values. The mean of each group is compared by statistical analysis using Anova 1 Tukey-HSD test. The criterion of protection is a statistically significant reduction in bacteraemia and meningitis (from CSF) compared with untreated animals. This procedure permitted us to reduce the detection limit from 10^2 or 10^3 cfu/mL (generally described for blood and CSF cultures) to $<10^2$ CFU/mL (log10 of 1.544 corresponding to 35 CFU/mL). The average (+/– 1 standard deviation) is calculated for each group, from the 8 individual animals.

Acknowledgments

Work at CAMR was funded by the UK Department of Health. Work at SBBio was sponsored by a grant from the Region Wallonne C-3754.

Table 2
Calculation of Weighted Mean CFU in Blood Samples

Strain H44/76 Chall. 10^7 Group 1	CFU found in the corrected volume at dilutions				SUM of CFU	SUM of added blood volumes	Individual mean	log10 of ind. mean	Weighted means (Log 10)	Standard deviation
	1/10 0.002*	1/100 0.0002*	1/1000 0.00002*	1/10000 0.000002*						
Animal 1	0	70	0	0	70	0.0002	350000	5.544	6.344	0.818
Animal 2	191	34	2	0	227	0.00222	102252	5.010		
Animal 3	0	0	256	35	291	0.000022	13227273	7.121		
Animal 4	0	191	30	0	221	0.00022	1004545	6.002		
Animal 5	0	0	0	48	48	0.000002	24000000	7.380		
Animal 6	0	0	185	4	189	0.000022	8590909	6.934		
Animal 7	0	288	17	2	307	0.000222	1382883	6.141		
Animal 8	0	0	90	2	92	0.000022	4181818	6.621		

*taking into account the correct blood volume.

References

1. Arko, R. J. (1989) Animal models for pathogenic *Neisseria* species. *Clin. Microbiol. Rev.* **2(Suppl.),** S56–S59.
2. Flexner, S. (1907) Experimental cerebro-spinal meningitis in monkeys. *J. Exp. Med.* **9,** 142–166.
3. Branham, S. E., Lillie, R. D., and Pabst, A. M. (1932) Observations on experimental meningitis in rabbits. *Public Health Rep.* **47,** 2137–2150.
4. Branham, S. E. and Lillie, R. D. (1937) Experimental meningitis in guinea pigs. *Public Health Rep.* **52,** 1135–1142.
5. Frasch, C. E. and Robbins, J. D. (1978) Protection against group B meningococcal disease. III. Immunogenicity of serotype 2 vaccines and specificity of protection in a guinea pig model. *J. Exp. Med.* **147,** 629–644.
6. Frasch, C. E., Parkes, L., McNelis, R. M., and Gotschlich, E. C. (1976) Protection against group B meningococcal disease. I. Comparison of group-specific and type-specific protection in the chick embryo model. *J. Exp. Med.* **144,** 319–329.
7. Pine, L., Quinn, F. D., Ewing, E. P. Jr, Birkness, K. A., White, E. H., Stephens, D. S., and Ribot, E. (1995) Evaluation of the chick embryo for the determination of relative virulence of *Neisseria meningitidis*. *FEMS Microbiol. Lett.* **130,** 37–44.
8. Miller, C. P. (1933) Experimental meningococcal infection in mice. *Science* **78,** 340–341.
9. Miller, C. P. and Castles, R. (1936) Experimental meningococcal infection in mice. *J. Infect. Dis.* **58,** 263–279.
10. Branham, S. E. and Pittman, M. (1940) Recommended procedure for mouse protection test in evaluation of anti-meningococcus serum. *Public Health Rep.* **55,** 2340–2346.
11. Gray-Owen, S. D. and Schryvers, A. B. (1996) Bacterial transferrin and lactoferrin receptors. *Trends Microbiol.* **4,** 185–191.
12. Holbein, B. E. (1980) Iron-controlled infection with *Neisseria meningitidis* in mice. *Infect. Immun.* **29,** 886–891.
13. Holbein, B. E. (1981) Enhancement of *Neisseria meningitidis* infection in mice by addition of iron bound to transferrin. *Infect. Immun.* **34,** 120–125.
14. Holbein, B. E. (1981) Differences in virulence for mice between disease and carrier strains of *Neisseria meningitidis*. *Can. J. Microbiol.* **27,** 738–741.
15. Holbein, B. E., Jericho, K. W., and Likes, G. C. (1979) *Neisseria meningitidis* infection in mice: influence of iron, variations in virulence among strains, and pathology. *Infect. Immun.* **24,** 545–551.
16. Schryvers, A. B. and Gonzalez, G. C. (1989) Comparison of the abilities of different protein sources of iron to enhance *Neisseria meningitidis* infection in mice. *Infect. Immun.* **57,** 2425–2429.
17. Brodeur, B. R., Tsang, P. S., Hamel, J., Larose, Y., and Montplaisir, S. (1986) Mouse models of infection for *Neisseria meningitidis* B,2b and *Haemophilus influenzae* type b diseases. *Can. J. Microbiol.* **32,** 33–37.

18. Woods, J. P., Frelinger, J. A., Warrack, G., and Cannon, J. G. (1988) Mouse genetic locus Lps influences susceptibility to *Neisseria meningitidis* infection. *Infect. Immun.* **56,** 1950–1955.
19. Wilks, K. E., Dunn, K. L., Farrant, J. L., Reddin, K. M., Gorringe, A. R., Langford, P. R., and Kroll, J. S. (1998) Periplasmic superoxide dismutase in meningococcal pathogenicity. *Infect. Immun.* **66,** 213–217.
20. Huet, M. and Suire, A. (1981) An animal model for testing the activity of meningococcal polysaccharide vaccine. *J. Biol. Stand.* **9,** 67–74.
21. Danve, B., Lissolo, L., Mignon, M., Colombani, S., Schryvers, A. B., and Quentin-Millet M-J. (1993) Transferrin binding proteins isolated from *Neisseria meningitidis* elicit protective and bactericidal antibodies in laboratory animals. *Vaccine* **11,** 1214–1220.
22. Martin, D., Cadieux, N., Hamel, J., and Brodeur, B. R. (1997) Highly conserved *Neisseria meningitidis* surface protein confers protection against experimental infection. *J. Exp. Med.* **185,** 1173–1183.
23. Brodeur, B. R., Larose, Y., Tsang, P., Hamel, J., Ashton, F., and Ryan, A. (1985) Protection against infection with *Neisseria meningitidis* group B serotype 2b by passive immunization with serotype-specific monoclonal antibody. *Infect. Immun.* **50,** 510–516.
24. Saukkonen, K., Abdillahi, H., Poolman, J. T., and Leinonen, M. (1987) Protective efficacy of monoclonal antibodies to class 1 and class 3 outer membrane proteins of *Neisseria meningitidis* B : 15 : P1.16 in infant rat infection model: prospects for vaccine development. *Microb. Pathog.* **3,** 261–267.
25. Saukkonen, K. (1988) Experimental meningococcal meningitis in the infant rat. *Microb. Pathog.* **4,** 203–211.
26. Saukkonen, K., Leinonen, M., Abdillahi, H., and Poolman, J. T. (1989) Comparative evaluation of potential components for group B meningococcal vaccine by passive protection in the infant rat and *in vitro* bactericidal assay. *Vaccine* **7,** 325–328.
27. Toropainen, M., Kayhty, H., Saarinen, L., Rosenqvist, E., Hoiby, E. A., Wedege, E., et al. (1999) The infant rat model adapted to evaluate human sera for protective immunity to group B meningococci. *Vaccine* **7,** 2677–2689.
28. Salit, I. E. and Tomalty, L. (1984) Experimental meningococcal infection in neonatal mice: differences in virulence between strains isolated from human cases and carriers. *Can. J. Microbiol.* **30,** 1042–1045.
29. Salit, I. E., Van Melle, E., and Tomalty, L. (1984) Experimental meningococcal infection in neonatal animals: models for mucosal invasiveness. *Can. J. Microbiol.* **30,** 1022–1029.
30. Mackinnon, F. G., Gorringe, A. R., Funnell, S. G., and Robinson, A. (1992) Intranasal infection of infant mice with *Neisseria meningitidis. Microb. Pathog.* **12,** 415–420.
31. Mackinnon, F. G., Borrow, R., Gorringe, A. R., Fox, A. J., Jones, D. M., and Robinson, A. (1993) Demonstration of lipooligosaccharide immunotype and cap-

sule as virulence factors for *Neisseria meningitidis* using an infant mouse intranasal infection model. *Microb. Pathog.* **15,** 359–366.

32. Gupta, R. K. and Siber, G. R. (1994) Comparison of adjuvant activities of aluminium phosphate, calcium phosphate and stearyl tyrosine for tetanus toxoid. *Biologicals* **22,** 53–63.

33. Seiler, A ., Reinhardt, R., Sarkari, J., Caugant, D. A., and Achtman, M. (1996) Allelic polymorphism and site-directed recombinantion in the opc locus of *Neisseria meningitidis*. *Mol. Microbiol.* **19,** 841–856.

18

Determination of Antibody Responses to Meningococcal Antigens by ELISA

Einar Rosenqvist, Helena Käyhty, and Andrew J. Pollard

1. Introduction

Enzyme-linked immunosorbent assay (ELISA, EIA) is a highly versatile and sensitive technique that can be used for quantitative as well as qualitative determination of almost any antigen or antibody. Reagents are stable, nonradioactive and, in most cases, commercially available. Owing to the simplicity and versatility of the method, ELISA represents probably one of the most used methods for studying antibody responses and antibody levels. Since Engvall and Perlman's first paper describing the ELISA in 1971 *(1)*, almost all laboratories working in serology or immunology have designed their own assays with different protocols for coating with antigens, incubation conditions, detecting systems, and ways of reporting of the results. In most cases, there is no need for strict interlaboratory standardization of ELISAs and each laboratory will develop a system that suits their needs. However, for some ELISAs, e.g., used in diagnostic laboratories and in vaccine trials, standardization is important, and this is considered in "Meningococcal Disease" Edited by AJ Pollard and MCJ Maiden, *(1a)*.

Noncompetitive ELISAs used to detect anti-meningococcal antibodies involve: 1) coating of a microtiter plate with the antigen to be studied; 2) blocking of unbound sites on the plate with an immunologically neutral protein; 3) addition of test sera and specific binding of antibodies to the solid-phase antigen on the plate; 4) addition of a detector antibody that recognizes the class or subclass of serum antibody; 5) generation of a color change on the ELISA plate linked to the amount of bound detector antibody; 6) calculation of concentration of specific antibodies in test sample.

From: *Methods in Molecular Medicine, vol. 66: Meningococcal Vaccines: Methods and Protocols*
Edited by: A. J. Pollard and M. C. J. Maiden © Humana Press Inc., Totowa, NJ

Essential to the success of any assay method is an understanding of the flexibility that can be allowed within the assay without compromising the consistency of the results. This chapter will outline general ELISA principles that will complement other chapters in this book and in "Meningococcal Disease" *(1a)*. We shall also discuss specific ELISA methods developed to examine human antibody responses against whole-cells or sub-components of meningococci and give references to some important published papers in the field, including specific details about examples that have been successful in our and others' laboratories.

A competitive, inhibition ELISA may be important for many purposes, e.g., to demonstrate the specificity of the antigen-antibody binding (see, e.g., refs. *2,3*) and the assay may also be used to quantitate antigens or epitopes. However, these methods will not be discussed in this chapter.

2. Materials

2.1. Microtiter Plates

Ideally the solid phase for ELISA should be hydrophilic and able to bind all kinds of molecules in a natural conformation and should not increase the assay background. The most commonly used solid phase for ELISA today is the 96-well polystyrene high-binding microtiter ELISA plate. Although different antigens may have a different binding affinity to the plastic, comparable results are obtained for most proteins using Immulon I plates obtained from Dynatech (Dynatech Laboratories Inc., Chantilly, VA), Greiner (Nurtingen, Germany or Stonehouse, UK), or MaxiSorp or PolySorp plates from Nunc (Roskilde, Denmark). Some antigens, such as meningococal capsular polysaccharides (CPS), bind poorly to polystyrene, and special high-binding plates, like MaxiSorp from Nunc or high-binding plates from Corning-Costar (distributed by Bibby Sterilin Ltd., UK) may be needed. Polyvinyl chloride (PVC) plates (Flow Laboratories, The Netherlands) have also been used, e.g., for the whole-cell ELISA, with satisfactory results *(4)*.

2.2. ELISA Readers

There are a variety of high-quality ELISA readers available commercially. Choose a reader that is able to read absorbances at several wavelengths (405–650 nm) and has the facility to communicate with and transfer data to a computer. Several manufacturers of ELISA readers do also provide good computer software for ELISA analysis.

2.3. Antigens

2.3.1. Whole Cells

For studies of the total antibody responses to infection or after vaccination, whole cells are often preferred as antigen in the ELISA. The most commonly used whole-cell preparations are heat-inactivated meningococci (4,5). Methods for preparing whole cells are considered in **Subheading 3.**

2.3.2. Outer-Membrane Vesicles

Outer-membrane vesicles (OMVs) are spheres of the meningococcal outer membrane that have been prepared from meningococci by several methods. These methods are described in **Subheading 3.** Native OMVs (nOMVs or blebs) are fragments of outer membranes and contain the outer-membrane proteins (OMPs), capsular polysaccharides (CPS), phospholipids, and 30–50% lipopolysaccharide (LPS), relative to protein. Detergent extracted outer-membrane vesicles (dOMV) are relatively similar to nOMV in major OMPs but contain less LPS (5–8% relative to protein), CPS and Opa proteins than nOMV. dOMVs may be prepared, e.g., by deoxycholate (DOC) extraction of whole cells at pH 8.6 (6). Preparation of dOMV for use as vaccine is described in Chapter 7.

2.3.3. Outer-Membrane Proteins

Several purified meningococcal OMPs have been used as antigens in ELISA. PorA (7); PorB (8); Opc (9,10); iron-regulated proteins (IRP), including transferrin-binding protein complex (Tbps) (11); and IgA1 protease (12) are examples of some important meningococcal proteins reported as antigens in ELISA studies. Purification procedures for these antigens are described in the original papers and methods for purification of porins and Tbps are presented in Chapters 6 and 8.

2.3.4. Liposomes

Some purified membrane proteins, e.g., Opc cannot be used as antigens to assay human antibodies directly because they stick nonspecifically to immunoglobulins, or they are denatured during the purification process. An alternative has been to incorporate the OMP into liposomes (9), as described in **Subheading 3.**

2.3.5. Lipopolysaccharides

Meningococcal LPS of different immunotypes may be prepared from cells by hot phenol-water extraction or from nOMVs by DOC-extraction and gelfiltration (Sephacryl S300) in a TRIS-DOC buffer, as described in **refs. 13–16.**

2.3.6. Capsular Polysaccharides

Meningococcal CPSs of serogroups A, B, C, Y, and W135 may be obtained either from NIBSC (National Institute for Biological Standards and Control, South Mimms, UK) or ATCC (American Tissue Culture Collection, Rockville, MD), or from various commercial vaccine manufacturers (e.g., BioMerieux), or produced locally by Cetavlon precipitation, as described (17) and in Chapter 3.

2.3.7. Protein Epitopes and Peptides

Studies of antibodies to specific epitopes or parts of meningococcal proteins may be performed by using synthetic peptides of varying size or recombinant proteins where epitopes from meningococcal proteins are inserted (*see* Chapter 13).

2.4. Buffers

2.4.1. Antigen-Coating Buffers (see **Note 1**)

Several buffers have been used for solutions with antigens, e.g.,

1. 0.1 M Tris-HCl, pH 8.6: 24.2 g (Sigma) Tris 7-9 (Sigma T-1378), 2 L distilled water, 13.5 mL 5 M HCl.
2. 0.1 M Carbonate buffer, pH 9.8: 10.6 g Na_2CO_3 (Sigma S-2127), 1 L distilled water, adjust with 5 M HCl.
3. 0.05 M Carbonate/bicarbonate buffer, pH 9.6: 1.59 g Na_2CO_3, 2.93 g $NaHCO_3$, 1 L distilled water. (Store at + 4°C for no more than 2 wk).
4. Phosphate-buffered saline (PBS), pH 7.4: 80 g NaCl, 11.6 g Na_2HPO_4, 2.0 g KH_2PO_4, 2.0 g KCl, 10 L distilled water.

2.4.2. Washing Buffer

PBS with 0.05% Tween-20 (PBST) or with 0.1% Brij-35 (*see* **Note 2**).

2.4.3. Blocking Buffer

PBST with 0.5–1% BSA, or 2–10% fetal or newborn bovine serum (NBBS), or 1% dried skimmed-milk powder.

2.4.4. Serum or Antibody Dilution Buffer

Same as blocking buffer.

2.4.5. Substrate Buffers

1. 0.2 M Citrate/phosphate buffer, pH 5.0: Make up stock solutions of 0.1 M (21.01 g/L) citric acid ($C_6H_8O_7 \cdot H_2O$) and 0.2 M (28.4 g/L) Na_2HPO_4. Just prior to use, add 48.5 mL 0.1 M citric acid to 51.5 mL of 0.2 M Na_2HPO_4. Check and adjust pH as necessary.
2. 10% diethanolamine buffer, pH 9.8: 97 mL Diethanolamine (note: toxic), 100 mg $MgCl_2 \cdot 6H_2O$, 25 mL 5 M HCl.

2.5. Substrates

2.5.1. Alkaline Phosphatase Substrate

PNPP: 10 mg p-nitrophenyl phosphate (Sigma 104, N9389) dissolved in 10 mL 10% diethanolamine buffer or in 0.05 M carbonate buffer, pH 9.8.

2.5.2. Peroxidase Substrates

OPD: 10 mg o-phenylenediamine dihydrochloride; (Sigma, P6912) dissolved in 50 mL citrate-phosphate buffer, pH 5.0, with 10 μL 30% hydrogen peroxide; or ABTS: 2,2'-Azino-bis(3ethylbenzthiaxoline-6-sulfonic acid) (Sigma A9941); or TMB: 3,3',5,5'-Tetramethylbenzidine (Sigma T3405, T5525).

2.6. Specific Antibodies and Conjugates

1. Alkaline phosphatase (AP)-conjugated or horse-radish peroxidase (HRP)-conjugated, affinity purified polyclonal or monoclonal anti-human IgG, IgM, or IgA are primarily used. There are several manufacturers with good products and every laboratory should evaluate which one best meets their needs.
2. IgG subclasses may be determined using subclass-specific mouse MAbs as the secondary antibody (e.g., anti IgG1 = HP6069; anti IgG2 = HP6002; anti IgG3 = HP6050; anti-IgG4 = HP6011) obtained from the International Union of Immunological Societies (IUIS), Immunoglobulin Subcommittee or WHO Collaborating Center for human Immunoglobulins (Centers for Disease Control), and HPR or AP enzyme conjugated anti-mouse antibodies as conjugate (e.g., Dakopatts, Sigma, but available from several suppliers). In addition, enzyme-labeled isotype specific antibodies (e.g., from ICN Biochemicals) can be used directly; thus no second detector antibody is needed *(5,18,19)*.

2.7. References and Control Sera

Internal standards ("house standards") with antibodies against the various antigens should be prepared from sera from blood donors or vaccinees or from convalescents after meningococcal disease. These sera may be arbitrarily assigned a certain U/mL for each antigen. If possible the specific antibody concentrations should be determined as gravimetrical units by other methods. Both sera with high, medium, and low ("negative") levels of antibodies should be collected. The reference sera should be dispensed in small volumes (100–500 μL) and frozen at –70°C. Reference serum CDC1992 with determined concentrations of specific IgG, IgM, and IgA for anti-C and anti-A-CPS is supplied by NIBSC *(20)*.

3. Methods
3.1. Preparation of Antigens
3.1.1. Whole Cells

1. Grow meningococci overnight on Tryptic soy agar (TSA) or supplemented (e.g., 1% isovitalex) GC medium base agar plates (Difco, Detriot) at 37°C in 5% CO_2.
2. Harvest bacteria with a loop or sterile glass slide and suspend them in PBS, pH 7.4, with 0.02% sodium azide (NaN_3) prior to killing by heating the container with the bacterial suspension in a water bath for 1 h at 56°C.

The whole cell preparation contains a mixture of intact and broken cells, native outer membrane vesicles (nOMV/"blebs") and CPS. This suspension can be stored for months or years at +4°C (*see* **Note 3**).

A modification of this method has been described *(21)*:

1. Incubate one-quarter of the growth from a plate of supplemented GC agar overnight at 37°C in 5% CO_2, and resuspend in 10 mL of PBS.
2. Incubate the suspension for 1 h at 56°C and allow to cool to room temperature.
3. Add sodium azide to a concentration of 0.02%.
4. Store the suspension at +4°C for at least 24 h to allow larger particles to settle, and use only the soluble supernatant for coating.

The antigen prepared by this method is mainly nOMVs and CPS. Quantitatively comparable results are obtained when such preparations are retested after storage at +4°C for 9 mo *(21)*.

3.1.2. Outer-Membrane Vesicles (nOMVs) (see also Chapter 7)

1. Grow cultures of *Neisseria meningitidis* overnight at 35°C either in baffled flasks with dialysed tryptic soy broth (TSB) (Difco Laboratories, Detroit, MI), on a rotatory shaker at 150 rpm, or on TSA, BHI, or Kellogg's agar plates in a 5% CO_2 atmosphere.
2. Harvest the cells by centrifugation of the liquid cultures at about 5000g for 10 min, or by scraping the bacteria from the agar plates with a loop or a sterile microscope slide.
3. Inactivate the bacteria by heating at 60°C for 30 min.
4. Prepare nOMVs by rapid shaking of the cell pellet with 3-mm glass beads for 30 min in a 0.2 *M* LiCl, 0.1 *M* NaAc buffer, pH 5.8.
5. Fractionate the preparation by centrifugation 15,000g for 15 min and then 2× ultracentrifugation (100,000g) for 90 min *(22)*.
6. Dissolve the membrane pellet in distilled water and determine the protein concentration by the Lowry technique, and adjust to a protein concentration of about 1 mg/mL.
7. Store the OMVs at –20°C. For preservation, sodium azide may be added to 0.02%.

3.1.3. Liposomes

To prepare Opc-liposomes, mix 27 mg phosphatidyl ethanolamine and 3.3 mg phosphatidyl choline (Avanti Polar Lipids, Birmingham, AL) dissolved in chloroform in a 25-mL glass flask, and dry by rotary evaporation under partial vacuum at 30°C for at least 1 h.

1. Resuspend 4 mg of Opc protein, purified as described *(10)*, in 1 mL of PBS containing 5% n-octyl α-D-glucanopyranoside (PBSO).
2. Add the protein solution to the dried phospholipids, and add PBSO until the solution is clear (total volume, 3 mL).

3. Dialyse the solution against PBS for 10 h at room temperature with five changes of buffer.
4. Homogenize the liposomes containing ~1 mg/mL of Opc in an ultrasonic water bath for 5 min, and add sodium azide to 0.02%.
5. Before coating ELISA plates, resuspend the liposomes by incubation in an ultrasonic water bath for 5 min and then dilute to 4 µg Opc/mL in 0.06 M carbonate buffer, pH 9.6.
6. Make control liposomes ("null liposomes") in the same way, except do not add protein.

Liposomes with other purified membrane proteins may be prepared in the same way.

3.1.4. Lipopolysaccharides

Pure meningococcal LPS in water gives poor or irregular coating on polystyrene ELISA plates. Therefore alternative preparations are required in order to facilitate binding to the ELISA plate.

1. LPS-BSA complexes *(23,24)*:
   a. To prepare complexes of LPS and BSA, sonicate LPS (1 mg/mL) dissolved in distilled water containing 0.5% triethylamine (TEA) for 30 s.
   b. Dissolve BSA (10 mg/mL) in distilled water containing 0.5% TEA.
   c. Mix one volume of the LPS solution with 1 volume of the BSA solution and dry by rotary evaporation.
   d. Redissolve the LPS/BSA complexes in 1 volume distilled water and store frozen at –20°C (1 mg LPS/mL).
2. LPS-PolymyxinB Complexes *(25)*:
   a. Mix equal volumes of 1 mg/mL of Polymyxin B sulphate (Sigma) with 10 µg/mL of LPS in pyrogen-free distilled water and stir for 30 min at room temperature.
   b. Place the mixture into a clean, boiled dialysis bag and dialyze overnight against distilled water to remove unbound Polymyxin.
   c. Dilute the dialyzed complex in 0.05 M carbonate buffer, pH 9.6.
3. LPS-DOC micelles *(26)*: Mix one volume of LPS (1 mg/mL) dissolved in distilled water with 1 volume of 0.1% deoxycholate (DOC) in PBS, pH 7.4, and shake rapidly with a Vortex mixer for 1–2 min.

3.1.5. Peptides and Protein Epitopes

Some examples using these antigens in ELISA are given here:

1. Synthetic peptides containing the VR1 and VR2 region from P1.7,16 meningococcal PorA have been used as antigens in ELISA by coating microtiter plates over night at 37°C with 8-mers peptides and multiple antigen peptides (MAPs), (1 µg/mL) in 0.05 M carbonate buffer, pH 9.6 *(27)*, or by coating polystyrene

microtiter plates (Dynatech, Immulon 2) for 2 h at 37°C with 18-mer peptides (5 μg/mL) in PBS, pH 7.2 *(28)*.

2. Antibodies to the VR1 (P1.7) and VR2 (P1.16) epitopes in PorA molecules have been determined in ELISA using as coating antigen the VR1 and VR2 loops inserted into the bacillar penicillinase as a carrier protein. The antigens were solubilized in 0.1% sodium dodecyl sulfate (SDS) and diluted to 5 μg/mL for coating ELISA plates over night *(29)*.

3. Antibodies to synthetic 104-mers and 16-mers peptides from meningococcal IgA1 protease have been studied by Brieske et al. *(11)* and Thiesen et al. *(12)*. The peptides were dissolved (6 μg/mL) in 0.05 *M* carbonate buffer and used to coat Nunc Maxisorb plates at 37°C overnight.

3.2. Samples to be Analyzed

ELISA may be used to determine antibody levels in many biological specimens including serum, plasma, ascites, spinal fluids, nasal fluids, saliva, milk, or feces. When analyzing saliva and nasal fluids, both specific and total antibody should be determined.

3.2.1. Serum Antibodies

1. Collect blood into plain glass vacutainer tubes with no anticoagulant and allow to clot for 60 min at room temperature, or overnight at 4°C.
2. Centrifuge the clotted samples at 1200*g* for 10 min and then aspirate serum and freeze in aliquots at –20°C or preferably –70°C (*see* **Note 4**).

3.2.2. Salivary Antibody *(30,31, and see* **Note 5***)*.

1. Oral test kits: Oral test kits (Malvern Medical Developments, Worcester, UK) are now widely used in the UK for saliva collection.
   a. Remove the foam swab from the collection device and rub over the gums for 1 min.
   b. Replace the swab in the tube, add 1 mL of transport medium (10% fetal calf serum [FCS], 0.2% Tween 20, PBS, pH 7.4) and vortex for 20 s.
   c. Invert the swab in the tube and centrifuge at 2,000*g* for 5 min.
2. Wicks:
   a. Collect saliva on wicks of synthetic fibers and cellulose (Polywicks (PFT#941925), Polyfiltronic Group Inc., Rockland, MA) placed in the mouth until soaked with saliva (2–3 min).
   b. Weigh the wicks before and after exposure and calculate the amount of absorbed saliva. Extract the absorbed secretion from the paper by 0.01 *M* PBST, pH 7.0 *(31)*.
3. Pipette: Saliva samples can also be collected with a flexible pipet directly from the oral cavity.

3.2.3. Nasal-Fluid Antibody

Spray approx 0.4 mL sterile, lukewarm PBS into each nostril and collect the fluid flowing out of the nostril by filter-paper wicks and extract absorbed secretion as for saliva. Extracts from saliva or nasal fluid are stored at –70°C (*see* **Note 5**).

3.3. Coating

Most proteins adsorb easily to solid polystyrene plastic surfaces. Generally the adsorption process is rapid. Reported times for the coating may vary from 1 h to several days and the temperature may vary from + 4°C to 37°C. The binding mechanism predominantly involves multiple hydrophobic interactions between the solid phase and the biomolecules. Passive adsorption may therefore interfere with the structure and function of adsorbed antigens. When establishing the ELISA for the first time it is recommended that a "checker-board" titration approach is adopted. Increasing concentrations of antigen are compared with increasing concentrations of immune or control serum. In this way, an ELISA is prepared that will find the optimum concentration of antigen and antibody for the ELISA.

3.3.1. Whole Cells

Coat ELISA plates with 100 µL of heat-killed meningococci (OD ≈ 0.1 at 600 nm) in PBS and let dry overnight in an incubator at 37°C without humidification (*4,5*). Dried plates may be stored for several weeks without affecting the results.

3.3.2. OMVs, Purified OMPs, and Liposomes

1. Add 100 µL of OMVs or OMPs to the wells of a 96-well plate at a concentration of 4 µg protein/mL in 0.05 M Tris-HCl, pH 8.6, or carbonate buffer, pH 9.6, and incubate overnight at 37°C.
2. The plates should be covered with a lid or plastic sheet and may be stored, for most antigens at + 4°C for several weeks.
3. For the Opc liposome ELISA, the plates are coated over night at + 4°C with Opc liposome suspension at a protein concentration of 4 µg/mL in 0.05 M carbonate-coating buffer.

3.3.3. Lipopolysaccharides (LPS)

1. Coat microtiter plates (e.g., Immunoplate II, (NUNC), or Immulon II, (Dynatech or Greiner) overnight at 37°C with 100 µL/well of 0.2 µg/mL of LPS-BSA complexes, or with 0.5–1 µg/mL of LPS-PolymyxinB complexes dissolved in 0.05 M carbonate/bicarbonate buffer, pH 9.8.
   or
2. Coat microtiter plates overnight at room temperature with 100 µL per well of LPS-DOC micelles (2 µg LPS/mL) dissolved in PBS with 0.1% DOC (*32*).

3.3.4. Capsular Polysaccharides

CPSs bind poorly to most of the polystyrene plates used for ELISA. Thus methods that produce more efficient binding have been explored. Several options are available for coating meningococcal CPSs onto the ELISA plate and are also discussed in Chapter 21 and in "Meningococcal Disease" Edited by AJ Pollard and MCJ Maiden. To increase the binding, the wells can be pre-coated with poly-L-lysine *(33)* or the CPS can be conjugated to poly-L-lysine *(34)*. However, this may also increase the nonspecific binding of antibodies. Recently a procedure using a mixture of methylated human serum albumin (mHSA) and CPS has been described and used widely in a consensus EIA for meningococcal group A and C responses *(35,36)*; *see* also **Notes 6** and **7**).

3.3.5. Peptides

Passive physical adsorption of peptides to the surface of conventional poly-styrene microtiter plates is relatively inefficient. However, some peptides may be used for coating of ELISA-plates by passive adsorption in the same way as with proteins, using concentrations of 0.5–10 µg/mL in an alkaline-coating buffer. Some peptides adsorb better if left to dry overnight in the wells on the microtiter plates. Alternatives has been to use peptides conjugated to a carrier protein like BSA or keyhole limpet hemocyanin (KLH), or to biotinylate the peptides at the N-terminus and use ELISA plates previously coated with streptavidin *(37)*. It is also possible to conjugate peptides directly to BSA adsorbed to the surface of microtiter plates *(38)* or to chemically modify the surface of the microtiter plates, e.g., by hydrocoating and covalently immobil-izaton of the peptides *(39)*. Peptides that were either undetectable or poorly recognized when adsorbed on coventional polystyrene plates were readily rec-ognized when immobilized by the hydrocoating technique.

The conformation of peptide epitopes may have a significant effect on anti-body binding. When small peptides are used they may not be in right confor-mation, as they tend to present only a linear sequence for antibody binding. This may partly be overcome by conjugation to carrier proteins or use of cyclic peptides *(40)*.

3.4. Blocking

To avoid nonspecific binding of antibodies, blocking with inert proteins may be advantageous, but often this process is unnecessary if the concentration of serum is not too high (*see* **Notes 8–10**).

1. After washing the coating buffer out of the wells, add 200 µL of blocking buffer per well for 1 h at 37°C.

2. Blocking material may be 0.5–5% of BSA, NBBS, skimmed milk, casein, or gelatin dissolved in PBST.

3.5. Serum Incubation

1. After blocking, wash the plates in PBST.
2. Incubate each well with 100 µL of serial dilutions of antibodies in blocking buffer.

In addition to the test samples, each ELISA plate should contain a two- or threefold dilution series of a standard serum for calibration. Two to three coated wells, incubated with buffer instead of antibodies, should be included as blanks and their average values subtracted from all standard curves and test values prior to further calculations. The test samples should also be tested in duplicates or triplicates using either single dilutions or twofold dilution series. Multiple sera from each individual should always be tested on the same plate. Test sera yielding values outside the measured range of the standard curves should be repeated using other dilutions. Undiluted serum or secretions should be avoided because of problems with interference from other constituents and too high viscosity. The times used for incubation with antibodies may vary from 1 h to overnight (*see* **Note 11**). Overnight incubation may be practical when a large number of samples and plates have to be analyzed, in order to reduce variations in incubation time. The temperature during antibody incubation may influence the results, particularly if the avidity of the antibodies is low (*see* **Note 12**).

3.6. Detection of Antibody Binding

After thorough washing (3–4 times) of the plates in PBST or in Tris-HCl saline, binding of specific antibodies are detected, either directly with enzyme-conjugated anti-antibodies as detector antibody, or in order to increase sensitivity, with a second enzyme-labeled antiglobulin antibody, directed against the detector antibody. It is also possible to use biotinylated detector antibodies and enzyme-labeled streptavidin *(19,41)*. The use of antibody-enzyme conjugates simplifies the assay and these are preferred.

Add 100 µL of anti-human immunoglobulin (class or subclass specific) HRP- or AP-conjugated antibody diluted in blocking buffer and incubate the plates for 1–2 h at room temperature or 37°C. For new batches of conjugate the optimum concentration of conjugate should be determined by titration.

3.6.1. Substrate

1. Wash the plates four times and add the freshly made ELISA substrate, at 100 µL/well.

2. Incubate the plates in the dark at room temperature for 15–60 min or until the OD reaches a predetermined level.
3. The reaction may be stopped with 25–100 µL 2 *M* sulphuric acid (for OPD and TMB) or with 4 M NaOH (for nitrophenyl phosphate [NPP]) prior to reading absorbance in the plate reader.

The most common enzyme conjugates are alkaline phosphatase (AP), in which case NPP in diethanol amine or carbonate buffer, pH 9.8, is used as enzyme substrate (reading at 405 nm), or HRP using either OPD (reading at 492 nm), TMB (reading at 450 nm), or ABTS (reading at 405 nm) in citrate-phosphate buffer, pH 5.0, and 0.01% H_2O_2 as soluble enzyme substrate.

3.7. Quantitation of Antibody Levels

Binding of antibodies in ELISA represent a combination of both concentration and affinity effects and the observed OD is not linear proportional with antibody concentration. There are at least three main ways of reporting the results from an ELISA study: 1) as OD values using a defined serum dilution, 2) as a titer (endpoint analysis), or 3) in quantitative units (as U/mL or µg/mL).

3.7.1. OD Values

In many cases it is not necessary to have a precise measure of the antibody concentration of a given sample. It may then be sufficient to report the results as positive or negative, or high, medium, or low, which is indeed the form in which many routine results are reported. It is then sufficient to give the results from ELISA as percentage of a reference serum or directly as OD values. This gives a better impression of the observed raw data than transformed data, and needs no extra calculations. A reference serum should be included on all plates and the absorbance should be read when the reference reaches a predetermined OD value. The absorbance should be corrected for day-to-day and plate-to-plate variations, according to the OD value of the reference serum. If different incubation times with substrate has been used, the OD/min or OD/100min should be given. The drawback of using the observed OD values is the lack of linearity between OD and antibody concentration (*see* **Fig. 1A–C**), and if the antibody concentrations in the samples vary a lot, one pre-set dilution may not be enough for all samples.

3.7.2 Titers

Serum titers may be calculated from linear regression plots (log OD vs log dilutions) as reciprocal of highest serum dilution giving an OD values above a defined value (**Fig. 1E,F**). This value may either be chosen as 2× background with a negative serum, or another arbitrarily defined value (e.g., OD = 0.3 or 0.1 h^{-1}).

Another method to calculate titers is to use a modified Scatchard plot for data analysis *(42)*. Here the absorbance (OD) is plotted as y-axis against the

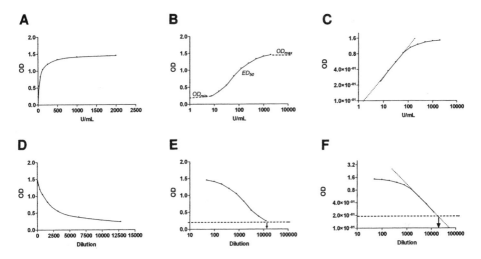

Fig. 1. Observed relationship between color developed in ELISA (OD) and antibody concentration (**A–C**) or serum dilution (**D–F**), with various transformations of the axes. A and D) linear vs linear; B and E) linear vs log; C and F) log vs log.

absorbance times the reciprocal dilution as x-axis. Under conditions of equilibrium and antibody excess a straight line is obtained for each serum, which is then extrapolated to the x-axis to yield the antibody titer. If the samples are compared with a reference serum with known U/mL on the same ELISA plate, also the U/mL in the test samples can be calculated.

3.7.3. Quantitative Units

The concentration of antigen-specific antibodies for each well are determined by comparison with a reference standard. It is then a requirement that the sample sera show parallel dose-response curves with the reference. Several attempts to represent the antibody concentration on a linear scale have been made (*see* **refs.** *43,44*). The standard curves may be fitted to straight lines after point to point curves, or by logarithmic transformation in the lower part of the data (**Fig. 1C**), or to sigmoidal curves (**Fig. 1B**) after fitting all the data to four-parameter fitting using the equation:

$$OD_{obs} = OD_{min} + \frac{OD_{max} - OD_{min}}{1 + (Conc_x/ED_{50})^{slope}}$$

$$Conc_x = Dilution \times ED_{50} \times \left(\frac{OD_{obs} - OD_{min}}{OD_{max} - OD_{obs}}\right)^{-slope}$$

where OD_{max} and OD_{min} represent the upper and lower asymptotes of the dilution curve, respectively. ED_{50} is the dilution associated with the point of symmetry of the sigmoid curve and is located at the midpoint of the assay found at the inflection point of the curve (**Fig. 1B**). $Conc_x$ is the actual concentration of antibodies related to the observed OD_{obs}.

The concentration of antigen-specific antibodies in each test serum should be calculated as the geometric mean of the values from those dilutions where the ODs were within the range of the standard curve, except for sera, which were excluded on the basis of lack of parallelism because the values calculated at different dilutions differed more than twofold.

In order to express the specific antibody concentrations as gravimetric units (µg or ng Ig/mL) each serum may be compared with a standard curve calculated from a separate ELISA, on the same microtiter plate, that uses anti-human IgG coated onto microtiter wells as a catching antigen, and a known concentration of an Ig (class or subclass) standard *(12)*. Alternatively, the concentration of specific antibodies in the reference serum may be determined separately, e.g., by use of chimeric mouse-human antibodies *(19)*.

4. Notes

1. It is important to pay attention to the quality of water when making the coating buffers; pyrogen-free water should be used.
2. PBST can affect the signal with AP conjugates in which case use Tris-buffered saline (TBS).
3. If the whole cells are to be used in ELISA immediately, the sodium azide can be omitted. Some degradation of CPS in whole cells stored at + 4°C has been observed over time (particularly group A-CPS), whereas protein epitopes seem to be stable for several years *(46)*.
4. Repeated freezing (–20°C) and thawing and heat inactivation of sera may influence the results in ELISA.
5. Antibodies in secretions can be destroyed by proteases, which are found in high concentration in the fluid. Furthermore, IgA is sensitive to repeated thawing and freezing. Thus, it has been recommended that saliva secretions are stored at –70°C, preferably in PBS with 50% glycerol *(46)* and with protease inhibitors (0.2 mM AEBSF (4-(2aminoethyl)-benzenesulfonylfluoride (Boehringer Mannheim GmbH, Germany), 0.1 µg/mL Aprotinin (Sigma), and 3.2 µM Bestatin (Sigma) *(31)*. However, other data indicate that the IgA antibodies in saliva are rather stable without protease inhibitors, even when frozen at –20°C in PBS. In addition, we have experienced recently that enzyme inhibitors could interfere in ELISAs (B. Haneberg, personal communication).
6. Purified serogroup A CPS alone is reported to bind efficiently to high-binding microtiter plates (Immulon I or MaxiSorp) without any additions and indeed,

coating with methylated HSA apparently increased the nonspecific binding of test sera *(12)*.

7. A modification of the previously described 2-d assay for anti-CPS antibodies *(36)* has been undertaken to permit analysis of antibodies to serogroup A CPS in human sera in 1 d and to be compatible with automation *(47)*. Antigen-coating parameters, ELISA-plate type, the kinetics of primary and secondary antibody-incubation steps, the buffer compositions, including detergents, serum require-ments, and the need for blocking steps, were examined. The results showed that the conditions for coating the A-CPS-methylated HSA antigen complex can be either overnight at +4°C or 90 min at 37°C with equivalent results. The modified 1-d assay involved the elimination of the 5% NBBS blocking step and incubation with the primary antibodies for 2 h at room temperature rather than at over night at +4°C. An excellent agreement with the standardized method *(35)* was observed.

8. No significant effect of blocking with 0.5% BSA was observed for OMV ELISA with human sera at dilutions higher than 1:50. Blocking with 10% FCS may be needed when sera from tropical countries (e.g., Africa and Brazil) are analyzed, owing to higher nonspecific binding of antibodies than observed with sera from, e.g., Norway or Iceland.

9. Commercial NBBS sometimes contains antibodies that give background and FCS has to be used.

10. Blocking with skimmed milk in LPS-ELISA removed the binding of anti-L8 LPS antibodies and should be avoided (S.R. Andersen, personal communication).

11. The diffusion of antibodies from aqueous solution to the solid phase may be a limiting factor for antibody binding. The effect of shaking the plates has been studied by incubating with serum with or without rapid shaking of the microtiter plates (600 rpm, Easyshaker, STL Labinstrument, Grödig). In the absence of shaking, 4-h incubation steps were needed to attain the same quantitative results as 1 h at room temperature with rapid shaking *(11)*.

12. When human-serum antibodies to serogroup B and C-CPS are assayed both at +4°C and +37°C, a significant higher binding was observed at +4°C than at 37°C for B-CPS but not for C-CPS *(34)*. This indicates that the anti-B antibodies are of lower avidity than the anti-C antibodies. For anti-A-CPS ELISA incubation with serum at 37°C is not recommended because it may result in a loss of sensitivity *(12)*.

Acknowledgment

The authors are very grateful to Ray Borrow for comments on the manuscript.

References

1. Engvall, E. and Perlman, P. (1971) Enzyme-linked immunosorbent assay (ELISA). Quantitative assay of immunoglobulin G. *Immunochemistry* **8,** 871–874.
1a. Pollard, A. J. and Maiden, M. C. J., eds. (2001) *Meningococcal Disease.* Humana Press, Totowa, NJ.

2. Blundell, K. R., Fox, A. J., Guiver, M., Jones, D. M., and Poolman, J. T. (1987) The development of an inhibition enzyme-linked immunosorbent assay to detect total antibody to the P1.16 subtype antigen of *Neisseria meningitidis* in human sera. *Serodiag. Immunother.* **1,** 353–361.

3. Akinwolere, O. A., Kumararatne, D. S., Bartlett, R., Goodall, D. M., and Catty, D. (1994) Two enzyme linked immunosorbent assays for detecting antibodies against meningococcal capsular polysaccharides A and C. *J. Clin. Pathol.* **47,** 405–410.

4. Abdillahi, H. and Poolman, J. T. (1988) Typing of group-B Neisseria meningitidis with monoclonal antibodies in the whole-cell ELISA. *J. Med. Microbiol.* **26,** 177–180.

5. Pollard, A. J., Galassini, R., van der Voort, E. M., Booy, R., Langford, P., Nadel, S., et al. (1999) Humoral immune responses to Neisseria meningitidis in children. *Infect. Immun.* **67,** 2441–2451.

6. Fredriksen, J. H., Rosenqvist, E., Wedege, E., Bryn, K., Bjune, G., Froholm, L. O., et al. (1991) Production, characterization and control of MenB-vaccine "Folkehelsa": an outer membrane vesicle vaccine against group B meningococcal disease. *NIPH Ann.* **14,** 67–79.

7. Guttormsen, H. K., Wetzler, L. M., and Solberg, C. O. (1994) Humoral immune response to class 1 outer membrane protein during the course of meningococcal disease. *Infect. Immun.* **62,** 1437–1443.

8. Guttormsen, H. K., Wetzler, L. M., and Naess, A. (1993) Humoral immune response to the class 3 outer membrane protein during the course of meningococcal disease. *Infect. Immun.* **61,** 4734–4742.

9. Rosenqvist, E., Hoiby, E. A., Wedege, E., Kusecek, B., and Achtman, M. (1993) The 5C protein of Neisseria meningitidis is highly immunogenic in humans and induces bactericidal antibodies. *J. Infect. Dis.* **167,** 1065–1073.

10. Achtman, M., Neibert, M., Crowe, B. A., Strittmatter, W., Kusecek, B., Weyse, E., et al. (1988) Purification and characterization of eight class 5 outer membrane protein variants from a clone of Neisseria meningitidis serogroup A. *J. Exp. Med.* **168,** 507–525.

11. Brieske, N., Schenker, M., Schnibbe, T., Quentin-Millet, M. J., and Achtman, M. (1999) Human antibody responses to A and C capsular polysaccharides, IgA1 protease and transferrin-binding protein complex stimulated by infection with Neisseria meningitidis of subgroup IV-1 or ET-37 complex. *Vaccine* **17,** 731–744.

12. Thiesen, B., Greenwood, B., Brieske, N., and Achtman, M. (1997) Persistence of antibodies to meningococcal IgA1 protease versus decay of antibodies to group A polysaccharide and Opc protein. *Vaccine* **15,** 209–219.

13. Tsai, C. M., Mocca, L. F., and Frasch, C. E. (1987) Immunotype epitopes of Neisseria meningitidis lipooligosaccharide types 1 through 8. *Infect. Immun.* **55,** 1652–1656.

14. Gu, X. X. and Tsai, C. M. (1993) Preparation, characterization, and immunogenicity of meningococcal lipooligosaccharide-derived oligosaccharide-protein conjugates. *Infect. Immun.* **61,** 1873–1880.

15. Wu, L. H., Tsai, C. M., and Frasch, C. E. (1987) A method for purification of bacterial R-type lipopolysaccharides (lipooligosaccharides). *Anal. Biochem.* **160,** 281–289.
16. Evans, J. S. and Maiden, M. C. (1996) Purification of meningococcal lipo-oligosaccharide by FPLC techniques. *Microbiology* **142,** 57–62.
17. Frasch, C. E. (1990) Production and control of Neisseria meningitidis vaccines. *Adv. Biotechnol. Proc.* **13,** 123–145.
18. Sjursen, H., Wedege, E., Rosenqvist, E., Naess, A., Halstensen, A., Matre, R., and Solberg, C. O. (1990) IgG subclass antibodies to serogroup B meningococcal outer membrane antigens following infection and vaccination. *APMIS* **98,** 1061–1069.
19. Naess, L. M., Rosenqvist, E., Hoiby, E. A., and Michaelsen, T. E. (1996) Quantitation of IgG subclass antibody responses after immunization with a group B meningococcal outer membrane vesicle vaccine, using monoclonal mouse-human chimeric antibodies as standards. *J. Immunol. Methods* **196,** 41–49.
20. Carlone, G. M., Frasch, C. E., Siber, G. R., Quataert, S., Gheesling, L. L., Turner, S. H., et al. (1992) Multicenter comparison of levels of antibody to the Neisseria meningitidis group A capsular polysaccharide measured by using an enzyme-linked immunosorbent assay. *J. Clin. Microbiol.* **30,** 154–159.
21. Achtman, M., Kusecek, B., Morelli, G., Eickmann, K., Wang, J. F., Crowe, B., et al. (1992) A comparison of the variable antigens expressed by clone IV-1 and subgroup III of Neisseria meningitidis serogroup A. *J. Infect. Dis.* **165,** 53–68.
22. Frasch, C. E. and Mocca, L. F. (1978) Heat-modifiable outer membrane proteins of Neisseria meningitidis and their organization within the membrane. *J. Bacteriol.* **136,** 1127–1134.
23. Appelmelk, B. J., Verweij-van Vught, A. M., MacLaren, D. M., and Thijs, L. G. (1985) An enzyme-linked immunosorbent assay (ELISA) for the measurement of antibodies to different parts of the gram-negative lipopolysaccharide core region. *J. Immunol. Methods* **82,** 199–207.
24. Andersen, S. R., Bjune, G., Hoiby, E. A., Michaelsen, T. E., Aase, A., Rye, U., and Jantzen, E. (1997) Outer membrane vesicle vaccines made from short-chain lipopolysaccharide mutants of serogroup B Neisseria meningitidis: effect of the carbohydrate chain length on the immune response. *Vaccine* **15,** 1225–1234.
25. Scott, B. B. and Barclay, G. R. (1987) Endotoxin-polymyxin complexes in an improved enzyme-linked immunosorbent assay for IgG antibodies in blood donor sera to gram-negative endotoxin core glycolipids. *Vox Sang.* **52,** 272–280.
26. Rosenqvist, E., Hoiby, E. A., Wedege, E., Bryn, K., Kolberg, J., Klem, A., et al. (1995) Human antibody responses to meningococcal outer membrane antigens after three doses of the Norwegian group B meningococcal vaccine. *Infect. Immun.* **63,** 4642–4652.
27. Christodoulides, M. and Heckels, J. E. (1994) Immunization with a multiple antigen peptide containing defined B- and T-cell epitopes: production of bactericidal antibodies against group B *Neisseria meningitidis. Microbiology* **140,** 2951–2960.
28. Rouppe van der Voort, E. M., Kuipers, B., Brugghe, H. F., van Unen, L. M., Timmermans, H. A., Hoogerhout, P., and Poolman, J. T. (1997) Epitope specific-

ity of murine and human bactericidal antibodies against PorA P1.7,16 induced with experimental meningococcal group B vaccines. *FEMS Immunol. Med. Microbiol.* **17,** 139–148.

29. Idanpaan-Heikkila, I., Hoiby, E. A., Chattopadhyay, P., Airaksinen, U., Michaelsen, T. M., and Wedege, E. (1995) Antibodies to meningococcal class 1 outer-membrane protein and its variable regions in patients with systemic meningococcal disease. *J. Med. Microbiol.* **43,** 335–343.

30. Borrow, R., Fox, A. J., Cartwright, K., Begg, N. T., and Jones, D. M. (1999) Salivary antibodies following parenteral immunization of infants with a meningococcal serogroup A and C conjugated vaccine. *Epidemiol. Infect.* **123,** 201–208.

31. Haneberg, B., Dalseg, R., Wedege, E., Hoiby, E. A., Haugen, I. L., Oftung, F., et al. (1998) Intranasal administration of a meningococcal outer membrane vesicle vaccine induces persistent local mucosal antibodies and serum antibodies with strong bactericidal activity in humans. *Infect. Immun.* **66,** 1334–1341.

32. Rosenqvist, E., Hoiby, E. A., Bjune, G., Bryn, K., Closs, O., Feiring, B., et al. (1991) Human antibody responses after vaccination with the Norwegian group B meningococcal outer membrane vesicle vaccine: results from ELISA studies. *NIPH Ann.* **14,** 169–179.

33. Leinonen, M. and Frasch, C. E. (1982) Class-specific antibody response to group B Neisseria meningitidis capsular polysaccharide: use of polylysine precoating in an enzyme-linked immunosorbent assay. *Infect. Immun.* **38,** 1203–1207.

34. Mandrell, R. E. and Zollinger, W. D. (1982) Measurement of antibodies to meningococcal group B polysaccharide: low avidity binding and equilibrium binding constants. *J. Immunol.* **129,** 2172–2178.

35. Carlone, G. M., Frasch, C. E., Siber, G. R., Quataert, S., Gheesling, L. L., Turner, S. H., et al. (1992) Multicenter comparison of levels of antibody to the Neisseria meningitidis group A capsular polysaccharide measured by using an enzyme-linked immunosorbent assay. *J. Clin. Microbiol.* **30,** 154–159.

36. Gheesling, L. L., Carlone, G. M., Pais, L. B., Holder, P. F., Maslanka, S. E., Plikaytis, B. D., et al. (1994) Multicenter comparison of Neisseria meningitidis serogroup C anti-capsular polysaccharide antibody levels measured by a standardized enzyme-linked immunosorbent assay. *J. Clin. Microbiol.* **32,** 1475–1482.

37. Saunders, N. B., Brandt, B. L., Warren, R. L., Hansen, B. D., and Zollinger, W. D. (1998) Immunological and molecular characterization of three variant subtype P1.14 strains of Neisseria meningitidis. *Infect. Immun.* **66,** 3218–3222.

38. Price, M. R., Sekowski, M., Hooi, D. S., Durrant, L. G., Hudecz, F., and Tendler, S. J. (1993) Measurement of antibody binding to antigenic peptides conjugated in situ to albumin-coated microtitre plates. *J. Immunol. Methods* **159,** 277–281.

39. Gregorius, K., Mouritsen, S., and Elsner, H. I. (1995) Hydrocoating: a new method for coupling biomolecules to solid phases. *J. Immunol. Methods* **181,** 65–73.

40. Hoogerhout, P., Donders, E. M., Gaans-van den Brink, J. A., Kuipers, B., Brugghe, H. F., van Unen, L. M., et al. (1995) Conjugates of synthetic cyclic peptides elicit bactericidal antibodies against a conformational epitope on a class 1 outer membrane protein of Neisseria meningitidis. *Infect. Immun.* **63,** 3473–3478.

41. Naess, L. M., Aarvak, T., Aase, A., Oftung, F., Hoiby, E. A., Sandin, R., and Michaelsen, T. E. (1999) Human IgG subclass responses in relation to serum bactericidal and opsonic activities after immunization with three doses of the Norwegian serogroup B meningococcal outer membrane vesicle vaccine. *Vaccine* **17,** 754–764.

42. Fusco, P. C., Michon, F., Laude-Sharp, M., Minetti, C. A., Huang, C. H., Heron, I., and Blake, M. S. (1998) Preclinical studies on a recombinant group B meningococcal porin as a carrier for a novel Haemophilus influenzae type b conjugate vaccine. *Vaccine* **16,** 1842–1849.

43. Plikaytis, B. D., Turner, S. H., Gheesling, L. L., and Carlone, G. M. (1991) Comparisons of standard curve-fitting methods to quantitate Neisseria meningitidis group A polysaccharide antibody levels by enzyme-linked immunosorbent assay. *J. Clin. Microbiol.* **29,** 1439–1446.

44. Plikaytis, B. D., Holder, P. F., Pais, L. B., Maslanka, S. E., Gheesling, L. L., and Carlone, G. M. (1994) Determination of parallelism and nonparallelism in bioassay dilution curves. *J. Clin. Microbiol.* **32,** 2441–2447.

45. Rosenqvist, E., Wedege, E., Hoiby, E. A., and Froholm, L. O. (1990) Serogroup determination of *Neisseria meningitidis* by whole-cell ELISA, dot-blotting and agglutination. *APMIS* **98,** 501–506.

46. Butler, J. E., Spradling, J. E., Rowat, J., Ekstrand, J., and Challacombe, S. J. (1990) Humoral immunity in root caries in an elderly population. 2. *Oral Microbiol. Immunol.* **5,** 113–120.

47. Diakun, K. R., Martin, D. C., Mininni, T., Skuse, J., Ziembiec, N., and Quataert, S. (1998) Immunoassay of human *Neisseria meningitidis* serogroup A antibody. *Immunol. Invest.* **27,** 203–220.

19

Immunoblot Analysis of Sera from Patients and Vaccinees

Elisabeth Wedege

1. Introduction

This chapter will describe the use of the immunoblotting method for analysing antibody specificities towards meningococcal antigens in sera from vaccinees, receiving group B meningococcal outer-membrane vesicle (OMV) vaccines, or from patients, falling ill with meningococcal disease. The power of the blotting technique lies in the simultaneous identification of many immunogenic components in a sample. Within the meningococcal field, this method has been employed in analyzes of antibody specificities of sera from vaccinees *(1–6)*, patients *(7–10)*, and carriers *(11,12)* as well as for characterization of OMV vaccines *(13,14)*. Some of these studies present various ways of quantifying the blotting results *(5,7,9,11)*.

The immunoblotting assay consists of several steps: 1) separation of meningococcal antigens in sodium dodecyl sulphate (SDS)-containing polyacrylamide gel; 2) electrotransfer of the separated components in the SDS-gel to a filter or membrane, 3) blocking of the remaining free protein-binding sites in the membrane, 4) incubation of the membrane with human sera (primary antibodies), 5) incubation of the membrane with antibodies directed against the primary antibodies (secondary antibodies), and 6) detection of antigen-antibody complexes.

SDS-polyacrylamide-gel electrophoresis (SDS-PAGE) is one of the most commonly used techniques in protein analysis. It gives information on the number of proteins in a mixture, their relative abundance and molecular weights, and, in combination with the blotting technique, also on protein antigenicity. For immunoblot studies of sera from vaccinees or patients, OMVs are

From: *Methods in Molecular Medicine, vol. 66: Meningococcal Vaccines: Methods and Protocols*
Edited by: A. J. Pollard and M. C. J. Maiden © Humana Press Inc., Totowa, NJ

most often used as antigens. Such antigens, consisting of the major outer-membrane proteins (OMPs) and lipopolysaccharide (LPS), give a less complex band pattern in SDS-gels than the corresponding whole-cell suspensions. The antigens can be denatured in various ways before application on the SDS-gel. Standard treatment is heating at 100°C for 5 min in a sample buffer containing SDS and a reducing reagent to break disulphide bridges (2-mercaptoethanol or dithiothreitol [DTT]). SDS, a negatively charged amphipatic molecule, complexes with nonpolar side chains and positively charged groups in the polypeptide chains and unfolds them by destroying noncovalent bindings *(15)*. The resulting rod-like negative protein-SDS complexes are loaded on a polyacrylamide gel cast between two glass plates. During electrophoresis (**step 1**) they move through the gel towards the anode so that proteins of low molecular weights move faster than those of higher molecular weights. An inverse relationship between the logarithm of molecular weights and the distance of migration is demonstrated *(16)*.

In **step 2**, the actual blotting procedure, the resolved OMV components in the gel are electrophoretically transferred to a nitrocellulose (NC) membrane filter, resulting in an exact replica (blot) of the protein pattern in the gel. The blotted proteins, retained to the filter mainly by hydrophobic forces *(17)*, are accessible to reactions with the primary antibodies (**step 4**), but to prevent unspecific binding the filter is incubated with a blocking reagent (**step 3**). The secondary antibodies (**step 5**) are labeled in various ways to detect their binding to the primary antibodies, most often by the enzyme horseradish peroxidase (HRP). Addition of enzyme substrates (**step 6**) will result in colored bands on the membrane where the secondary antibodies have detected complexes between the primary antibodies and one or more of the blotted antigens.

Because the optimal conditions for antigen-antibody formation may vary from sample to sample, as reflected in the many articles published on the blotting method, this immunoassay in many respects can be considered as "an art." The method described in this chapter is based on that reported by Towbin et al. *(18)*. This method was later renamed Western blotting by Burnette *(19)*; however, several review articles advise against this dubious geographical jargon *(17,20–23)*, and I will use the term immunoblotting.

The aim of the described immmunoassay is to analyze IgG antibody specificities of sera from many patients or vaccinees against the same meningococcal antigen.

The protocol below describes the casting of two 12% acrylamide mini-gels of thickness 0.75 mm, following the method of Laemmli *(24)*, which are loaded with OMVs on the whole gel surface without using well-forming combs. From the two resulting blots, each cut into about 25 strips, this experimental set-up may allow detection of the OMV antibody specificities of about 50 different sera. However, it is recommended to analyze each serum both without and with a detergent, such as Empigen BB *(25,26)*, which may partially refold conformational epitopes lost during boiling of the OMVs in SDS-sample buffer; thus about 25 different sera may be analyzed in the protocol (*see* **Note 1**). By including the detergent in the assay, the blotting results reflect the antibody levels measured in ELISA *(9,27)*.

2. Materials
2.1. SDS-PAGE

1. Solution A: 30% acrylamide. Dissolve 29.2 g acrylamide and 0.8 g N,N'-methylene-bis-acrylamide in water to a total volume of 100 mL (*see* **Note 2**). The reagents are toxic, avoid contact by using gloves, mask, and a fume cupboard when weighing. Polymerized gels are not toxic. Store solution in a dark bottle at 4°C for not more than 1–2 mo.
2. Solution B: 1.5 *M* Tris-HCl, pH 8.8. Dissolve 18.2 g Tris-base in about 60 mL water; adjust to pH 8.8 with 4 *N* HCl; add water to 100 mL total volume.
3. Solution C: 0.5 *M* Tris-HCl, pH 6.8. Dissolve 6.0 g Tris-base in about 60 mL water; adjust pH to 6.8 with 4 *N* HCl; add water to 100 mL total volume.
4. 10% (w/v) SDS. Dissolve 10 g SDS in water to a total volume of 100 mL. Store in a bottle at room temperature to avoid precipitation. Stable for about 1 yr.
5. 10% (w/v) ammonium persulphate. Dissolve 1 g in water to a total volume of 10 mL. Distribute small aliquots into small plastic tubes to be stored at –20°C. Freshly made or thawed samples are stable at 4°C for about 1 wk.
6. Electrode buffer: 0.025 *M* Tris, 0.192 *M* glycine, 0.1% SDS, pH 8.3. Dissolve 3.0 g Tris-base, 14.4 g glycine, and 1.0 g SDS in water to a total volume of 1 L. Do not adjust pH.
7. Sample buffer: 0.0625 *M* Tris, 0.7 *M* mercaptoethanol, 2% SDS. Mix 4.2 mL water, 1.0 mL solution C, 0.8 mL glycerol, 1.6 mL 10% SDS, and 0.4 mL 2-mercaptoethanol.
8. TEMED: N,N,N,'N'-tetramethylenediamine. Toxic.
9. 0.2 % Pyronin Y. Dissolve 20 mg in 10 mL water. Store at –20°C.
10. Staining solution. Dissolve 1 g Coomassie brilliant blue in 500 mL methanol; add 100 mL 100% acetic acid and water to 1 L *(28)*. Stable at room temperature for about 1 yr. The solution can be reused several times.
11. Destaining solution. Mix 100 mL methanol and 100 mL 100% acetic acid with water to 1 L.
12. Gel-electrophoretic apparatus for two mini-gels with glass plates, spacers, clamp assemblies, and casting stand.
13. Power supply.
14. Horizontal rotating platform.
15. Suction pump.

16. Vacuum bottle (100–250 mL volume), graduated pipets, micropipets with disposable tips, gloves.

2.2. Immunoblotting

1. Transfer buffer: 0.025 M Tris, 0.192 M glycine, pH 8.3. Dissolve 3.0 g Tris-base and 14.4 g glycine in about 500 mL water, add 200 mL methanol, bring to 1 L with water. pH is about 8.3; do not adjust.
2. Phosphate-buffered saline (PBS), pH 7.2. Dissolve 1.5 g $Na_2 HPO_4 \cdot 2H_2O$, 0.4 g KH_2PO_4, and 6.8 g NaCl in 1 L water. Other recipes for PBS can also be used.
3. Blocking buffer: 3% bovine serum albumin (BSA) in PBS. Dissolve 3 g BSA (Sigma, fraction V) in a total volume of 100 mL PBS. Store frozen; smaller volumes can be kept at 4°C for about 1 wk. This solution is used for blocking and dilution of primary and secondary antibodies.
4. 0.05 M sodium acetate buffer, pH 5.0. Dissolve 6.8 g Na-acetate·3H$_2$O in 900 mL water, bring to pH 5.0 with 100% acetic acid. Adjust volume to 1 L with water.
5. 0.05 M 3-amino-9-ethyl-carbazole (AEC). Dissolve 0.5 g AEC in 50 mL dimethylformamide. Store in a dark bottle at 4°C for not more than 3–4 mo. Toxic.
6. 30% Empigen BB (lauryl-betaine) (Albright & Wilson Ltd, Whitehaven, Cumbria, UK). Stable at room temperature for more than 1 yr.
7. 30% hydrogen peroxide. Caustic.
8. Amido black staining solution. Dissolve 0.1 g amido black in 25 mL isopropanol, 10 mL 100% acetic acid, and 65 mL water. Stable at room temperature for about 1 yr. The solution can be reused several times.
9. Destaining solution. 250 mL isopropanol, 100 mL 100% acetic acid, and water to 1 L. Stable at room temperature for about 1 yr.
10. Blotting apparatus: The blot electrode module to be inserted into the gel-electrophoretic tank, gel-holder cassettes, cooling unit, and 4 fiber pads (8 × 11 cm).
11. Filters: For blotting of two gels, two NC-filters (pore size 0.45 µm; cut to size 7 × 9.5 cm with scissors or scalpel), 4 filter papers 0.5-mm thick (size 8 × 10 cm).
12. Power supply.
13. Horizontal rotating platform.
14. Smaller equipments: Pen that can write on wet NC-filters, soft pencil, suitable plastic boxes for incubations and soaking of filters, glass or plastic plates (dimensions approx 12 × 20 cm), scalpel, clean ruler, flat tweezers, graduated pipets, Pasteur pipets, micropipets with disposable tips, dispenser bottle, gloves, vortex mixer.

2.3. Protein Samples

1. OMVs prepared by deoxycholate- or LiCl-extraction (*13,29, see* also **Chapters 7** and **18**).

2.4. Primary and Secondary Antibodies

1. Human sera: Sera from vaccinees, receiving meningococcal OMV vaccines, or from patients with meningococcal disease. Stable at –20°C or lower for

years. Use gloves and sterile tips; vortex the tubes before taking out the samples.

2. Mouse monoclonal antibodies (MAbs): MAbs specific for the major outer-membrane proteins (OMPs) (class 1 [PorA], 2/3 [PorB], 4 and 5 [Opc]) of the OMV antigen used for immunoblotting. Stable at –20°C or lower for years. PorA and PorB MAbs may be obtained from National Institute for Biological Standards and Controls, South Mimms, Potters Bar, UK.

3. Peroxidase-conjugated rabbit anti-human IgG: Stable for years at 4°C (DAKO A/S, Denmark).

4. Peroxidase-conjugated rabbit anti-mouse Ig: Stable for years at 4°C (DAKO A/S).

3. Methods

3.1. SDS-PAGE

Each vertical polyacrylamide mini-gel (about 7 × 6 cm) is cast between two glass plates of different heights and consists of two layers, a separating gel in the bottom overlaid by a stacking gel of lower acrylamide concentration; its thickness is determined by vertical spacers separating the plates. As there are many different gel-electrophoretic equipments available, the reader is referred to the manual supplied with their mini-gel system on how to assemble the glass plates. The important thing is to use clean glass plates without chipped ends to prevent leakage of the acrylamide-gel solution during casting. Because polymerization of acrylamide is temperature-dependent, reagents, glass plates, and other parts of the equipment in contact with the plates should be at room temperature (20–25°C) in order to obtain optimal polymerization and reproducible gels. Use gloves when handling acrylamide solutions.

3.1.1. Casting of the Separating Gel (12% Acrylamide)

1. Assemble two sets, each consisting of two glass plates with 0.75-mm spacers, and attach them to the casting stand. Put a mark on the smallest plates about 2 cm from the top with a marker pen to indicate the height of the separating gel.

2. Mix 3.4 mL water, 2.5 mL solution B, and 4.0 mL solution A in a small vacuum flask. De-gas the stoppered bottle for about 1 min, or until bubbling stops, while slowly shaking the contents to remove oxygen that inhibits polymerization.

3. Add 100 μL 10% SDS, 50 μL 10% ammonium persulphate, and 5 μL TEMED and swirl the contents gently. Apply the solution between the glass plates up to the mark using a graduated or a Pasteur pipet.

4. Repeat casting for the second gel.

5. Use a syringe or Pasteur pipet to overlay the gel solutions with water by gently letting it run down the sides of each of the spacers to a height of about 1 cm. This overlay will result in a flat gel surface and prevent entry of oxygen. Polymeriza-

tion, detected as a sharp water-gel front, starts within minutes once TEMED is added, but is only completed after 60–90 min (*see* **Note 3**).

3.1.2. Casting of the Stacking Gel

1. Pour out the water on top of the separating gels, rinse the gel surface with water, and remove all drops by tilting the casting stand.
2. Mix 6.1 mL water, 2.5 mL solution C, and 1.3 mL solution A in the vacuum flask to obtain a 4 % stacking gel. De-gas for about 1 min.
3. Add 100 µL 10% SDS, 50 µL 10% ammonium persulphate, and 10 µL TEMED while shaking gently. Apply the solution on top of the two separating gels to a height of about 1 cm.
4. Overlay with water as described in **Subheading 3.1.1., step 5** (*see* **Note 4**). Leave gels at room temperature for about 30–45 min.
5. Rinse the surface of the stacking gels with water; remove all water drops with tissue paper.
6. Remove the plates with the gels from the casting stand and insert them into the electrode assembly according to the manufacturer's instructions.

3.1.3. Sample Preparation

1. In a small plastic tube, dilute OMVs in sample buffer so that the final SDS concentration of the sample is not below 1%. For two gels, it is suitable to mix 100 µL OMVs (about 1 mg/mL) with 250 µL sample buffer.
2. Boil the tube in a water bath for 5 min (*see* **Note 5**). To prevent overboiling, pierce the lid beforehand with a map pin.
3. Following boiling, add a few µL of the Pyronin Y solution to color the sample purple (*see* **Note 6**).

3.1.4. Sample Application

1. Overlay the stacking gels with electrode buffer.
2. Use a Hamilton microsyringe, positioned closely to the gel surface, to gently load under the electrode buffer 150 µL of the dense sample solution to each gel (corresponding to about 50 µg OMV protein per gel).
3. Label the gel holders to differentiate gel 1 from gel 2.

3.1.5. Electrophoresis

1. Fill electrode buffer in the upper and lower buffer chamber according to manufacturer's instructions. Do not splash to avoid distortion of the samples.
2. Remove air bubbles attached to the bottom ends of the glass plates with a bent Pasteur pipet or stainless wire, put the lid on the tank and connect it to a power supply ensuring proper polarity (+ electrode at the bottom), usually assisted by color-coded plugs.
3. Run the gels at 200 V for 30–45 min until the tracking dye is about 0.3 cm from the bottom of the plates.

3.1.6. Removal of SDS-Gels

1. Turn off the power supply, lift out the electrode assembly, and remove the plates from the clamps.
2. Twist the upper plate gently away from the gel according to the manufacturer's instructions. Cut off the stacking gel and also a tiny corner from one of the gels to differentiate gel 1 from gel 2. Use gloves when handling the gels.
3. Pull each gel gently away from the lower glass plate and transfer it to the tray with transfer buffer and filters (*see* **Subheading 3.2.1., step 1**).

3.2. Electrotransfer

3.2.1. Preparation of Blots

1. While the SDS-PAGE electrophoresis is running, soak NC-filters (labeled with a pen in one corner), paper filters, and fiber pads (*see* **Subheading 2.2., items 10 and 11**) in a plastic tray filled with transfer buffer for 15 min or more.
2. Place one open gel cassette holder in the tray with the anode side bottom-down. Onto the anode panel, build a sandwich in the buffer of the following components in this order: 1) fiber pad, 2) filter paper, 3) NC-filter with label facing upwards, 4) SDS gel, 5) filter paper, and 6) fiber pad. Use gloves during this procedure and make sure that no air bubbles are trapped between the NC-filter and gel.
3. Center the sandwich components in the holder, fold the cathode panel over, and lock the holder carefully without twisting, taking care that the two plates of the holder are aligned.
4. Repeat procedure with the second gel.

3.2.2. Transfer Conditions

1. Place the blotting electrode assembly in the buffer tank as instructed in the manufacturer's manual, fill the tank half way up with cold transfer buffer. Slide the gel-cassette holders gently into the tracks of the electrode assembly, so that the anode panel of the holder is facing the anode side of the electrode assembly.
2. Insert the cooling unit as instructed in the manual, add transfer buffer just to cover the gel holders and replace the lid.
3. Put the tank into a bucket filled with crushed ice so that it is covered up to the lid.
4. Connect the plugs to the power supply and perform the electrotransfer at 100 V for 1 h.
5. Turn off the power supply, disconnect plugs, and remove gel holders from the electrode assembly.
6. Open the holder with the anode side facing down, carefully remove the upper fiber pad and filter paper; then mark the outline of the gel on the NC-filter with a soft pencil. Pyronin Y is visible as a purple band at the lower end of the filter. Use gloves when handling the filters.

7. Peel the blotted gel from the NC-filter, stain it in Coomassie brilliant blue (*see* **Note 7**) as described in **Subheading 3.2.4.** Place the NC-filters on a clean glass or plastic plate.

3.2.3. Staining of NC-filters with Amido Black

1. Place the ruler along one of the short sides of the wet NC-filter, using the pencilled outline of the gel as a guide, and cut off a strip of 0.5 cm width or less with the scalpel. Dry the strip at room temperature for about 15 min.
2. Transfer the strip to a box filled with Amido black staining solution by means of the tweezers and stain for about 1 min while shaking.
3. Rinse the strip in tap water, destain in destaining solution for 2 min, rinse in tap water, and let it dry flat on a glass or plastic plate at room temperature (*see* **Note 8**).
4. Place the remaining part of the NC-filter horizontally over the edge of a box or lid so that it does not stick flat to the surface, let it dry at room temperature for 15 min or more to increase fixation of the proteins to the filter.

3.2.4. Staining of SDS-Gels

1. Stain the blotted gels in a suitable container filled with Coomassie brilliant blue solution for about 1 h at room temperature on a rotary platform.
2. Pour off the staining solution, rinse the gels with tap water, and destain with destaining solution for about 1 h until clear background or visible bands are seen (*see* **Note 9**).

3.3. Blocking

1. Transfer the dried NC-filters to a box filled with blocking buffer and incubate for 30 min on a rotary platform. Use a plastic or glass box of dimensions suited to the filters and cover the filters with blocking buffer so they are fully wetted with solution during this step (*see* **Note 10**).

3.4. Incubation with Primary Antibodies

3.4.1. Postvaccination or Patient Sera

1. Following blocking, place the NC-filters on a plate and use a ruler and scalpel to cut each filter into 3 mm-wide vertical strips. From each blot about 25 strips can be obtained, each containing 2 µg or less of OMVs. Number the strips on the top or bottom with a pen that does not smear on wet paper.
2. Use tweezers to transfer each strip into a suitable incubation tray, such as mini-trays with 8 wells (dimensions 0.7 × 10.5 cm) available from several manufacturers. Add 1 mL blocking buffer to each well either before or after inserting the strips, but keep the strips wetted all the time to prevent them from breaking (*see* **Note 11**).
3. Add human sera to the wells. A dilution of 1:200 for vaccination and patient sera is often suitable (5 µL to 1 mL blocking buffer), but the serum amount has to be determined by trial and error (*see* **Note 12**). When testing new antigens, it is

advisable to include control strips incubated either without primary or secondary antibodies.

3.4.2. Effect of Renaturating Detergent

1. For each serum, incubate one strip without and one with Empigen BB to a final concentration of 0.15% (5 µL to 1 mL blocking buffer) (*see* **Note 13**).

3.4.3. Guide Strips with MAbs

1. To identify the exact positions of the various OMV proteins on the blots, incubate at least one strip from each blot with a combination of different MAbs to such proteins. The MAbs are usually diluted 1:5,000 or more in the blocking buffer; notice that most PorB-specific MAbs need about 0.25% Empigen BB for binding (8 µL to 1 mL blocking buffer).
2. Put the lid on the trays and incubate the strips overnight at room temperature on a rotary platform (*see* **Note 14**).

3.4.4. Washing

1. Next morning, suck off the antibody solutions from the wells with a pipet tip attached to a suction pump or similar set-up. Rinse the pipet tip in water between each aspiration to prevent transfer of antibodies between the wells.
2. Add 1–2 mL PBS to each well using, e.g., a dispenser bottle to wash off unbound antibodies. Incubate for about 5 min on the rotary platform.
3. Aspirate and repeat the washing procedure twice.

3.5. Incubation with Secondary Antibodies

1. Dilute 100 µL peroxidase-conjugated anti-human IgG in 50 mL blocking buffer (1:500 dilution) and add 1 ml of this solution to each of the strips that were incubated with the human sera (*see* **Note 15**).
2. Dilute 10 µL peroxidase-conjugated anti-mouse Ig in 10 mL blocking buffer (1:1,000 dilution) and add 1 mL to the guide strips that were incubated with the MAbs.
3. Incubate the strips for 2 h at room temperature on the rotary platform. Control that the strips are covered by liquid during the incubation.
4. Wash off unbound secondary antibodies as described in **Subheading 3.4.4.**, but substitute PBS with 0.05 *M* Na-acetate buffer in the final wash (*see* **Note 16**).

3.6. Detection of Antibody Specificities

3.6.1. Staining

1. Mix 50 mL 0.05 *M* Na-acetate buffer and 2 mL AEC solution in a suitable container; transfer all strips from one blot, that were incubated with the human sera, into this staining solution.
2. Transfer all guide strips with the MAbs to a separate box with staining solution.
3. Shake the strips for a few minutes on a rotary platform to saturate them with the stain.

4. Add 25 µL 30% H_2O_2 per 50 mL staining solution and continue incubation until red-brown immunoreactive bands are detected on the strips. Take care that all strips move freely in the staining solution. For comparative purposes, stain all strips for the same time, usually 10 min; guide strips need only a few min staining. The brownish precipitate that is often formed does not affect the staining.
5. Discard the staining solution and rinse the strips in tap water a few times.
6. Repeat the staining procedure with the strips from the other blot.
7. With the tweezers, align the strips closely side by side on a glass or plastic plate using the Pyronin Y marker and the gel outline on the filter as a guide. Align the strip, previously stained with Amido black, with the others. Tilt the plate slightly, let the strips dry at room temperature (*see* **Note 17**) and store them on the plate in a dark cupboard until recording.

3.6.2. Recording

1. Record the immunoblot results with a camera, using black and white film, or with a video camera equipped with a video printer. Band contrast is improved with a green filter.
2. Photograph the blotted SDS gels, stained with Coomassie blue, with an orange filter.
3. Identify the major bands on the strips by comparison with the patterns on the Amido black-stained strip and the guide strips (*see* **Note 18**). The pattern on the SDS gels may also help in the identification (*see* **Note 7**).

3.6.3. Quantitation of Immunoreactive Bands

1. Scan the bands on the blots with a suitable computer software program (e.g., as shown in **ref. 9**). The program should allow manipulation of the baseline used in integration of the peak areas of the scans; some programs with fixed baseline functions may underestimate the density of highly stained neighbor bands, e.g., PorA and PorB bands (*see* **Note 19**). Strips may also be analyzed with a gel scanner (*see* **Note 20**).
2. Scan the strips, incubated with Empigen BB, only when they visually demonstrate bands of higher densities compared to the corresponding strips incubated without detergent. The detergent-treated strips usually have a higher background.

3.6.4. Storage

1. After recording, use tweezers to align the strips loosely into a plastic pocket that can be taped in the journal. Under such conditions, the strips show no visible fading for years. The strips are brittle and break easily; therefore do not glue or tape the strips themselves as this makes it more difficult later to pick out strips that are suitable for publication figures.

4. Notes

1. The total time of the experiment is about 1.5 d. An experienced worker may run 4 gels simultaneously, thus doubling the amount of sera to be analyzed.

2. Because contaminants may interfere with acrylamide polymerization, it is important to use reagents of analytical grade in the gel-casting solutions. If not otherwise stated, all solutions are made with distilled water and are stable at 4°C for about 1 yr.

3. To save time, cast the separation gel the day before and the stacking gel next morning. Cast separation gels can be stored in the cold room for several days taking care that the water overlay does not dry out. The stacking gel has to be cast on the day the gel electrophoresis will be performed.

4. If combs are used to make wells in the stacking gel, the water overlay is omitted.

5. The reduction-modifiable class 4 protein can be identified by a slightly lower molecular weight if 2-mercaptoethanol is omitted from the sample buffer during boiling. Milder denaturation of OMVs can be performed by incubation with sample buffer at room temperature or on ice; alternatively at 45°C for 30 min in a sample buffer with 0.5% SDS and 0.5% Triton X-100 *(30)*. These conditions will allow detection of the trimeric forms of PorA and PorB and the lower molecular weight form of the heat-modifiable class 5 proteins.

6. Pyronin Y is used as tracking dye instead of bromophenol blue as this stain will bind to the NC-filter. If unboiled samples are investigated, beware that high concentrations of Pyronin Y may depolymerize several OMPs in the same way as boiling. Pyronin B shows similar effects.

7. Weak protein bands are always left in the gel after blotting. Staining of the blotted gel will check if irregularities occurred during the SDS-PAGE.

8. Perform the staining procedure rapidly to avoid shrinkage of the NC-strip *(31)*.

9. Reduce destaining time by immersing a piece of rubber foam into the destaining solution. Destained gels can be stored in destaining solution or in water for weeks.

10. Blocked or unblocked filters can be dried and stored at 4°C for some months or more with little loss in antigenicity.

11. The minimum incubation volume for one strip is about 0.5 mL. Up to four strips can be incubated in a 2-mL volume, taking care that they are fully wetted with blocking buffer.

12. A simple way of estimating suitable dilutions of primary and secondary antibodies is to dot the boiled antigen on NC-filters and incubate the dot blots with a range of different antibody dilutions (*see* Chapter 9 of "Meningococcal Disease" Edited by A. J. Pollard and M. C. J. Maiden.

13. Empigen BB may partially refold some conformational epitopes on outer membrane proteins, that were destroyed during heat-treatment with SDS sample buffer, and so allow antibody binding. However, as this and other detergents displace antigens of lower molecular weight from the filter *(26)*, one strip has always to be incubated without detergent. Other agents present during the incubation, such as the primary antibodies *(32,33)* and BSA in the blocking buffer *(34)*, may also have renaturating effects. Because of the displacing effect of detergents, they should not routinely be included in blocking and washing buffers without proper testing.

14. Adjust rotation so that the solutions do not seep over the walls of the wells. Always leave an empty well in the incubation tray between the guide strips

with the MAbs and the strips with the human sera to avoid transfer of the antibodies.

15. Do not use sodium azide in the blocking buffer or in other solutions as this agent inhibits the peroxidase activity.

16. The Na-acetate buffer will lower the pH of the strips to the more optimal pH range of the peroxidase.

17. The background staining of the strips will fade rapidly once the strips are dried.

18. Beware that aspartyl-prolyl peptide bonds may be cleaved in hot SDS sample buffer giving rise to proteolytic fragments *(35)*. For PorA, probed with PorA-specific MAbs, such products may be seen as distinct immunoreactive bands in the class 5 protein range *(13)*.

19. Heavily stained bands may also demonstrate a prozone phenomenon in that IgG binding intensity will be higher at serum dilutions above the standard 1:200 dilutions *(27)*.

20. Use of a gel scanner requires the strips to be turned around with the immunoreactive bands facing the scanner, which is cumbersome when dealing with many strips. Owing to their static nature, the loose strips will easily move when closing the lid of the scanner.

Acknowledgments

Karin Bolstad is thanked for her valuable comments on the manuscript.

References

1. Boslego, J., Garcia, J., Cruz, C., Zollinger, W., Brandt, B., Ruiz, S., et al., and the Chilean National Committee for Meningococcal Disease. (1995) Efficacy, safety, and immunogenicity of a meningococcal group B (15:P1.3) outer membrane protein vaccine in Iquique, Chile. *Vaccine* **9,** 821–829.

2. Milagres, L. G., Ramos, S. R., Sacchi, C. T., Melles, C. A. E., Vieira, V. S. D., Sato, H., et al. (1994) Immune response of Brazilian children to a *Neisseria meningitidis* serogroup B outer membrane protein vaccine: comparison with efficacy. *Infect. Immun.* **62,** 4419–4424.

3. Peeters, C. C. A. M., Rümke, H. C., Sunderman, L. C., Rouppe van der Voort, E. M., Meulenbelt, J., Schuller, M., et al. (1996) Phase I clinical trial with a hexavalent PorA containing meningococcal outer membrane vesicle vaccine. *Vaccine* **14,** 1009–1015.

4. Rosenqvist, E., Høiby, E. A., Wedege, E., Kusceck, B., and Achtman, M. (1993) The 5C protein of *Neisseria meningitidis* is highly immunogenic in humans and induces bactericidal antibodies. *J. Infect. Dis.* **167,** 1065–1073.

5. Rosenqvist, E., Høiby, E. A., Wedege, E., Bryn, K., Kolberg, J., Klem, A., et al. (1995) Human antibody responses to meningococcal outer membrane antigens after three doses of the Norwegian group B meningococcal vaccine. *Infect. Immun.* **63,** 4642–4652.

6. Wedege, E. and Frøholm., L. O. (1986) Human antibody response to a group B serotype 2a meningococcal vaccine determined by immunoblotting. *Infect. Immun.* **51,** 571–578.

7. Idänpään-Heikkilä, I., Høiby, E. A., Chattopadhyay, P., Airaksinen, U., Michaelsen, T. E., and Wedege, E. (1995) Antibodies to meningococcal class 1 outer-membrane protein and its variable regions in patients with systemic meningococcal disease. *J. Med. Microbiol.* **43,** 335–343.

8. Mæland, J. A. and Wedege, E. (1989) Serum antibodies to cross-reactive *Neisseria* outer membrane antigens in healthy persons and patients with meningococcal disease. *APMIS* **97,** 774–780.

9. Wedege, E., Høiby, E. A., Rosenqvist, E., and Bjune, G. (1998) Immune responses against major outer membrane antigens of *Neisseria meningitidis* in vaccinees and controls who contracted meningococcal disease during the Norwegian serogroup B protection trial. *Infect. Immun.* **66,** 3223–3231.

10. Zollinger, W. D., Boslego, J. W., Moran, E. E., Brandt, B. L., Cruz, C., Martinez, M., and Garcia, J. (1994) Effect of vaccination with meningococcal outer membrane protein vaccine on subsequent antibody reponses to carriage and natural infections, in *Pathobiology and Immunobiology of Neisseriaceae* (Conde-Glez, C. J., Morse, S., Rice, P., Sparling, R., and Calderon, E., eds.), Instituto Nacional de Salud Publica. Cuernavaca, Morelos, Mexico, pp. 954–960.

11. Jones, G. R., Christodoulides, M., Brooks, J. L., Miller, A. R. O., Cartwright, K. A. V., and Heckels, J. E. (1998) Dynamics of carriage of *Neisseria meningitidis* in a group of military recruits: Subtype stability and specificity of the immune response following colonization. *J. Infect. Dis.* **178,** 451–459.

12. Woods, J. P. and Cannon, J. G. (1990) Variation in expression of class 1 and class 5 outer membrane proteins during nasopharyngeal carriage of *Neisseria meningitidis*. *Infect. Immun.* **58,** 569–572.

13. Fredriksen, J. H., Rosenqvist, E., Wedege, E., Bryn, K., Bjune, G., Frøholm, L. O., et al. (1991) Production, characterization and control of MenB-vaccine "Folkehelsa": an outer membrane vesicle vaccine against group B meningococcal disease. *NIPH Ann.* **14,** 67–80.

14. van der Ley, P., van der Biezen, J., and Poolman, J. T. (1995) Construction of *Neisseria meningitidis* strains carrying multiple chromosomal copies of the *porA* gene for use in the production of a multivalent outer membrane vesicle vaccine. *Vaccine* **13,** 401–407.

15. Waehneldt, T. V. (1975) Sodium dodecyl sulfate in protein chemistry. *BioSystems* **6,** 176–187.

16. Shapiro, A. L., Vinuela, E., and Maizel, J. V., Jr. (1967) Molecular weight estimation of polypeptide chains by electrophoresis in SDS-polyacrylamide gels. *Biochem. Biophys. Res. Comm.* **28,** 815–820.

17. Gershoni, J. M. and Palade, G. E. (1983) Protein blotting: Principles and applications. *Anal. Biochem.* **131,** 1–15.

18. Towbin, H., Staehelin, T., and Gordon, J. (1979) Electrophoretic transfer of proteins from polyacrylamide gels to nitrocellulose sheets: procedures and some applications. *Proc. Natl. Acad. Sci. USA* **76,** 4350–4354.

19. Burnette, W. N. (1981) "Western blotting": Electrophoretic transfer of proteins from sodium dodecyl sulfate-polyacrylamide gels to unmodified nitrocellulose

and radiographic detection with antibody and radioiodinated Protein A. *Anal. Biochem.* **112,** 195–203.

20. Beisiegel, U. (1986) Protein blotting. *Electrophoresis* **7,** 1–18.
21. Huisman, J. G. (1986) Immunoblotting: An emerging technique in immunohematology. *Vox Sang.* **50,** 129–136.
22. Gershoni, J. M. (1988) Protein blotting: a manual, in *Methods of Biochemical Analysis,* vol 33 (Glick, D., ed.), John Wiley and Sons, New York, pp. 1–58.
23. Stott, D. I. (1989) Immunoblotting and dot blotting. *J. Immunol. Methods* **119,** 153–187.
24. Laemmli, U. K. (1970) Cleavage of structural proteins during the assembly of the head of bacteriophage T4. *Nature* **227,** 680–685.
25. Mandrell, R. E. and Zollinger, W. D. (1984) Use of a zwitterionic detergent for the restoration of the antibody-binding capacity of electroblotted meningococcal outer membrane proteins. *J. Immunol. Methods* **67,** 1–11.
26. Wedege, E., Bryn, K., and Frøholm, L. O. (1988) Restoration of antibody binding to blotted meningococcal outer membrane proteins using various detergents. *J. Immunol. Methods* **113,** 51–59.
27. Wedege, E., Bolstad, K., Wetzler, L. M., and Guttormsen, H. K. (2000) IgG antibody levels to meningococcal porins in patient sera: comparison of immunoblotting and ELISA measurements. *J. Immunol. Methods* **244,** 9–15.
28. Nicolas, R. H., and Goodwin, G. H. (1982) Isolation and analysis, in *The HMG Chromosomal Proteins* (Johns, E. W., ed.), Academic Press, London, pp. 41–68.
29. Frasch, C. E. and Mocca, L. F. (1978) Heat-modifiable outer membrane antigens of *Neisseria meningitidis* and their organization within the membrane. *J. Bacteriol.* **136,** 1127–1134.
30. Abdillahi, H., Crowe, B. A., Achtman, M., and Poolman, J. T. (1988) Two monoclonal antibodies specific for serotype-4 antigen of *Neisseria meningitidis. Eur. J. Clin. Microbiol. Infect. Dis.* **7,** 293–296.
31. Gershoni, J. M. and Palade, G. E. (1982) Electrophoretic transfer of proteins from sodium-dodecyl-sulfate-polyacrylamide gels to a positively charged membrane filter. *Anal. Biochem.* **124,** 396–405.
32. Chavez, L. G. and Benjamin, D. G. (1978) Antibody as an immunological probe for studying the refolding of bovine serum albumin. *J. Biol. Chem.* **253,** 8081–8086.
33. Carlson, J. D. and Yarmush, M. L. (1992) Antibody assisted protein refolding. *Biotechnology* **10,** 86–91.
34. Tomáska, L. and Nosek, J. (1995) Several polymers enhance the sensitivity of the Southwestern assay. *Anal. Biochem.* **227,** 387–389.
35. Rittenhouse, J. and Marcus, F. (1984) Peptide mapping by polyacrylamide gel electrophoresis after cleavage at aspartyl-prolyl bonds in sodium dodecyl sulfate-containing buffers. *Anal. Biochem.* **138,** 442–448.

20

Serogroup B and C Serum Bactericidal Assays

Ray Borrow and George M. Carlone

1. Introduction

Meningococci are usually classified based on serological reactivity of their polysaccharide capsules with serogroups A, B, and C, currently the most common causes of disease. Serogroup A meningococci can cause massive outbreaks particularly in areas such as the African meningitis belt, whereas other areas such as in the Americas and Europe, serogroups B and C predominate. Although licensed vaccines for serogroups A and C exist, based on the polysaccharide capsules, no such vaccine exists thus far for serogroup B owing to its poor immunogenicity in humans. This chapter discusses and details serum bactericidal assay protocols for measuring the complement-mediated lysis of serogroups B and C meningococci by human sera following vaccination or disease.

Neisseria meningitidis serogroup C polysaccharide vaccines, developed at the Walter Reed Army Institute of Research and tested in military recruits, have been shown to be immunogenic in humans by Gotschlich et al. 1969 *(1)*. These vaccines elicited both haemagglutinating and bactericidal antibodies. Antibody responses to these capsular polysaccharide (CPS) vaccines have been measured by various serologic methods: capillary precipitation, haemagglutination, immunofluorescence, radial immunodiffusion, latex agglutination, opsonizing antibody, complement fixing antibody, bactericidal antibody, radioimmunoassay (RIA), and enzyme-linked immunosorbent assay (ELISA) *(1–5)*. Meningococcal polysaccharide vaccines were licensed using data obtained by RIA and bactericidal assays. Of the "quantitative" procedures reported, only RIA and ELISA accurately measure CPS antibody levels with the serum volumes typically obtained from young children, and a serum bacte-

From: *Methods in Molecular Medicine, vol. 66: Meningococcal Vaccines: Methods and Protocols*
Edited by: A. J. Pollard and M. C. J. Maiden © Humana Press Inc., Totowa, NJ

ricidal assay (SBA) has historically *(1,2)* been used to measure functional antibody titers. Both of these serologic surrogates, and possibly others, will likely be used to license the new generation of protein-polysaccharide conjugate meningococcal vaccines without the need of a classical efficacy trial. However, questions still remain as to the exact laboratory protocols necessary to accurately predict clinical protection.

The role of circulating antibody and complement in protection from meningococcal disease was demonstrated in the 1900s *(1)* and reviewed recently *(5)*. Serum bactericidal antibody activity has been shown to highly correlate with immunity to meningococcal disease *(1,6)*. An inverse correlation was observed between the age-related incidence of disease and the age-specific prevalence of complement-dependent serum bactericidal activity *(1)*. Induction of complement-dependent bactericidal antibodies after vaccination with meningococcal polysaccharide or protein conjugate vaccines is regarded as acceptable evidence of the potential efficacy of these vaccines *(2)*.

In 1976, the World Health Organization (WHO) Expert Committee on Biological Standardization recommended a SBA to satisfy the requirements for production and release of meningococcal polysaccharide vaccine *(4)*. These SBA requirements have also been used to support vaccine licensure. In order for a vaccine to be acceptable for licensure, ≥90% of the immunized adult subjects must have a fourfold rise (increase of 2 dilutions) in SBA titer when tested against target strains by the specified SBA *(4)*. A fourfold or greater rise in SBA titer is currently used to estimate the potential efficacy of meningococcal vaccines during field trials, as well as to determine seroconversion after immunization with the currently licensed polysaccharide vaccine or protein-polysaccharide conjugate vaccines *(7)*. Care must be taken when looking at fourfold rises in titer with infants' sera owing to pre-immunization sera for this age group containing maternal antibodies. Numerous procedures have been used to evaluate meningococcal serum bactericidal activity *(7)*. These procedures differ by a number of factors from the recommended WHO SBA. Some of these methods were published prior to the WHO recommendations; however, some researchers continue to use and reference these earlier versions of SBA. In most cases, these various assays are being used without an apparent comparison to the procedure recommended by WHO. It is apparent that a standard protocol must be used and adopted for comparison and evaluation of new and developing meningococcal vaccines. Inter-laboratory comparisons, which will be necessary for conjugate vaccine licensure, are virtually impossible to interpret unless reagents and target strains are shared among laboratories using similar procedures. The use of nonstandardized SBAs to measure functional activities of potential vaccines may lead to over- or underestimation of prediction of potential vaccine efficacy and possibly to premature release or delay of field trials and licensure *(7)*.

The complement source used in the SBA appears to be of critical importance. Unlike the reported serogroup B SBAs that use human complement, the WHO recommended procedure for serogroups A and C uses baby rabbit serum as a complement source. Intuitively, a normal human complement source would be desirable; however, in practice, large volumes of a suitable human source are not available or difficult to obtain; agammaglobulinemic sera is also not available in large volumes as a complement source.

When SBA titers have been compared after using baby rabbit and human serum as a complement source, significant differences in antibody titers have been observed; human complement tends to give lower titers *(7)*. The original assays that associated bactericidal antibody with protection used normal human serum that lacked bactericidal activity to strains used in the study as a complement source with test sera from individuals after natural infection *(1)*. Vaccine licensure, however, was supported using SBA titers obtained using baby rabbit complement with sera before and after vaccination.

A recent multi-laboratory study standardized the serogroup C SBA and compared it to the recommended WHO procedure *(7)*. The standardized assay and the WHO recommended assay differed only by selection of the target strains, growth of the target strains, and the final well volume. The modified assay will facilitate inter-laboratory comparisons of the functional antibody produced in response to current or developing serogroup C meningococcal vaccines. However, a decision still needs to be made regarding the complement source to be used in this protocol.

The SBA can be used to measure large numbers of sera in an immunogenicity study. Semi-automation can be achieved by the use of colony counters and dilutors. In fact, more sera can be assayed by SBA than by ELISA in the same amount of time. Therefore, the choice of assay to access vaccine immunogenicity is not a limiting factor for large-scale immunogenicity studies or manufacturing consistency testing.

There are two standardized ELISA that can reproducibly measure serum anti-capsular antibody concentrations; a standard IgG ELISA that measures both high- and low-avidity antibodies *(8)* and a modified ELISA that measures predominately high-avidity IgG antibodies *(9)*. Results from these assays are, in general, not in good agreement when IgG antibody levels are compared after one or two doses of polysaccharide, or one or two doses of protein-conjugate vaccine. IgG ELISA levels after a single dose of either vaccine generally has a low correlation with SBA, presumably owing to low-avidity antibodies. Correlation of the standard IgG ELISA and SBA is in good agreement after the primary vaccination series and after a booster dose. The use of a human complement source in the SBA tends to give much lower antibody titers than when baby rabbit complement is used. Large volumes of suitable human source complement preserved sera are not available and are difficult to procure owing to the occurrence of naturally occurring anti-meningococcal antibodies from oropharyngeal carriage of meningococci or other Neisserial species. In the absence of a commercial source, the standardization of assays between laboratories, each of whom using their own in-house source of human complement, is difficult. Commercially available heterologous complement has the advantage of being manufactured and supplied to a high standard of consistency. The optimal choice of complement source in the serogroup C SBA, however, still needs to be determined.

A standard reference serum (available from the National Institute for Biological Standards and Control [NIBSC], Potters Bar, Herts, UK) and 12 quality-control sera (Centers for Disease Control and Prevention [CDC], Atlanta, GA) are available for use in SBA assays. The reference serum and quality control sera were prepared in adults using polysaccharide vaccine; however, it appears that this serum is suitable for determining antibody levels and SBA titers in infant and toddler sera from individuals vaccinated with the protein conjugate vaccine. In conclusion, for the serogroup C SBA, questions still need to be answered and some research may need to be completed before we can confidently substitute these laboratory surrogates for clinical-efficacy trials. Caution should be observed particularly with the selection or rejection of new meningococcal serogroup C polysaccharide-based vaccine formulations when based predominately on results obtained from the current iteration of these laboratory protocols.

Due to the poor immunogenicity of the serogroup B polysaccharide in humans, serogroup B vaccine research has focused mainly on other bacterial components, especially on preparations of outer-membrane proteins (OMPs) or vesicles (OMVs). Three such vaccines have now been thoroughly evaluated (two in response to national epidemics): the Norwegian and Cuban OMP vaccines (10,11), and the third for the phenotypically diverse serogroup B disease as seen in the UK and elsewhere (12). All these vaccines contain phenotypically different major OMPs, the PorA (or class 1) OMP is believed to be an important determinant of OMP-induced immunity. As for serogroup C, the SBA has become the primary serologic assay used to assess protective immunity stimulated by serogroup B meningococcal vaccine components a number of SBA assays have been described which differ greatly (12–22).

Unlike serogroup C SBAs, the choice of complement is clear for serogroup B SBAs; human complement. Human post-vaccination antibody to meningococcal serogroup B polysaccharide has been shown to be strongly bactericidal with rabbit complement, but to have little or no bactericidal activity in conjunction with human complement *(23)*. The specificity of human antibodies that are bactericidal for serogroup B meningococci have been investigated in a number of studies, often with conflicting results *(6,12–22,24–28)*. Some discrepancies may be attributable to the use of different complement sources and to differences in the assays used. It is again significant that the studies of Goldschneider et al. *(2,6)* which established the correlation between serum bactericidal activity and immunity to meningococcal disease were done with human complement. In those studies, the presence of bactericidal antibody with specificity for serogroup B polysaccharide was not specifically demonstrated. Since that time, a number of studies utilizing bactericidal assays employed rabbit complement *(27,28–30)*. Bactericidal antibodies with serogroup B specificity have been demonstrated by several workers by using rabbit complement *(27,28)*. In some of these studies the bactericidal activity appeared to be directed against the serogroup B polysaccharide *(28,30)* but in other studies anti-serogroup B polysaccharide antibodies were found to lack bactericidal activity *(27)*. Anti-serogroup B polysaccharide antibodies are almost all of the IgM isotype *(30)* and are of relatively low avidity *(31)* thus are especially sensitive to variables such as complement source.

Depending on the antigen/antigens being studied, a variety of serogroup B isolates may be used as target strains in the serogroup B SBA. It has been demonstrated that there are a number of immunogenic antigens of which the phenotypic expression should be monitored to ensure intra- and inter-laboratory. For example, these include the PorA OMP *(14,18)* and the Opc *(15)*.

The protocol described below for serogroup B and C SBAs is recommended so the number of variables that can occur in this assay may be kept to a minimum to ensure ease of comparison of serum bactericidal titers between various meningococcal vaccine trials in the global campaign to license effective vaccines for the control of meningococcal disease.

1.1. Principle of Assay

N. meningitidis target strains are lysed in the presence of meningococcal-specific antibody and complement (antibody-mediated, complement-dependent killing). Serial dilutions of human sera are incubated with appropriate target strains and complement. Meningococcal-specific antibody binds to the target-cell surface via meningococcal-specific protein or carbohydrate moieties. The C1q subunit of C1 binds to the Fc portion of the surface-bound Ig. The binding of C1q to Ig activates the classical pathway of complement that ultimately results in death of the target cell. The serum bactericidal titer for each unknown serum is expressed as the reciprocal serum dilution yielding ≥50% killing as compared to the number of target cells present before incubation with serum and complement.

1.2. Safety

1.2.1. Sera

All human sera may contain HIV, hepatitis B, and/or human pathogens. Use universal precautions when handling any specimen from a human source. Immunization with hepatitis B vaccine is highly recommended.

1.2.2. N. meningitidis Isolates

Biosafety level 2 practices are generally recommended when working with *N. meningitidis*. However the potential for generating aerosols using this bactericidal procedure increases the risk of exposure, so biosafety level 3 practices should be considered and an appropriate microbiological safety cabinet is essential. Immunization with serogroup A and C polysaccharide or serogroup C protein-polysaccharide conjugate vaccine should be considered but should only be used with, not in place of, the aforementioned recommendations. Laboratory-acquired infections have been reported *(32–37)*.

2. Materials

2.1. Serum Samples

1. A positive serum sample of known SBA titer should be assayed on each run. Quality-control sera should be collected by the testing laboratories. The CDC can provide a limited amount of quality-control sera. A standard reference serum (CDC1992) collected from adults immunized with a quadrivalent polysaccharide vaccine is available from the NIBSC *(38)*.
2. The minimum volume of serum needed is 30 μL. This volume will allow one measurement of bactericidal activity for each serum.
3. Serum samples to be assayed should be stored frozen at –70°C and not be freeze/thawed more than four times.
4. When using very opaque sera (e.g., hyperlipemic), counting colonies in the microtiter plate using the 'agar overlay' method can be difficult. The 'agar overlay' method is not recommended in these instances and the 'tilt' method is advised (*see* **Note 1**).

2.2. Bacteria

See **Note 2** for storage of strain aliquots.

1. Serogroup C target strain. C11 (phenotype C : 16 : P1.7ᵃ,1) (also known as 60E) *(1)* may be obtained from the Food and Drug Administration (FDA, Rockville,

MD), the American Type Culture Collection (ATCC) (10801 University Blvd., Manassas, VA), CDC, or Public Health Laboratory Service (PHLS) Meningococcal Reference Unit (MRU) (Manchester, UK).

2. Serogroup B or OMP/OMV vaccine target strains. Depending on the vaccine composition being investigated, the target strain(s) may vary. Serogroup B strains may be obtained from most Meningococcal Reference Units and National Collections of Typing Strains, for example in the US from the CDC, in the UK from NCTC, or PHLS MRU. Classical strains such as H44/76 (B : 15 : P1.7,16) may be obtained from NIH (Norway).

2.3. Complement

1. Rabbit complement. Pooled baby rabbit serum (Pel Freeze Inc, Brown Deer, Wisconsin, US; distributors in the UK are MAST Group Ltd., Mast House, Derby Road, Bootle, Merseyside, L20 1EA, UK) may be used for serogroup C SBA but not serogroup B *(23)*. Keep at –70°C and transport on dry ice. Aliquot bottles, which must only be defrosted for a minimum of time, into small volumes (1–3 mL) that must also be kept frozen at –70°C and defrosted only immediately prior to use. If thawed complement must be refrozen, quick-freeze with ethanol and dry ice is recommended. New lots of rabbit complement must be assayed with low, medium, and high quality-control sera (*see* **Subheading 2.1.1.**) and titers must fall within one dilution either side of the established SBA titer. Previously tested sera (in addition to quality controls) may also be assayed with titers being within one dilution of their previously established SBA titer. Assays should be performed in duplicate for this validation. All normal controls should still be checked.

2. Human complement. Can be used in either serogroup B or C SBA. Keep as for rabbit complement. *See* **Note 3** for collection and qualification of human complement.

2.4. Bactericidal Buffer

A variety of bactericidal buffers may be used though either of the following may be used. With all new batches of bactericidal buffer it should be determined that there is no decrease in viable cell count after 60 min.

1. Geys balanced salts solution (Gibco BRL, Cat. no. 24260-028 or equivalent) with 0.5% bovine serum albumin (BSA) (fraction V) (Sigma, Cat. no. A7906 or equivalent). Filter-sterilize (0.22 μM) and store at +4°C.

2. Dulbecco's phosphate-buffered saline (PBS) containing 0.5 mM MgCl$_2$ and 0.9 mM CaCl$_2$; pH 7.4) (Life Technologies, Cat. no. 14080 or equivalent) with 0.1% glucose (Sigma, Cat. no. G7528, or equivalent). Filter-sterilize (0.22 μM) and store at +4°C.

3. Hanks balanced salt solution (HBSS), pH 7.2, containing 4 mM NaHCO$_3$ (Gibco BRL, Cat. no. 14175-046 or equivalent) and 0.1% BSA (fraction V) (Sigma, Cat. no. A7906 or equivalent). Filter-sterilize (0.22 μM) and store at +4°C.

2.5. Agar Plates

See **Note 4** for discussion on the choice of broth vs agar and different types of agar. A number of agar media are suitable. Either of the two listed below are recommended.

1. Blood agar (Blood agar base no 2 with defibrinated horse blood (5%); Oxoid, Cat. no. CM331 or equivalent.)
2. Brain-heart infusion (Becton Dickenson, Cat. no. 4311065 or equivalent) with 1% horse serum (Life Technologies, Cat. no. 16050-098 or equivalent).
3. Tryptic Soy Broth (TSB) with 0.9% Noble Agar (for 'agar overlay' method). TSB (Becton Dickenson, Cat. no. 211825 or equivalent) 30 g, Noble Agar (Becton Dickenson, Cat. no. 0142-17-0 or equivalent) 9 g, Type 1 water or endotoxin-free water 1 L.

2.6. 96-Well Tissue-Culture Plates

1. For the tilt method, U-bottomed plates are recommended because small volumes collect at the center of each well, making plating out easier. 96-well, U-bottomed tissue-culture plates (Sterilin, Cat. no. 611U96 or equivalent).
2. For the agar-overlay method, flat-bottomed plates are recommended because this aids with visualization and light scatter. 96-well, flat-bottomed tissue-culture plates (Costar Inc., Cat. no. 3596 or equivalent).

2.7. Specialized Equipment

1. Appropriate microbiological safety cabinet (Biosafety level 2 safety cabinet).
2. Colony counter (for tilt method) (Perceptive Instruments, Haverhill, Suffolk, UK or equivalent) (A modification of the Cardinal Automatic Colony Counting System).
3. Microscope: (For agar overlay or tilt method if colony counter unavailable). Dissecting microscope with optics capable of 10–15× magnification.
4. Spectrophotometer: For adjusting meningococcal-cell suspensions.
5. Incubators: Both +37°C incubators and 5% CO_2, +37°C incubators.

3. Methods
3.1. Day 1

1. Preparation of target strain: An aliquot of the target strain should be defrosted and plated out overnight at 37°C with 5% CO_2 on blood agar or brain heart infusion (with 1% horse serum) agar.

3.2. Day 2

1. Approximately 10–20 meningococcal colonies are picked from the overnight culture and spread out over an agar plate and cultured for 3–4 h at 37°C with 5% CO_2.
2. Working in the safety cabinet, cells are suspended in bactericidal buffer at an optical density (OD) of 0.1 at 650 nm, with a cuvet of path length 10 mm or an

OD of 0.3 at 600 nm with a cuvet of path length 16 mm. The cell suspension is then diluted in 5-mL bactericidal buffer (*see* **Subheading 4.4.**) to yield approx 50–60 CFU/10 μL. Fill wells of columns 1–11 of a sterile, U-bottomed, 96-well plate with 20 μL of bactericidal buffer (equilibrated to room temperature). Add 10 μL of buffer to column 12. *See* **Table 1** for microtitration plate template.

3. Following the template (**Fig. 1**), add 20 μL of heat-inactivated (56°C for 30 min) sera to column 1. Using a multi-channel pipet, serially dilute the 8 test sera two-fold in the microtiter wells by removing 20 μL from the wells of column 1 and transferring to the wells of column 2 and mixing 6 times. Continue diluting through to column 9. Withdraw 20 μL from column 9 and discard.
4. Add 10 μL of test serum (heat-inactivated) to the corresponding well of column 12.
5. Add 10 μL of the working solution of bacteria to every well.
6. Add 10 μL of heat-inactivated (56°C for 30 min) complement to all wells of columns 11 and 12.
7. Add 10 μL of complement (removed 10 min previously from the –70°C freezer) to columns 1 to 10 and gently tap plates to mix.
8. Using the tilt method (*see* **Note 1**), plate out 10 μL from all wells of column 11 to determine T_0.
9. Seal the plates with plate sealers before transferring to the 37°C incubator.
10. Incubate the plates for 1 h at 37°C (without CO_2).
11. For the tilt method, in which the agar plate is tilted through 45°C to allow the drops to run down the plate, 10 μL drops are plated out from every well and incubated overnight at 37°C with 5% CO_2 for T_{60}.

For the 'agar overlay' method TSB containing 0.9% Noble Agar (100 μL) equilibrated to 48°C (liquefied by heating to 100°C) is added to each well and the plate incubated overnight at 37°C with 5% CO_2 for T_{60}.

3.3. Day 3

1. Count the number of colonies for T_0 and T_{60}. The number of colonies in column 11 is the number of viable cells. Column 12 is a test for complement-independent killing (*see* **Note 5**). Column 10 is a complement control (*see* **Note 6**).
2. The serum bactericidal titer is reported as the reciprocal serum dilution yielding ≥50% killing at T_{60} as compared with the number of viable cells.
3. In order to assign a titer, the following conditions must be met.
   a. Target cell growth in column 12 (the serum control well) is ≥80% of the CFU in column 11.
   b. The test serum must have a clearly defined SBA titer. In order to assign a titer at 50% reduction in CFU, at least two consecutive serial dilutions of the test serum must have a cell count <20% of the CFU per well compared to the CFU in column 11.

Serum, which does not fulfill condition (a.) should be retested. If growth in the serum control well is <20% of the CFU per well compared to the CFU in

Table 1
Microtitration Plate Template

Assay	1	2	3	4	5	6	7	8	9	10	11	12
Bactericidal buffer (µL)	20	20	20	20	20	20	20	20	20	20	20	See below
Patient serum (µL)	Nine twofold serial serum dilutions									0	0	
	Transfer 20 µL from column 1–9, mix 6 times, and discard 20 µL from column 9											
Complement (µL)	10	10	10	10	10	10	10	10	10	10	10[a]	
Cells (µL)	10	10	10	10	10	10	10	10	10	10	10	
Final volume (µL)	40	40	40	40	40	40	40	40	40	40	40	
Reciprocal final serum dilution	4	8	16	32	64	128	256	512	1024			

Column 11, [a]heat-inactivated complement.
Column 12, Add 10 µL of bactericidal buffer, 10 µL of heat-inactivated serum, 10 µL of heat-inactivated complement, and 10 µL of working solution of organisms (*see* **Note 5**).

column 11 after repeat testing, then the titer must be reported as "Not determined due to reduction in the control well" (*see* **Note 5**). A serum that does not fulfill condition (b.) should be retested. If there are not at least two consecutive serial dilutions of the test serum with cell counts <20%, then the titer should be reported as <8.

Sera that give >50% of CFU per well compared to the CFU in column 11 in the test serial dilution must be reported to have a SBA titer of <4. Reproducibility of the assay is poor, including target cell growth in serum control wells, with serum dilutions <1:4.

4. Notes

1. Methods for culturing target-cell survivors. Few differences have been noted when comparing different methods of growth by the tilt method, agar overlay (in which 100 mL of TSB containing 0.9% Noble agar is overlaid in each well of the plate before overnight incubation at 37°C with 5% CO_2), or the spot method (*7*) though the latter is the least accurate. For ease of automation with semi-automated colony counters, the tilt method is generally preferred.

2. Target-strain stocks. Multiple aliquots (0.5 mL) of the target strain(s) must be stored to prevent sub-culturing. Recommended storage media is Nutrient broth (Becton Dickenson, Cat. no. 4311479 or equivalent) with 15% glycerol. The stock of glycerol broth was prepared by taking a swab of an overnight meningococcal culture from a blood-agar plate or brain-heart infusion (with 1% horse serum) plating and emulsifying in the glycerol broth to make a heavy suspension. This is then divided into 0.5-mL volumes in sterile plastic vials and immediately stored frozen at –70°C.

3. Collection and testing of human complement donor sera. The ideal complement source for use in the meningococcal bactericidal assay is serum from a human with agammaglobulinemia because this serum does not contain antibodies that might contribute to bacteriolysis in the bactericidal assay. Most patients with this disease now receive exogenous replacement immunoglobulin making such serum hard to find. A small percentage of healthy adults lack serum antibodies against either or both serogroup B and/or C strains of meningococci and their sera may serve as a complement source for the bactericidal assay.

Draw blood in Vacutainer tubes with either red or red/black tops used for collecting clotted blood samples. A volume for collection of serum for complement is 250 mL, which will typically yield approx 150 × 1 mL aliquots of serum complement. Allow the blood to clot at room temperature for 30 min. Centrifuge for 10 min at 12,000*g* and aliquot the sera into 1–3 mL sterile tubes.

Freeze the tubes immediately at –70°C. On no account freeze/thaw tubes or let temperature drop below –70°C. Snap-freezing with ethanol and dry ice may be used.

Prospective donor sera for serogroup C SBA are first screened for IgG and IgM anti-capsular antibodies by ELISA *(8,9)*. Donor sera that are negative in the ELISA (<0.8 µg/mL for **ref.** *[8]* or <0.4 U/mL for **ref.** *[9]* of antibody) are tested at final concentrations of 25 and 50% for intrinsic bactericidal in the absence of exogenous antibody. Donor sera are selected if they are negative (complement does not kill bacteria to a level greater than ~15% of the T_0 plated control) when tested at both 25 and 50%. The target strain used for screening should be the same as to be used in the SBA assay as sera may contain anti-OMP antibodies, which are bactericidal only against particular strains. Serum from complement donors should also be tested for hemolytic complement activity (CH_{50}). The testing laboratory establishes the normal range with an in-house population. For serum stored at –70°C for more than 6 mo, this assay should be repeated.

If using human plasma as complement source, a 0.5 U/mL (final) concentration of heparin is required to prevent clotting in assay.

4. Choice of media. Care should be taken with using agar media other than the blood and brain-heart infusion agar listed above. Certain media result in complement sensitive bacteria and media incorporating antibiotics should be avoided. Broths such as Mueller-Hinton (Cat. no. CM405) (with 2% Vitox supplement, Cat. no. SR090A) may be used for target-strain culture, but this results in lower SBA titers, possibly owing to loss of capsule on centrifugation to remove broth prior to assay or owing to clumping of cells.

5. Decrease in CFU in column 12. Column 12 is a control column to measure noncomplement mediated lysis of cells. Serum samples may contain antibiotics with a result the number of CFUs in column 12 is decreased. The β lactam family (containing penicillin) can be overcome with the use of β lactamase (Merck Ltd., Cat. no. 39084 3G or equivalent). The dilution in this serum control well must always be 1;4 regardless of the initial dilution in the serial diluted serum wells. The serum used in this control well must be heat-inactivated.

6. Decrease in CFU in column 10. Column 10 is a control column to measure the complement resistance of the target strain. If the number of CFUs decreases as compared with column 11, this is owing to the target strain becoming complement-sensitive, which may be affected by many things. These include density and thickness of the capsule *(39)* or sialylation status of the lipooligosaccharide *(40)* usually incurred due to incorrect storage, multiple subculturing, or inappropriate growth media (*see* **Note 4**).

Acknowledgments

Many thanks to Carl Frasch (Center for Biologics Evaluation and Research, Food and Drug Administration) for critically reviewing the content and understanding of this chapter and Derrick Lake (CDC) for his comments on the technical aspects.

References

1. Gotschlich, E. C., Goldschneider, I., and Artenstein M. S. (1969) Human immunity to the meningococcus IV. Immunogenicity of serogroup A and serogroup C polysaccharides in human volunteers. *J. Exp. Med.* **129,** 1367–1384.
2. Goldschneider, I., Gotschlich, E. C, and Artenstein, M. S. (1969) Human immunity to the meningococcus. I. The role of humoral antibodies. *J. Exp. Med.* **129,** 1307–1326.
3. Arakere, G. A. and Frasch, C. E. (1991) Specificity of antibodies to O-acetyl-positive and O-acetyl-negative group C meningococcal polysaccharides in sera from vaccinees and carriers. *Infect. Immun.* **59,** 4349–4356.
4. World Health Organization (1976) Requirements for meningococcal polysaccharide vaccine. World Health Organization technical report series, no. 594. World Health Organization, Geneva.
5. Frasch, C. E. (1995) Meningococcal vaccines: past, present and future, in *Meningococcal Disease* (Cartwright, K. A. V., ed.), John Wiley and Sons Ltd., Chichester, UK.
6. Goldschneider, I, Gotschlich, E. C., and Artenstein, M. S. (1969) Human immunity to the meningococcus II. Development of natural immunity. *J. Exp. Med.* **129,** 1327–1348.
7. Maslanka, S. E., Gheesling, L. L., LiButti, D. E., Donaldson, K. B. J., Harakeh, H. S., Dykes, J. K., et al. (1997) Standardization and a multilaboratory comparison of *Neisseria meningitidis* serogroup A and C serum bactericidal assays. *Clin. Diagn. Lab. Immunol.* **4,** 156–167.
8. Gheesling, L. L., Carlone, G. M., Pais, L., Holder, P. F., Maslanka, S. E., Plikaytis, B. D., et al. (1994) Multicenter comparison of *Neisseria meningitidis* serogroup C anti-capsular polysaccharide antibody levels measured by a standardized enzyme-linked immunosorbent assay. *J. Clin. Microbiol.* **32,** 1475–1482.
9. Granoff, D. M., Maslanka, S. E., Carlone, G. M., Plikaytis, B. D., Santos, G. F., Mokatrin, A., and Raff, H. V. (1998). A modified enzyme-linked immunosorbent assay for measurement of antibody responses to meningococcal C polysaccharide that correlate with bactericidal responses. *Clin. Diagn. Lab. Immunol.* **5,** 479–485.
10. Bjune, G., Høiby, E. A., Grønnesby, J. K. Arnesen, O., Fredriksen, J. H., Halstensen, A., et al. (1991) Effect of outer membrane vesicle vaccine against group B meningococcal disease in Norway. *Lancet* **338,** 1093–1096.
11. Sierra, G. V. G., Campa, H. C., Varcacel, N. M., Garcia, I. L., Izquierdo, P. L., Sotolongo, P. F., et al. (1991) Vaccine against group B *Neisseria meningitidis*: protection trial and mass vaccination results in Cuba. *NIPH Ann.* **4,** 195–210.

12. Cartwright, K. A. V., Richmond, P., Morris, R., Rümke, H., Fox, A. J., Borrow, R., et al. (1999) Immunogenicity and reactogenicity in UK infants of a novel meningococcal vesicle vaccine containing multiple class 1 outer membrane proteins. *Vaccine* **17,** 2612–2619.

13. Boslego, J., Garcia, J., Cruz, C., Zollinger, W., Brandt, B., Ruiz, S., et al. (1995) Efficacy, safety, and immunogenicity of a meningococcal vaccine group B (15:P1.3) outer membrane protein vaccine in Iquique, Chile. Chilean National Committee for Meningococcal Disease. *Vaccine* **13,** 821–829.

14. Høiby, E. A., Rosenqvist, E., Frøholm, L. O., Bjune, G., Feiring, H., Nøkleby, H., and Rønnild, E. (1991) Bactericidal antibodies after vaccination with the Norwegian meningococcal serogroup B outer membrane vesicle vaccine: a brief survey. *NIPH Ann.* **14,** 147–156.

15. Rosenqvist, E., Høiby, E. A., Wedege, E., Kusecek, B., and Achtman, M. (1993) The 5C protein of *Neisseria meningitidis* is highly immunogenic in humans and induces bactericidal antibodies. *J. Infect. Dis.* **167,** 1065–1073.

16. Milagres, L. G., Ramos, S. R., Sacchi, C. T., Melles, C. E., Vieira, V. S., Sato, H., et al. (1994) Immune response of Brazilian children to a *Neisseria meningitidis* serogroup B outer membrane protein vaccine: comparison with efficacy. *Infect. Immun.* **62,** 4419–4424.

17. Aase, A., Bjune, G., Høiby, E. A., Rosenqvist, E., Pedersen, A. K., and Michaelsen, T. E. (1995) Comparison among opsonic activity, antimeningococcal immunoglobulin G response, and serum bactericidal activity against meningococci in sera from vaccinees after immunization with a serogroup B outer membrane vesicle vaccine. *Infect. Immun.* **63,** 3531–3536.

18. Rosenqvist, E., Høiby, E. A., Wedege, E., Bryn, K., Kolberg, J., Klem, A., et al. (1995) Human antibody responses to meningococcal outer membrane antigens after three doses of the Norwegian group B meningococcal vaccine. *Infect. Immun.* **63,** 4642–4652.

19. van der Ley, P., van der Biezen, J., and Poolman, J. T. (1995) Construction of *Neisseria meningitidis* strains carrying multiple chromosomal copies of the porA gene for use in the production of a multivalent outer membrane vesicle vaccine. *Vaccine* **13,** 401–407.

20. van der Voort, E. R., van der Ley, P., van der Biezen, J., George, S., Tunnela, O., van Dijken, H., et al. (1996) Specificity of human bactericidal antibodies against PorA P1.7,16 induced with a hexavalent meningococcal outer membrane protein vesicle vaccine. *Infect. Immun.* **64,** 2745–2751.

21. Perkins, B. A., Jonsdottir, K., Briem H., Griffiths, E., Plikaytis, B. D., Høiby, E. A., et al. (1998) Immunogenicity of two efficacious outer membrane protein-based serogroup B meningococcal vaccines among young adults in Iceland. *J. Infect. Dis.* **177,** 683–691.

22. Tappero, J. W., Lagos, R., Ballesteros, A. M., Plikaytis, B., Williams, D., Dykes, J., et al. (1999) Immunogenicity of two outer membrane protein serogroup B meningococcal vaccines: a randomised, controlled trial in Chile. *JAMA* **281,** 1520–1527.

23. Zollinger, W. D. and Mandrell, R. E. (1983) Importance of complement source in bactericidal activity of human antibody and murine monoclonal antibody to meningococcal group B polysaccharide. *Infect. Immun.* **40,** 257–264.

24. Craven, D. E., Shen, K. T., and Frasch, C. E. (1982) Natural bactericidal activity of human serum against *Neisseria meningitidis* isolates of different serogroups and serotypes. *Infect. Immun.* **37,** 132–137.

25. Holten, E., Vaage, L., and Jyssum, K. (1970) Bactericidal activity in sera from carriers of sulphonamide-resistant meningococci. *Scand. J. Infect.* **2,** 201–204.

26. Jones, D. M. and Eldridge, J. (1979) Development of antibodies to meningococcal protein and lipopolysaccharide serotype antigens in healthy carriers. *J. Med. Microbiol.* **12,** 107–111.

27. Kasper, D. L., Winklehake, B. L., Brandt, B. L., and Artenstein, M. S. (1973) Antigenic specificity of bactericidal antibodies in antisera to *Neisseria meningitidis. J. Infect. Dis.* **127,** 378–387.

28. Zollinger, W. D., Mandrell, R. E., Altieri, P., Berman, S., Lowenthal, J., and Artenstein, M. S. (1978) Safety and immunogenicity of a *Neisseria meningitidis* type 2 protein vaccine in animals and humans. *J. Infect. Dis.* **137,** 728–739.

29. Griffiss, J. M. and Betram, M. A. (1977) Immunoepidemiology of meningococcal disease in military recruits. II. Blocking of serum bactericidal activity by circulating IgA early in the course of invasive disease. *J. Infect. Dis.* **136,** 733–739.

30. Zollinger, W. D., Mandrell, R. E., Griffiss, J. M., Altieri, P., and Berman, S. (1979) Complex of meningococcal group B polysaccharide and outer membrane protein immunogenic in man. *J. Clin. Invest.* **63,** 836–848.

31. Mandrell, R. E. and Zollinger, W. D. (1982) Measurement of antibodies to meningococcal group B polysaccharide: low avidity binding and equilibrium binding constants. *J. Immunol.* **129,** 2172–2178.

32. Bhatti, A. R., DiNinno, V. L., Ashton, F. E., and White, L. A. (1982) A laboratory-acquired infection with *Neisseria meningitidis. J. Infect.* **4,** 247–252.

33. Centers for Disease Control (1991) Laboratory-acquired meningococcemia: California and Massachusetts. *MMWR.* **40,** 46–47.

34. Bremner, D. A. (1992) Laboratory acquired meningococcal septicaemia (Abst.) *Aust. Microbiol.* **13,** A106.

35. Anonymous (1992) Laboratory-acquired meningococcal infection. *Commun. Dis. Rep. Wkly.* **2,** 39.

36. Guibourdenche, M., Darchis, J. P., Boisivon, A., Collatz, E., and Riou, J. Y. (1994) Enzyme electrophoresis, sero- and subtyping, and outer membrane protein characterisation of two *Neisseria meningitidis* strains involved in laboratory-acquired infections. *J. Clin. Microbiol.* **32,** 701–704.

37. Paradis, J. F. and Grimard, D. (1994) Laboratory-acquired invasive meningococcus: Quebec. *Can. Commun. Dis. Rep.* **20,** 12–14.

38. Holder, P. K., Maslanka, S. E., Pais, L. B., Dykes, J., Plikaytis, B. D., and Carlone, G. M. (1995) Assignment of *Neisseria meningitidis* serogroup A and C class-

specific anticapsular antibody concentrations to the new standard reference serum CDC 1992. *Clin. Diag. Lab. Immunol.* **2,** 132–137.

39. Masson, L., Holbein, B. E., and Ashton, F. E. (1982) Virulence linked to polysaccharide production in serogroup B *Neisseria meningitidis. FEMS Microbiol. Lett.* **13,** 187–190.

40. Vogel, U., Claus, H., Heinze, G., and Frosch, M. (1999) Role of lipopolysaccharide sialylation in serum resistance of serogroup B and C meningococcal disease isolates. *Infect. Immun.* **67,** 954–957.

21

A Modified ELISA for Measurement of High-Avidity IgG Antibodies to Meningococcal Serogroup C Polysaccharide that Correlate with Bactericidal Titers

Dan M. Granoff and John J. Donnelly

1. Introduction

This chapter describes a modified enzyme-linked immunosorbent assay (ELISA) employing assay conditions that ensure specificity of antibody binding and favor detection primarily of high-avidity serum IgG antibodies to meningococcal serogroup C polysaccharide (1). Antibody-binding assays such as the ELISA offer a convenient and reproducible method for quantifying anticapsular antibody responses to vaccination or disease. However, the results do not always correlate well with assays of antibody functional activity, such as bactericidal activity. For example, a standardized ELISA for measurement of antibody responses to meningococcal C polysaccharide has been described (2). When used to assay relatively homogenous populations of serum antibodies, for example in sera from immunized adults (3), or from younger individuals given a single vaccine (4), the results of the standard ELISA correlated well with serum bactericidal titers. In contrast, much lower correlations were observed when assaying heterologous populations of serum antibodies from vaccinated infants or toddlers (5,6), particularly from clinical studies comparing antibody responses of different age groups (6), or studies comparing responses to a polysaccharide and conjugate vaccines (7,8).

In studies of the function of antibodies to *Haemophilus influenzae* type b and *Streptococcus pneumoniae* polysaccharides, high-avidity antibodies were more active than low-avidity antibodies in eliciting complement-mediated bac-

From: *Methods in Molecular Medicine, vol. 66: Meningococcal Vaccines: Methods and Protocols*
Edited by: A. J. Pollard and M. C. J. Maiden © Humana Press Inc., Totowa, NJ

teriolysis and opsonization and conferring passive protection in animal models of bacteremia *(9–12)*. Therefore, the most likely explanation for the poor performance of the standard IgG ELISA for predicting meningococcal serogroup C bactericidal-antibody responses is that the assay detects both high- and low-avidity antibodies, and the high-avidity population is more active in eliciting bacteriolysis than the low-avidity antibodies. In an attempt to improve the correlation between measurements of IgG anticapsular antibody concentrations and bactericidal titers in sera from subjects receiving different meningococcal serogroup C vaccines, we developed a modified ELISA that employs conditions that minimize detection of low-avidity anticapsular antibodies (i.e., detects primarily high-avidity antibodies) *(1)*. The results from the modified ELISA, but not the standard ELISA, closely parallel the magnitude of the respective bactericidal titers elicited in toddlers by different meningococcal vaccines *(1)*.

The modified ELISA described herein uses adipic acid-derivitized polysaccharide as the solid-phase coating antigen, a blocking buffer consisting of 1% BSA (radioimmunoassay reagent grade), and a serum diluting buffer containing a fixed concentration of the chaotropic agent ammonium thiocyanate (SCN), which inhibits antigen-antibody interactions in a dose-dependent fashion *(13)*.

1.1. Choice of Coating Antigen

For the modified assay, we needed a solid-phase antigen that is: 1) efficiently absorbed to the microtiter plates, 2) unaffected by the presence of SCN in the serum diluting buffer, and 3) associated with minimal nonspecific binding of Ig. In pilot studies, meningococcal C polysaccharide mixed with methylated human albumin was adsorbed to microtiter wells, as described for the standard ELISA *(2)*. With this antigen preparation, it was unclear whether some polysaccharide might enter the soluble phase during incubation with test sera diluted with buffer containing SCN. Furthermore, with the use of meningococcal C polysaccharide mixed with methylated human albumin as the solid-phase antigen, high absorbance values were observed when assaying serum samples from some unvaccinated children or adults, and this binding activity was not inhibitable upon the addition of soluble meningococcal C polysaccharide *(1)*. Therefore, to ensure antibody-binding specificity, we developed an alternative solid-phase antigen consisting of adipic acid-derivatized polysaccharide, described in detail in **Note 1**. Binding of this antigen to the solid phase appeared to be stable when incubated with sera diluted in buffer containing SCN. Also, specificity of antibody binding to this solid-phase antigen was very high, as determined by dose-response inhibition of antibody binding of a variety of pre-

or post-vaccination serum pools in the presence of soluble meningococcal C polysaccharide *(1)*.

1.2. Blocking Buffer

Several blocking buffers were evaluated to determine which yielded the lowest background titers when non-immune sera were assayed in different microtiter plates. Among the different blocking buffers tested, 1% bovine serum albumin (BSA); radioimmunoassay reagent grade) in the absence of a nonionic detergent, such as Brij (used in the standard ELISA; *2*), was equivalent or superior to other blocking buffers, as determined by the lowest background optical density (OD) values.

1.3. Use of SCN in the Serum Diluting Buffer

Antibody binding in the presence of increasing concentrations of chaotropic salts has been reported to correlate directly with antibody avidity *(13)*. Therefore, in the modified ELISA the chaotropic agent SCN, which inhibits antigen-antibody interactions in a concentration-dependent fashion, was included in the serum dilution buffer to minimize binding of low-avidity antibody. A concentration of SCN was sought that would minimally decrease the IgG ELISA binding of a toddler serum pool containing vaccine-induced meningococcal serogroup C anticapsular antibodies that were active in a complement-mediated bactericidal assay, while significantly decreasing the ELISA titers of a second toddler pool containing poorly functional, vaccine-induced anticapsular antibodies *(1)*. The desired results occurred at a concentration of approx 75 mM SCN *(1)*, which was selected for use in the serum diluting buffer in the modified IgG ELISA.

1.4. Control of Specificity of Antibody Binding

As originally described *(1)*, the modified IgG ELISA employs replicate microtiter plates in which specificity of antibody binding is assessed by subtracting the respective absorbance values obtained with each serum sample diluted with buffer containing competing soluble meningococcal polysaccharide from the corresponding value obtained from the sample diluted with buffer alone. This analysis was performed to correct for signal from antibodies binding to epitopes that might have been created when the polysaccharide was derivatized and attached to the ELISA plates. However, in subsequent studies, we found that the routine use of soluble meningococcal serogroup C polysaccharide inhibitor as a control for IgG antibody-binding specificity proved not to be universally necessary, because >90% inhibition was observed for virtually all test samples. Therefore, this step is no longer included routinely in performing the modified ELISA. However, as described in **Note 3**, this inhibition control is important when the modified ELISA is used to measure IgM or total Ig anticapsular antibody concentrations, where nonspecific binding is more of a problem (unpublished data).

1.5. Comparison of Performance of Modified and Standard ELISA

The modified and standard assays were compared for measuring IgG antibody concentrations in sera of toddlers vaccinated with meningococcal polysaccharide vaccine or a meningococcal serogroup C conjugate vaccine (*1*). The results were compared to the respective complement-mediated bactericidal antibody titers measured with human complement. In sera obtained after one or two doses of vaccine, the correlation coefficients, r, for comparison of the antibody concentrations measured by the standard ELISA to the respective bactericidal-antibody titers, were 0.45 and 0.29. In contrast, the correlation coefficients for comparison of the antibody concentrations measured by the modified ELISA and the respective bactericidal titers after one or two doses of vaccine were 0.85 and 0.87. As shown in **Table 1**, with the standard assay there were no significant differences between the geometric mean antibody responses of the two vaccine groups. In contrast, with the modified assay the conjugate vaccine group had 5- to 20-fold higher post-vaccination serum antibody concentrations than in the polysaccharide group. Importantly, the results of the modified assay, but not the standard ELISA, paralleled the respective geometric mean bactericidal-antibody titers. Thus, by employing conditions that favor detection of higher-avidity IgG antibody, the modified ELISA provides results that correlate closely with measurements of antibody functional activity that are thought to be important in protection against meningococcal disease.

2. Materials and Equipment

2.1. Equipment

1. Automated plate washer, Skatron SkanWasher 300 automated plate washer or equivalent.
2. Bio-Tek Microplate Reader, Model EL312e using dual wavelength reading at 405/630 nm or equivalent.
3. Gilson P20, P200, and P1000 automatic pipets or equivalent, calibrated every 6 mo.
4. $37 \pm 1°C$ humidified incubator box.
5. Bench-top vortex mixer.
6. 2–8°C refrigerator for storage of sera and reagents.
7. –15°C to –25°C freezer for storage of sera and reagents.
8. –70°C to –90°C freezer for storage of sera and reagents.

Table 1
Antibody Concentrations in Sera of Toddlers Vaccinated with Meningococcal C Conjugate Vaccine or Meningococcal Polysaccharide Vaccine, as Assessed by Different Assays[a]

Assay, method, and vaccine	Geometric mean			Probability[b]	
	Preimmunization	Post-dose 1	Post-dose 2	Post-dose 1	Post-dose 2
IgG anticapsular antibody					
Standard ELISA (µg/mL)					
Polysaccharide vaccine	0.12	7.0	9.7		
				0.11	0.81
Conjugate vaccine	0.18	5.1	9.3		
Modified ELISA (U/mL)					
Polysaccharide vaccine	0.22	1.0	1.2		
				<0.001	<0.001
Conjugate vaccine	0.20	4.8	21.0		
Bactericidal antibody (1/Titer)					
Polysaccharide vaccine	4.2	14	16		
				<0.001	<0.001
Conjugate vaccine	4.4	74	761		

[a]Serum samples were selected from toddlers showing a wide range of IgG antibody responses to vaccination. There were 35 subjects in the polysaccharide group and 35 in the conjugate group *(1)*.
[b]Comparing respective geometric mean antibody concentrations or titers elicited by the two vaccines.
Reprinted by permission from *(1)*.

2.2. Lot-Validated Materials

1. 96-well, U-bottom polystyrene ELISA plates (Dynatech Immulon 2 microtitration plates lot NT320516 or equivalent, Fisher Cat. no. 14-245-79).
2. *Neisseria meningitidis* serogroup C capsular polysaccharide (MenC PS) derivatized with adipic acid dihydrazide (ADH) in the presence of ethyl-3-(3-dimethylaminopropyl) carbodiimide-HCl (EDC) (*see* **Note 1**). Store working aliquots of derivatized MenC PS-ADH at 2°C to 8°C. MenC PS-ADH is stable for at least 1 yr at –15°C to –25°C.
3. Reference serum (lot A289 or equivalent), calibrated for MenC PS IgG antibodies against the MenC reference serum (CDC1992; *see* **Note 2**; Centers for Disease Control and Prevention, Atlanta, GA). Storage of serum aliquots is at –15°C or below. Serial twofold dilutions are prepared from in-house reference serum A289, beginning at a dilution of 1:400 and extending to 1:51,200. This pool was prepared from post-vaccination sera of adults immunized with meningococcal

polysaccharide vaccine. The concentration of IgG antibody to meningococcal C polysaccharide in pool A289 was assigned a value of 39 U/mL when assayed by an ELISA (without SCN in the serum-diluting buffer). This value was obtained by comparison to the titration curve generated with CDC1992 reference serum (assigned a concentration of 24.1 µg/mL IgG anti-meningococcal C polysaccharide antibody) *(14)*. When the in-house reference pool, A289, was re-assayed in replicate in an IgG ELISA performed with and without 75 m*M* SCN in the serum-diluting buffer, approx 25% less antibody binding was detected in the presence of SCN. Therefore, for use as a reference serum in the modified ELISA, this pool was assigned an IgG value of 30.8 U of antibodies per mL detected in the presence of SCN.

2.3. Internal Quality Controls

These controls were prepared by pooling sera or plasma from subjects with no detectable MenC IgG antibodies (negative control) or with varying concentrations (low-positive and high-positive control) of MenC IgG antibodies. Working aliquots of control sera are stored at 2°C to 8°C for up to 1 mo.

1. Negative control, lot 10–13 or equivalent. Lot 10–13 has a concentration of IgG antibodies against MenC capsular polysaccharide below the level of detection (less than 0.4 U/mL).
2. Low-positive control, lot 10–03 or equivalent. Lot 10–03 has a mean MenC IgG antibody concentration of 1.4 U/mL (95% CI = 1.0, 1.9 U/mL).
3. High-positive control, lot 10–04 or equivalent. Lot 10–04 has a mean MenC IgG antibody concentration of 19.4 U/mL (95% CI = 10.2, 28.7 U/mL).

2.4. Conjugate

Alkaline phosphatase-conjugated anti-human IgG (lot CC608, American Qualex or equivalent). The conjugate is a mouse monoclonal anti-human IgG Fc-specific (clone #HP6043) conjugated to alkaline phosphatase. This lot of conjugate is stored at a concentration of approx 1 mg/mL in 0.05 *M* Tris-HCl buffer, pH 8.0, 1 m*M* MgCl$_2$, and 50% glycerol in 0.5-mL aliquots. Store working aliquots at 2°C to 8°C. The conjugate is stable at –15°C to –25°C for up to 1 yr. Conjugate lot #CC608 is used at a dilution of 1:5000. Each new lot must be titered and appropriate bridging studies performed to determine the optimum dilution used in the assay.

2.5. Alkaline Phosphatase Substrate Tablets

Sigma 104 alkaline phosphatase substrate, 20 mg tablets (Sigma Cat. No. N-2765 or equivalent. Store according to manufacturer's instructions.

2.6. Prepared Solutions and Reagents

1. Sterile water for reagent preparation, nonpyrogenic water for irrigation (Baxter #2F7115, VWR catalog #68100-012), or sterile water for injection. Store at room temperature. Expiration date is noted on the bottle label.
2. Phosphate buffered saline (1X PBS), pH 7.3 ± 0.1, 20X stock solution. Store at room temperature. Expiration date is noted on the bottle label. Dilute 20X in sterile water for 1X.
3. 7.5 *M* stock ammonium thiocyanate (SCN) solution (Sigma catalog #A-3020), prepared in PBS. Store at room temperature. Expires 2 wk from date of preparation.
4. 3 *N* NaOH solution. Store at room temperature. Expiration date is noted on the bottle label.
5. Substrate buffer: 5X diethanolamine concentrate solution (Pierce catalog #34064). Store concentrate according to manufacturer's instructions. Dilute to 1X in water immediately before use.
6. Blocking buffer: 1X PBS, 1% bovine serum albumin (BSA) RIA grade, Fraction V, 96–99% albumin (Sigma Cat. No. A-7888), 0.02% sodium azide, pH 7.3 ± 0.1. Store at 2°C to 8°C. Expires 3 mo from date of preparation.
7. Wash buffer: 1X PBS, 0.1% Tween 20 (Sigma #P-1739), 0.02% sodium azide, pH 7.3 ± 0.1. Store at room temperature. Expires 3 mo from date of preparation.
8. Diluent for conjugate: 1X PBS, 1% BSA, 0.1% Tween 20, 0.02% sodium azide, pH 7.3 ± 0.1. Store at 2°C to 8°C. Expires 3 mo from date of preparation.
9. Serum dilution buffer: dilute 7.5 *M* SCN 1 : 100 in diluent for conjugate. Prepare on day of use.
10. 10% sodium azide. Store at room temperature. Expiration date is noted on the bottle. Diluted and used as described above to prepare buffers.

2.7. Disposables

1. Reservoir troughs, Matrix Technologies Corp. or equivalent.
2. Polypropylene tubes, sterile 1–50 mL volume capacity.
3. Well polypropylene 0.5 mL deep-well plates for pre-dilutions or equivalent.
4. Glassware and pipettes for reagent preparation.
5. Plastic wash bottles (Fisher Cat. No. 03-409-10D) or equivalent.

3. Method

3.1. ELISA Method

1. Coat microtiter plate wells with 100 µL of 1 µg/mL test antigen and incubate for 1 h at 37°C in a humidified box.
2. Aspirate the solution, wash the wells three times with wash buffer, and block for 1 h at room temperature with 1% BSA (Sigma) in blocking buffer.
3. Wash the plates three times with wash buffer.

4. Predilute test and reference sera with serum diluting buffer.
5. To the first row of wells, add 200 μL of prediluted test sera or samples of an in-house reference serum pool (A289) or quality-control sera (described in **Subheading 2.3.**). The remaining wells should contain 100 μL of serum-diluting buffer. Assay all sera in duplicate. Prepare serial twofold dilutions of the serum samples in the microtiter plates, resulting in a 100-μL final volume in each well.
6. Maintain the microtiter plates overnight (16–18 h) at 4°C in a humidified box.
7. On the following day, aspirate wells, and wash five times with PBS. To each well, add 100 μL of alkaline phosphatase-conjugated, murine monoclonal anti-human IgG.
8. After 1 h at 37°C, wash the plates with PBS, and add 100 μL of 1 mg/mL substrate prepared in diethanolamine solution (Pierce).
9. After 30 min, stop the colorimetric reaction by addition of 25 μL of 3 N NaOH.
10. Measure absorbance at 405 nm with a 630-nm background filter and a Bio-Tek 312e Microplate Reader (Bio-Tek Instruments Inc., Winooski, VT).

3.2. Calculation of Antibody Concentrations in Serum

1. Prepare the standard curve using serial twofold dilutions of in-house reference serum A289, beginning at a dilution of 1:400 and extending to 1:51,200. The best fit for the resulting titration curve is obtained by using a four-parameter logistic equation in the KC-3 software package (Bio Tek Instruments, Inc.). IgG anticapsular antibody concentrations in the test sera are assigned by comparison to the reference curve (*see* **Note 3**).
2. To calculate the antibody concentration, average individual antibody concentrations are obtained from dilutions of test sera that yield OD values in the linear portion of the curve (OD, 0.5–1.5). Samples with OD values between 0.14 and 0.49 at the lowest dilution tested (1:50) are considered positive, because an OD of 0.14 is >4 standard deviations above the background value. For these low-titer samples, the assigned values are extrapolated directly from a single point on the standard curve. The average of the IgG concentrations from replicate titration curves of each test serum is determined and reported in IgG U/mL. The lower limit of antibody detection with this modified ELISA is 0.4 U/mL (*see* **Note 4**).

4. Notes

1. Derivatization of meningococcal C polysaccharide. Vaccine grade meningococcal serogroup C polysaccharide (lot 84) was provided by Chiron Vaccines S.p.A. (Siena, Italy). The polysaccharide is derivatized with adipic acid dihydrazide (ADH) by the carbodiimide method *(15)*. Briefly, 5 mg/mL polysaccharide was reacted with 0.5 *M* ADH (Sigma, St. Louis, MO) in the presence of 0.1 *M* 1-ethyl-3-(3-dimethylaminopropyl) carbodiimide-HCl (Pierce, Rockford, IL) for 15 min at room temperature while the pH was maintained between 6.5 and 7.0. The derivatized polysaccharide was dialyzed against phosphate-buffered saline (PBS) and stored at 20°C. Acid ninhydrin 2 reagent (Sigma) was used to deter-

mine the concentration of the polysaccharide in the final product (*16*), and the extent of ADH incorporation was measured by using the trinitrobenzene sulfonic acid (Sigma) assay (*17*). The typical antigen lots used had a polysaccharide-to-ADH ratio of 25 ng of ADH per μg of meningococcal C polysaccharide.

2. Assignment of antibody concentrations in quality-control antiserum. The CDC1992 MenC PS IgG reference serum has a reported IgG MenC PS antibody concentration of 24.1 μg/mL (*14*). Based on the CDC reference sera, Chiron reference lot A289 was assigned a titer value of 39 U/mL of MenC IgG antibodies. Lot A289 reference serum was further calibrated against itself in the presence of thiocyanate (SCN) for high-avidity MenC IgG antibodies, and was assigned a titer value of 30.8 U/mL of MenC high-avidity IgG antibodies.

3. Measuring IgM or total Ig anticapsular antibodies by the modified ELISA. When assaying IgM or total antibody concentrations to serogroup C polysaccharide, specificity of antibody binding is determined by assaying replicate microtiter plates containing test sera diluted with diluting buffer containing soluble meningococcal C polysaccharide (final concentration, 25 μg/mL) as an inhibitor of antibody binding on one plate, and test sera diluted with serum-diluting buffer alone on the other plate. Absorbance values for wells containing dilutions of serum incubated with soluble meningococcal C polysaccharide are subtracted as background from the corresponding values for the wells in which sera are diluted with buffer alone (*18*). This procedure is no longer used for assaying IgG antibody concentrations (*see* above).

4. Assay validation. With a series of dilutions of high-titer serum samples, the results of the modified ELISA were linear within a range of 0.4–300 U/mL. There was no significant effect of varying incubation times or incubation temperatures ± 10% on the assigned antibody concentration. The coefficient of variation of the modified ELISA performed by different operators on different days was <10%.

Acknowledgments

We are indebted to the following individuals who provided important technical and intellectual contributions in the development of the modified ELISA: Howard Raff, George Santos, William Wacknov, R. Randall Deck, and Rose Sekulovich.

References

1. Granoff, D. M., Maslanka, S. E., Carlone, G. M., Plikaytis, B. D., Santos, G. F., Mokatrin, A., and Raff, H. V. (1998) A modified enzyme-linked immunosorbent assay for measurement of antibody responses to meningococcal C polysaccharide that correlate with bactericidal responses. *Clin. Diagn. Lab. Immunol.* **5,** 479–485.
2. Gheesling, L. L., Carlone, G. M., Pais, L. B., Holder, P. F., Maslanka, S. E., Plikaytis, B. D., et al. (1994) Multicenter comparison of *Neisseria meningitidis*

serogroup C anti-capsular polysaccharide antibody levels measured by a standardized enzyme-linked immunosorbent assay. *J. Clin. Microbiol.* **32,** 1475–1482.

3. Anderson, E. L., Bowers, T., Mink, C. M., Kennedy, D. J., Belshe, R. B., Harakeh, H., et al. (1994) Safety and immunogenicity of meningococcal A and C polysaccharide conjugate vaccine in adults. *Infect. Immun.* **62,** 3391–3395.

4. King, W. J., MacDonald, N. E., Wells, G., Huang, J., Allen, U., Chan, F., et al. (1996) Total and functional antibody response to a quadrivalent meningococcal polysaccharide vaccine among children. *J. Pediatr.* **128,** 196–202.

5. Leach, A., Twumasi, P. A., Kumah, S., Banya, W. S., Jaffar, S., Forrest, B. D., et al. (1997) Induction of immunologic memory in Gambian children by vaccination in infancy with a group A plus group C meningococcal polysaccharide-protein conjugate vaccine. *J. Infect. Dis.* **175,** 200–204.

6. Maslanka, S. E., Tappero, J. W., Plikaytis, B. D., Brumberg, R. S., Dykes, J. K., Gheesling, L. L., et al. (1998) Age-dependent *Neisseria meningitidis* serogroup C class-specific antibody concentrations and bactericidal titers in sera from young children from Montana immunized with a licensed polysaccharide vaccine. *Infect. Immun.* **66,** 2453–2459.

7. Campagne, G., Garba, A., Fabre, P., Schuchat, A., Ryall, B., Boulanger, D., Bybel, M., Carlone, G., Briantais, P., Ivanoff, B., Xerri, B., and Chippaux, J. P. (1997) Safety and immunogenicity of three doses of a *Neisseria meningitidis* A + C diphtheria conjugate vaccine in infants in Niger. *Pediatr. Infect. Dis. J.* **19,** 144–150.

8. Lieberman, J. M., Chiu, S. S., Wong, V. K., Partidge, S., Chang, S. J., Chiu, C. Y., et al. (1996) Safety and immunogenicity of a serogroups A/C *Neisseria meningitidis* oligosaccharide-protein conjugate vaccine in young children. A randomized controlled trial. *JAMA* **275,** 1499–1503.

9. Amir, J., Liang, X., and Granoff, D. M. (1990) Variability in the functional activity of vaccine-induced antibody to *Haemophilus influenzae* type b. *Pediatr. Res.* **27,** 358–364.

10. Lucas, A. H. and Granoff, D. M. (1995) Functional differences in idiotypically defined IgG1 anti-polysaccharide antibodies elicited by vaccination with Haemophilus influenzae type B polysaccharide-protein conjugates. *J. Immunol.* **154,** 4195–4202.

11. Schlesinger, Y. and Granoff, D. M. (1992) Avidity and bactericidal activity of antibody elicited by different *Haemophilus influenzae* type b conjugate vaccines. The Vaccine Study Group. *JAMA* **267,** 1489–1494.

12. Usinger, W. R. and Lucas, A. H. (1999) Avidity as a determinant of the protective efficacy of human antibodies to pneumococcal capsular polysaccharides. *Infect. Immun.* **67,** 2366–2370.

13. Macdonald, R. A., Hosking, C. S., and Jones, C. L. (1988) The measurement of relative antibody affinity by ELISA using thiocyanate elution. *J. Immunol. Methods* **106,** 191–194.

14. Holder, P. K., Maslanka, S. E., Pais, L. B., Dykes, J., Plikaytis, B. D., and Carlone, G. M. (1995) Assignment of *Neisseria meningitidis* serogroup A and C class-

specific anticapsular antibody concentrations to the new standard reference serum CDC1992. *Clin. Diagn. Lab. Immunol.* **2,** 132–137.

15. Bartoloni, A., Norelli, F., Ceccarini, C., Rappuoli, R., and Costantino, P. (1995) Immunogenicity of meningococcal B polysaccharide conjugated to tetanus toxoid or CRM197 via adipic acid dihydrazide. *Vaccine* **13,** 463–470.

16. Yao, K. and Ubuka, T. (1987) Determination of sialic acids by acidic ninhydrin reaction. *Acta Med. Okayama* **41,** 237–241.

17. Schneerson, R., Barrera, O., Sutton, A., and Robbins, J. B. (1980) Preparation, characterization, and immunogenicity of *Haemophilus influenzae* type b polysaccharide-protein conjugates. *J. Exp. Med.* **152,** 361–376.

18. Granoff, D. M., Kelsey, S. K., Bijlmer, H. A., Van Alphen, L., Dankert, J., Mandrell, R. E., et al. (1995) Antibody responses to the capsular polysaccharide of *Neisseria meningitidis* serogroup B in patients with meningococcal disease. *Clin. Diagn. Lab. Immunol.* **2,** 574–582.

22

Whole-Blood Model

Catherine A. Ison

1. Introduction

Neisseria meningitidis is an obligate human pathogen. When it interacts with the host, it can establish a commensal relationship or can, on a minority of occasions, invade and cause systemic disease. Protection against systemic disease, particularly for serogroup A and C infections, has been equated with the presence of bactericidal antibody directed against the capsular polysaccharide (CPS) *(1)*. In serogroup B infections, the CPS resembles host-cell moieties, is non-immunogenic, and does not induce protection *(2)*. Hence other components of the bacterial-cell envelope, such as outer-membrane proteins (OMPs), and cellular mechanisms of host defense, such as phagocytosis, have been implicated in immunity to serogroup B infections *(3,4)*.

Interaction between the host and bacteria have largely been studied using serum alone or isolated polymorphs. However, particularly in serogroup B infections, it is likely that both elements of the immune response are important and so this chapter describes the use of whole blood in an ex vivo model of meningococcal bacteraemia. Whole-blood assays have been used to measure the bactericidal power of blood in early studies *(5)* including against meningococci *(6,7)* and was used by Heist et al. in 1921 *(5)* to demonstrate differences between the ability of blood from healthy adults to kill meningococci. The whole-blood assay (WBA) assesses the complete bactericidal activity of blood and allows simultaneous analysis of bactericidal activity, neutrophil activation, cytokine production, and bacterial-antigen expression. The whole-blood model has shown enormous potential as an ex vivo model to examine a number of the parameters that are likely to be important in the cascade of events associated with systemic infection, which can lead to septic shock and death.

From: *Methods in Molecular Medicine, vol. 66: Meningococcal Vaccines: Methods and Protocols*
Edited by: A. J. Pollard and M. C. J. Maiden © Humana Press Inc., Totowa, NJ

1.2. Uses of the Whole-Blood Model

1.2.1. Development of the Whole-Blood Model

A number of parameters are important to consider in order to establish a reproducible and robust assay; volume of blood, container used, rotating speed, anticoagulant, and bacterial-growth conditions. It is imperative that the container for the blood, the volume used, and the rotation speed chosen allows mixing without activation of the neutrophils, as determined by the production of tumor necrosis factor (TNF) and expression of L-selectin and CD11b. The bactericidal effect of the blood will also be dependent on adequate mixing. The volume of blood used is dependent on the population being studied and can vary between 1–5 mL. The original assay used 3–5 mL of blood from an adult volunteer with a rotation speed of 9 rpm *(8)* but the current assay for use on blood from children uses 1.0 mL volume rotated at 20 rpm *(9)*. The reproducibility of the assay can be determined by testing 5×1.0 mL of blood from the same donor with the same meningococcal isolate on three occasions. The coefficient of variation can then be calculated and should be <25%.

In early studies the effect of anticoagulant, heparin, or citrate, on the bactericidal effect of blood was shown to vary among isolates *(8)*. Citrate chelates divalent cations and hence would be expected to interfere with complement and inflammatory-cell function, both of which would be expected to play a role in killing of meningococci. Consequently in all current studies heparinized blood is being used. The bactericidal activity of the blood will also be influenced by the bacterial-growth conditions prior to inoculation into the blood. Differences have been found between the ability of blood from a single donor to kill organisms prepared from solid or in liquid medium. This probably reflects differences in the heterogeneity of the populations and in the bacterial antigens expressed. This is supported by our finding that organisms grown on solid medium overnight express transferrin-binding proteins (Tbp) whereas those grown into log phase in liquid culture for 4 hr do not express Tbp.

1.2.2. Bactericidal Activity

The immune response of children to their infecting strain has been studied in convalescent children 8–12 wk after meningococcal disease. Children previously infected with meningococci expressing either serogroup B or serogroup C capsules invariably showed bactericidal activity against their infecting strain irrespective of the age of the child, indicating that children under 2 yr of age possess an immune response to their infecting strain *(9)*. In addition, blood from these children was also shown to have bactericidal activity against other meningococci, albeit at a lower level. These results suggest that children who have suffered systemic meningococcal disease can produce both a specific and cross-reactive immune response. Children who had not suffered from systemic meningococcal disease also showed bactericidal activity against a panel of serogroup B isolates and a serogroup C isolate. The level of activity was lower than in convalescent children and showed a tendency to increase with age *(9)*.

1.2.3. Comparison of WBA and SBA

The 'gold' standard for measuring bactericidal activity has been the serum bactericidal assay (SBA), which detects the presence of antibody to CPS *(10)*. A fourfold increase in the SBA titer has been shown to correlate with protection induced by serogroup A and C polysaccharide vaccines *(1)*. The SBA has also been used to assess the immune response to serogroup B vaccines *(11)*, but the correlation with efficacy has been poor, in that the presence of a raised titer was indicative of protection but the absence of a raised titre did not imply a lack of protection *(11,12)*. In our studies we have compared bactericidal activity in both convalescent and normal children detected by the SBA and the WBA. Although the methods are not directly comparable the WBA appears to detect bactericidal activity in more children than the SBA. This could be simply because the use of freshly taken whole blood with its own complement source is more sensitive than serum and an exogenous complement source as used in the SBA. Alternatively, it is possible that killing of serogroup B meningococci requires the presence of other constituents of the blood including phagocytic cells. It has also been suggested that the immune response to serogroup B infections involves other antigens in the cell envelope that may be more easily detected by whole blood rather than serum alone.

1.2.4. Relationship of Neutrophil Activation, Killing, and Phaogocytosis

Polymorphonuclear leukocytes (PMNL) are thought to play a role in bacterial clearance in meningococcal infection, which contributes to host defense. However, PMNL activation and accumulation contributes to vascular and tissue damage that is deleterious to the host. The whole-blood model allows simultaneous determination of bactericidal activity and neutrophil activation, and has shown that meningococci are potent activators of neutrophils in this model *(8,13)*. It has also been possible using a series of isogenic mutants of *N. meningitidis* B1940 to demonstrate the contribution of the bacterial capsule and sialylation of lipopolysaccharide (LPS) to killing and neutrophil activation. The parent strain, which was capsulated and the LPS was sialylated, showed reduced shedding of L-selectin but the greatest survival, whereas the unencapsulated, nonsialylated mutant showed greater shedding of L-selectin but the least survival *(13)*. However, the relationship between bacterial killing and neutrophil adhesion molecule expression is still uncertain (8,13). It is not clear whether bacterial death, with the resultant release of cell-wall products such as LPS, initiates neutrophil activation or whether activated neutrophils have a greater capacity for bacterial killing. In this model shedding of L-selectin and upregulation of CD11b occurs very early, within the first 15 min after inoculation, and is followed by PMNL association or internalization of meningococci. However, in the same studies, it was not possible to demonstrate a clear relationship between bacterial death and phagocytosis, although we did not examine PMNL-mediated bacterial killing directly (14).

1.2.5. Antigen Expression in WBA

Meningococcal antigens that have been implicated in disease have mostly been studied using organisms grown in vitro rather than in vivo during infection because of the lack of a suitable animal model. The WBA provides an alternative system where bacteria can grow in an environment similar to that it encounters in vivo. In combination with detection by flow cytometry, bacteria can be examined directly without the need for growth on culture media, which may alter expression. To explore this approach, a procedure has been developed to isolate bacteria after growth in whole blood that does not disturb recognition of known antigens by monoclonal antibodies (MAbs). The expression of PorA, PorB, capsule, LPS, and Tbps has been monitored over 3 h and while expression of PorA, PorB, and LPS remained constant, capsule and Tbps varied. The use of the WBA to monitor bacterial-antigen expression could give valuable information about antigens that are associated with resistance to bactericidal activity and changes in environmental conditions.

2. Materials
2.1. Preparation of the Inoculum

1. Meningococcal isolates (reference strains or clinical isolates).
2. 15% glycerol (Prod. No. 101184, Merck Ltd, Poole, Dorset, UK) in dextrose broth (Prod. No. 0063-175, Difco Laboratories, East Moseley, UK). Mix the glycerol with the dextrose broth, aliquot into appropriate volumes, and sterilize at 121°C for 15 min. Store at room temperature for 2–3 mo.
3. GC agar (36 g/L GC agar base, Prod. No. 0289-17-3, Difco Laboratories, supplemented with 1% IsoVitaleX, (Becton Dickinson UK Ltd., Oxford, UK) or Vitox, Oxoid Ltd, Basingstoke, UK). Dissolve the GC agar in water, sterilize at 121°C for 15 min, and allow to cool to 50°C. Add the IsoVitaleX immediately prior to pouring the medium into petri dishes. Prepared GC agar can be stored at 4°C for up to 1 wk but are best freshly prepared.
4. Oxidase reagent (1% NNN'N'-tetramethyl-p-phenylenediamine dihydrochloride, Prod. No. 30386, Merck) should be prepared immediately prior to use.

5. Gram stains (Crystal Violet, Prod.No. PL8000; Gram's Iodine, Prod. No. PL8001; 15% Neutral Red, Prod. No. 8002 in Dilute Carbol Fuchsin, Prod. No. PL8004, Prolab, South Wirral, UK).

6. RapIDNH Haemophilus and Neisseria panel (Prod. No. ID1-1001) and RapID Inoculation fluid (Prod. No. ID25-1-2, Prolab). Store according to manufacturer's instructions.

7. Serogroup and serotype specific MAbs (National Institute of Biological Standards and Control, Potters Bar, UK).

8. GC Broth consisting of 15 g/L proteose peptone, No.3, (Prod. No. 0122-01, Difco Laboratories), 4 g/L dipotassium hydrogen phosphate (Prod. No. 10436, Merck), 1 g/L potassium dihydrogen phosphate (Prod. No. 10203, Merck), 5 g/L sodium chloride (Prod. No. 10241, Merck) supplement with 1% IsoVitaleX or Vitox.

9. RPMI-1640 (Prod. No. 32404, Life Technologies, Paisley, Scotland). Store at 4°C until required and prewarm before use by incubation at 37°C.

2.2. Collection of Blood

1. Heparin, use 10 U/mL of blood.
2. Sterilin 30 mL Universal container (Prod. No. 128B, Merck).
3. Sterilin 7 mL Bijoux container (Prod. No. 129B, Merck).

2.3. WBA Procedure

1. Heparinized blood.
2. Log phase-grown meningococci.
3. Platform shaker STR6 (Stuart Scientific).

2.4. Bactericidal Activity

1. Microtiter tray (Micro-Plate Cellstar, Greiner).
2. Multichannel pipet (8-channel, Anachem, Beds, UK).
3. RPMI-1640 (Life Technologies).
4. GC agar.

2.5. Determination of TNF-α Levels

1. MicroTest III™ Flexible assay plate (Falcon 3912, Becton Dickinson).
2. 0.1 M Bicarbonate buffer pH 9.6.
3. Bovine serum albumin (BSA) Factor V (Prod. No. A9647, Sigma).
4. 0.01 M Phosphate-buffered saline (PBS; Oxoid).
5. Tween 20 (Prod. No. 66368, Merck).
6. Mouse anti-human TNF-α (Pharmigen Prod. No. 18631D, Becton Dickinson UK Ltd.).
7. Recombinant human TNF-α (Pharmigen Prod. No. 19761T).
8. Biotinylated mouse anti-human TNF-α (Pharmigen Prod. No. 18642D).
9. Streptavidin-peroxidase (Prod. No. S-5512, Sigma).
10. Substrate: 0.4 mg/L ortho-phenyl-diamine (Prod. No. P-7288, Sigma), in 0.1 M

citric acid buffer, pH 5.0. For every 50 mL of substrate, add 20 µL fresh 30% hydrogen peroxide.
11. 2 *M* sulphuric acid (Prod. No. 10276, Merck).

2.6. Neutrophil Activation

1. Mouse anti-human CD11b conjugated to FITC (Prod. No. MCA551F, Serotec, Oxford, UK).
2. Mouse anti-human L-selectin, CD26L:RPE, conjugated to phycoerythrin (Prod. No. MCA1076PE, Serotec).
3. 5 mL polystyrene round bottom tube (Falcon 2054, Becton Dickinson UK, Ltd).
4. FACSLYSE (FACS™ Lysing solution, Prod. No 349202, Becton-Dickinson UK Ltd).
5. 0.01 *M* PBS (Prod. No. BR/4a, Oxoid).
6. FACSFIX (2% [w/v] formaldehyde + 2% [w/v] glucose).

2.7. Phagocytosis of Bacteria

2.7.1. Preparation of FITC-Labeled Bacteria

1. Meningococci (reference strains or clinical siolates).
2. Fluoroscein isothiocyanate (FITC, Prod. No. F-7250, Sigma).
3. 0.01 *M* PBS (Oxoid).
4. Sterilin 30-mL Universal container.
5. Parafilm.

2.7.2. Phagocytosis Assay

1. Anticoagulated (heparinized) blood.
2. FITC-labeled meningococci.
3. FACSLYSE. (*see* **item 4, Subheading 2.6.**)
4. 0.01 *M* PBS.
5. FACSFIX.
6. Flow cytometer (e.g., FACS Calibur, Becton Dickinson UK Ltd.).
7. Trypan blue (0.4% solution, Prod. No. T-8154, Sigma).

2.8. Bacterial Antigen Expression

2.8.1. Retrieval of Bacteria by a Nonculture Method

1. 30 mL Universal container.
2. Lysis solution: 1% saponin [w/v] in 1 m*M* PBS.
3. 20 m*M* PBS.
4. 10 m*M* PBS.

2.8.2. Indirect Immunofluorescent Labeling of Surface-Exposed Antigens

1. MAbs (as appropriate; *see* **Subheading 3.8.2.**).
2. 0.01 *M* PBS (Sigma).

3. Anti-mouse immunoglobulin conjugated to FITC (Prod. No. F0261, Dako, Denmark).
4. FACSFIX.

2.8.3. Analysis by Flow Cytometry

1. Propidium iodide (Prod. No. P4170, Sigma).
2. Flow cytometer
3. Cell Quest analysis and acquisition software.

3. Methods
3.1. Preparation of the Inoculum

1. The inoculum used routinely in this assay is meningococci grown into log-phase on either solid or in liquid medium.
2. Store strains of meningococci to be used in the assay either in the vapor phase of liquid nitrogen in 15% glycerol broth or freeze-dried. If a meningococcal strain is to be used in repeated experiments grow the organism, check for purity and store in multiple vials at one time to serve as a stock. Retrieve strains freshly each week from the stock and subculture a maximum of five times (*see* **Note 1**).
3. Retrieve the strains by growth on GC agar and incubate at 36°C in 5–7% carbon dioxide for 24 h. Subculture each strain at least once onto fresh GC agar before use in the assay, and incubate at 36°C in 5–7% carbon dioxide for 18 h.
4. Check the organisms for purity by performing the oxidase test and Gram stain to indicate the presence of *Neisseria* spp., which are oxidase-positive Gram-negative cocci. If the strain has not been fully identified previously, determine the identity by biochemical reactions using a kit such as RapidNH.
5. Check the serogroup of the strains prior to use in each assay by mixing a suspension of the meningococci with serogroup-specific antisera on a glass slide.
6. At regular intervals, check the serotype and serosubtype of the strains using specific MAbs in a dot-blot immunoassay, to detect mixing of strains during subculture.
7. Prepare log-phase meningococci using solid media by inoculating a small amount of growth from an overnight culture onto a fresh GC-agar plate and incubate at 36°C with 5–7% CO_2 in >90% humidity for 4 h.
8. Alternatively, prepare log-phase organisms in liquid medium. Prepare a suspension of each meningococcus from growth on an overnight culture on GC agar, and inoculate into GC broth to a final concentration of 5×10^6 cfu/mL. Incubate the broth at 36°C and shake at 280 rpm for 3.5 h.
9. Prior to use in the assay, harvest the mid-log phase from solid or liquid medium and prepare a suspension in RPMI-1640 medium at a concentration of approx 10^8 cfu/mL ($OD_{540nm} = 1.0$).

3.2. Collection of Blood

1. Collect whole venous blood without stasis and anticoagulate with heparin at 10 U/mL.

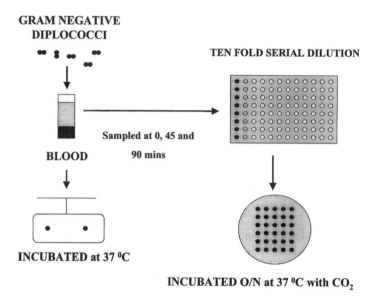

Fig. 1. Whole-blood assay.

2. Take sufficient blood for 1 mL per meningococcus to be tested and 1 mL as an uninoculated control for activation studies.
3. Place blood into a plastic universal container and mix gently to prevent clotting.
4. Aliquot the blood into 1 mL volumes in 7 mL plastic bijoux containers.

3.3. WBA Procedure

1. For each meningococcus to be tested inoculate 10 µL of a suspension of 10^8 cfu/mL into 1 mL of anticoagulated blood (final concentration 10^6 cfu/mL).
2. Gently mix the bacteria and blood and remove samples for bactericidal activity and neutrophil activation prior to incubation.
3. Place each blood sample on a rocking table at 20 rpm at 37°C.
4. Remove samples at intervals, as desired, over a period of 1.5 h for bactericidal activity and neutrophil activation.
5. Incubate the blood for a total of 3 h and then separate plasma for TNF levels (*see* **Subheading 3.5.**)

3.4. Bactericidal Activity

1. Remove samples in duplicate from each 1 mL of blood and perform a viable count to determine the bactericidal activity of the blood (**Fig. 1**).
2. Prepare a microtiter tray with 2 sets of 4 wells containing 90 µL of RPMI-1640 per strain.
3. Place 10 µL of blood into the first of the wells in each set.

4. Using a multi-channel pipet and a fresh tip, mix the blood and RPMI in the first well and transfer 10 µL to the second well and discard the tip to prevent any carry over of blood.

5. Using a fresh tip, repeat for wells 2–4. This will dilute the blood in 10-fold dilutions from 10^{-1} to 10^{-4}.

6. Transfer 5×10 µL from each dilution onto one fresh GC-agar plate per dilution.

7. Allow drops to dry into the agar and then incubate at 36°C in 5–7% carbon dioxide for 24 h (*see* **Note 2**).

8. After incubation, count the colonies on each of the five drops at the dilution giving between 10–30 colonies.

9. Express the viable count as cfu/mL (i.e., number of colonies counted $\times 20 \times$ dilution).

3.5. Determination of TNF-α Levels

1. After 3 h incubation, centrifuge the tubes containing blood and meningococci at 3000g for 15 min.

2. Transfer plasma to a fresh cryotube and store at –80°C until required for analysis.

3. Thaw plasma and use in the Pharmingen cytokine ELISA system to detect TNF released by cells during incubation with meningococci. All reagents are supplied by Pharmingen, unless otherwise stated.

4. Coat microtiter plates with 50 µL of anti-TNF antibody, (2 µg/mL), in 0.1 M bicarbonate buffer, pH9.6. Incubate for 6 h at room temperature.

5. Wash twice with PBS +0.05% Tween 20 (PBS-Tween).

6. Block the tray by adding 200 µL/per well of 3% BSA in PBS and incubate overnight at +4°C.

7. Wash twice with PBS-Tween.

8. Dilute test samples and standards (50–2000 pg/mL) in PBS + 3% BSA.

9. Add 100 µL of the test samples and standards to the microtiter tray in duplicate wells and incubate at room temperature for 4 h.

10. Wash 4 times with PBS-Tween.

11. Add 100 µL of biotinylated anti-TNF antibody, (1 µg/mL in 3% BSA in PBS) to each well and incubate for 45 min at room temperature.

12. Wash 6 times with PBS-Tween.

13. Add 100 µL of avidin-peroxidase 1:2000 diluted in 3% BSA in PBS, to each well and incubate in the dark for 1 h at room temperature.

14. Wash 8 times with PBS-Tween.

15. Add substrate to each well, incubate in the dark for 15–20 min and then stop reaction with 100 µL of 2 M H$_2$SO$_4$.

16. Read absorbence at 490 nm.

3.6. Neutrophil Activation

1. Double immunostain neutrophils for L-selectin and CD11b. Place 5 µL of both mouse anti-human CD11b conjugated to FITC and mouse anti-human L-selectin,

CD26L : RPE, conjugated to phycoerythrin in a 5 mL polystyrene round-bottom tube.

2. Remove 50 µL from the WBA, add to the antibodies, and incubate at room temperature for 10 min.
3. Lyse the red cells by the addition of 2 mL of FACSLYSE diluted 1:10 in distilled water (Becton Dickinson) and allow to stand for a further 10 min.
4. Pellet the cells by centrifugation at 1500*g* for 10 min.
5. Wash the pellet by the addition of PBS, repeat centrifugation, and then resuspend in 100 µL of filter-sterilized PBS.
6. Fix the cells by adding 100 µL of x2 FACSFIX (2% [w/v] formaldehyde + 2% [w/v] glucose) and store at +4°C for analysis by flow cytometry.

3.7. Phagocytosis of Bacteria

3.7.1. Preparation of FITC-Labeled Bacteria

1. Prepare a solution of 1 mg/mL of FITC in PBS and allow to stand at room temperature for 10–15 min (*see* **Note 3**).
2. Filter the solution through a 0.45-µm membrane filter to remove any particulate matter and FITC that has not completely dissolved.
3. Prepare a heavy suspension of meningococci in 1 mL of PBS in a 20-mL universal and then add an equal volume of the FITC solution.
4. Seal the tubes with parafilm and rotate at 20 rpm in 37°C incubator for 30 min.
5. Wash the bacteria twice by the addition of PBS followed by centrifugation at 2500*g*.
6. Finally, resuspend the pellet of FITC-labeled bacteria in 1 mL of PBS and adjust the resulting suspension to OD_{540nm} to 1.0 (approx 10^8 cfu/mL).

3.7.2. Phagocytosis Assay

1. Add 10 µL of OD = 1.0 FITC-labeled bacteria to 1 mL of anticoagulated blood and perform the assay as described in **Subheading 3.3.**
2. Monitor the uptake of bacteria by neutrophils by removing 50 µL samples of blood at 0, 30, and 60 min and lyse the red cells by adding 2 mL of FACSLYSE solution (diluted 1:10 in distilled water) and allow to stand at room temperature for 10 min.
3. Pellet the cells by centrifugation at 1500*g* for 10 min and wash twice in PBS.
4. Resuspend the cells in 100 µL of PBS, fix by the addition of 100 µL of FACSFIX, and store at 4°C until analyzed by flow cytometry (*see* **Note 4**).

3.8. Bacterial-Antigen Expression

3.8.1. Retrieval of Bacteria by a Nonculture Method

1. Perform the WBA as described in **Subheading 3.3.**
2. To retrieve bacteria from the assay, transfer each 1-mL volume of blood and meningococci to a 30 mL universal, add 9 mL of lysis solution (1% saponin [w/v] in 1 m*M* PBS) and allow to stand at room temperature for 5 min.

3. Stop the lysis by the addition of 10 mL of neutralizing solution (20 m*M* PBS) and centrifuge gently at 3000*g* for 10 min.
4. Resuspend the resulting pellet in 1 mL of 10 m*M* PBS, transfer to a microfuge tube, and centrifuge for 30 sec to pellet host-cell debris.
5. Remove the supernatant, place in a fresh tube, and centrifuge at 13,000*g* for 5 min to pellet the cells.
6. Finally wash the bacterial cells by the addition of 1 mL of filter-sterilized 10 m*M* PBS, collect by centrifugation, and resuspend in 210 μL of 10 m*M* PBS.
7. The number of viable bacteria recovered is determined by performing a viable colony count. The results are expressed as CFU/mL as the percentage of meningococci recovered determined using the following formula:

$$\frac{\text{Number of bacteria post isolation (CFU/mL) at each time point}}{\text{Number of bacteria present pre isolation (CFU/mL) at each time point}} \times 100$$

3.8.2. Indirect Immunofluorescent Labeling of Surface-Exposed Antigens

1. Centrifuge the resultant bacterial suspension at 13,000*g* for 5 min to pellet the cells, and resuspend in 100 μL of the MAb of choice at the appropriate dilution.
2. Incubate the bacteria: antibody mixture at 37°C for 30 min (*see* **Note 5**).
3. Retrieve the bacteria by centrifugation at 13,000*g* for 5 min, wash the pellet as described earlier, and incubate with 100 μL of diluted (1 : 50 in PBS) anti-mouse immunoglobulin conjugated to FITC at 37°C for a further 30 min.
4. Retrieve the cells again by centrifugation, wash and fix in 1% formaldehyde/ glucose solution, and hold at +4°C in the dark for analysis using flow cytometry (*see* **Notes 6, 7,** and **8**).

3.8.3. Analysis by Flow Cytometry

1. Add propidium iodide (PI), a nucleic acid stain, at a final concentration of 20 ng prior to acquisition.
2. To discriminate bacteria from other particles in the suspension use combined measurements of forward angle scatter (FSC) and side-angle scatter (SSC) and staining with PI, detected on an FL3 channel. Analyze organisms that satisfy these parameters and gate based on FSC, SSC, and PI staining. A total of 10,000 events (cells) are acquired and the amount of FITC present on the surface of each cell is registered on the FL1 channel using a logarithmic scale (*see* **Note 9**).
3. Express the results as frequency histograms with the relative median intensity fluorescence on the x-axis and events (number of cells) on the y-axis.

4. Notes

1. Probing of organisms grown into mid-log-phase in liquid or on solid medium with MAbs to PorA, Por B, and capsule demonstrated no difference in expression

of these antigens between the growth medium or during two to five subcultures (*see* **Subheading 3.1.**).

2. For reproducible results, prepare the culture medium used for determining the viable count freshly and dry in closed petri dishes overnight at 37°C in an incubator (*see* **Subheading 3.4.**).
3. Always use PBS and not water to prepare FITC solution (*see* **Subheading 3.7.1.**).
4. Add trypan blue to a final concentration of 2 µg/mL before analysis to quench fluorescence from bacteria attached to the surface of the cells (*see* **Subheading 3.7.2.**).
5. Nonspecific binding of the conjugate to the surface of the bacteria, which may give rise to a false-positive result, is determined by incubating the bacteria with the conjugate in the absence of the MAb (*see* **Subheading 3.8.2.**).
6. Unlabeled bacteria are also analyzed in order to determine levels of autofluorescence (*see* **Subheading 3.8.2.**).
7. Filter all solutions used in flow cytometry experiments through 0.2-µM filters (*see* **Subheading 3.8.2.**).
8. Antibodies that detect epitopes on surface exposed antigens are usually suitable for use with this technique (*see* **Subheading 3.8.2.**).
9. The analysis in this laboratory was performed on a FACS Calibur using the Cell Quest analysis and acquisition software (*see* **Subheading 3.8.3.**).

Acknowledgments

The work described in this chapter was supported by the Meningitis Research Foundation. I am grateful to Natasha Anwar for unpublished data and to Nigel Klein and Robert Heyderman for their support during collaborative studies.

References

1. Gotschlich, E. C., Goldschneider, I., and Artenstein, M. S. (1969) Human immunity to the meningococcus. IV. Immunogenicity of group A and group C meningococcal polysaccharides in human volunteers. *J. Exp. Med.* **129,** 1367–1384.
2. Wyle, F. A., Artenstein, M. S., Brandt, B. L., et al. (1972) Immunologic response of man to serogroup B meningococcal polysaccharide vaccines. *J. Infect. Dis.* **126,** 514–522.
3. Ross, S., Crosenthal, P. J., Berberich, H. M., and Densen, P. (1987) Killing of *Neisseria meningitidis* by human neutrophils: implications for normal and complement-deficient individuals. *J. Infect. Dis.* **155,** 1266–1275.
4. Estabrook, M. M., Christopher, N. C., Grifiss, J. M., Baker, C. J., and Mandrell, R. E. (1992) Sialylation and human neutrophil killing of group C *Neisseria meningitidis. J. Infect. Dis.* **166,** 1079–1088.
5. Heist, G. D., Solis-Cohen, S., and Solis-Cohen, M. (1922) A study of the virluence of meningococci for man and of human susceptibility to meningococcic infection. *J. Immunol.* **7,** 1–33.

6. Matsunami, T. and Kolmer, J. (1918) The relation of the meningococcidal activity of the blood to resistance to virulent meningococci. *J. Immunol.* **3,** 201–212.
7. Matsunami, T. and Kolmer, J. (1920) Studies on the meningococcidal activity of blood. *J. Immunol.* **5,** 51.
8. Ison, C. A., Heyderman, R. S., Klein, N. L., Peakman, M., and Levin, M. (1995) Whole blood model of meningococcal bacteraemia: a method for exploring host-bacterial interactions. *Microb. Pathog.* **18,** 97–107.
9. Ison, C. A., Anwar, N., Cole, M. J., Galassini, R., Heyderman, R. S., Klein, N. J., et al. and the Meningococcal Research Group (1999) Assessment of immune response to meningococcal disease: comparison of a whole-blood assay and the serum bactericidal assay. *Microb. Pathog.* **27,** 207–214.
10. Goldschneider, I., Gotschlich, E. C., and Artenstein, M. S. (1969) Human immunity to the meningococcus. I. The role of humoral antibodies. *J. Exp. Med.* **129,** 1307–1326.
11. Hoiby, E. A., Rosenqvist, E., Froholm, L. O., et al. (1991) Bactericidal antibodies after vaccination with the Norwegian meningococcal serogroup B outer membrane vesicle vaccine: a brief survey. *NIPH Ann.* **14,** 147–155.
12. Perkins, B. A., Jonsdottir, K., Briem, H., et al. (1998) Immunogenicity of two efficacious outer membrane protein-based serogroup B meningococcal vaccines among young adults in Iceland. *J. Infect. Dis.* **177,** 683–691.
13. Klein, N. J., Ison, C. A., Peakman, M., Levin, M., Hammerschmidt, S., Frosch, M., and Heyderman, R. S. (1996) The influence of capsulation and lipooligosaccharide structure on neutrophil adhesion molecule expression and endothelial injury by *Neisseria meningitidis. J. Infect. Dis.* **173,** 172–179.
14. Heyderman, R. S., Ison, C. A., Peakman, M., Levin, M., and Klein, N. J. (1999) Neutrophil response to *Neisseria meningitidis*: inhibition of adhesion molecule expression and phagocytosis by recombinant bactericidial/permeability-increasing protein (rBPI21). *J. Infect. Dis.* **179,** 1288–1292.

23

Antibody-Induced Opsonophagocytosis of Serogroup B Meningococci Measured by Flow Cytometry

Terje E. Michaelsen and Audun Aase

1. Introduction

Antibodies can protect against meningococcal infection by at least two mechanisms: complement-dependent serum bactericidal activity (SBA), and/or opsonophagocytosis (OP), leading to destruction of the bacteria *(1–4)*. Regarding group C meningococci, there seems to be a correlation between SBA activity and protection *(1)*, whereas OP has been less well-studied. This function may have a supplementary or even major role in protection against group B meningococci.

The traditional way of measuring opsonophagocytosis is fluorescence microscopy and visual inspection for fluorescent bacteria within the phagocytes. This method is rather laborious and not suitable for analyzing large serum samples. Two other procedures have been reported for opsonophagocytic measurements of antibodies against serogroup B meningococci, namely chemiluminescence *(5)* and flow cytometry *(2,4,6)*. The effector cells used in these experiments have most often been human peripheral-blood polymorphonuclear cells (PMNs), or monocytes *(4)*. As complement source, homologous complement *(2)* or external human serum without antibodies against meningococci *(4,6)* have been used. Using homologous complement, the sera must be analyzed at high concentration to avoid diluting out the complement. The target for measuring OP has either been ethanol-treated meningococci *(1,4)*, viable meningococci *(6)*, or latex particles coated with purified outer-membrane proteins (OMPs) *(7)*.

From: *Methods in Molecular Medicine, vol. 66: Meningococcal Vaccines: Methods and Protocols*
Edited by: A. J. Pollard and M. C. J. Maiden © Humana Press Inc., Totowa, NJ

We describe here a respiratory burst (RB) assay using effector cells from donors heterozygous for the FcγRIIa allels *(8)* for measuring the opsonophagocytic activity against group B meningococci. RB is a late event of the phagocytic process *(9)*, and is probably more related to meningococcal killing than internalization *(10)*. We use live meningococci as target, human PMNs as effector cells, and external human serum as a complement source. The RB activity is detected by flow cytometry and the results are recorded as the highest dilution of antibody preparations or serum giving a positive RB of the PMNs.

1.1. Flow Cytometry Assay for OP Activity

1.2.1. Principle

Antibody-induced phagocytosis of PMNs is followed by excessive oxygen consumption by the effector cells, known as the RB. This reaction can be detected using the cell-permeant probe, dihydrorhodamine 123 (DHR), that is converted to the fluorescent rhodamine 123 during the RB.

Test sera are mixed with meningococci and incubated to allow binding of specific antibodies to the bacteria (*see* **Note 1**). Next, a fixed amount of external human serum as complement source is added. Finally, DHR primed leukocytes are added to the mixture. If the test serum contains antibodies against meningococci, the complement cascade might be activated, leading to deposition of complement activation products on the meningococci. The effector cells might be triggered to phagocytize the opsonized meningococci both through Fcγ- and complement receptors. This dual triggering causes a synergistic response of the PMNs that are readily detected as fluorescence by the flow cytometer.

The meningococci may be either viable or ethanol-killed; however, we favor the use of viable log phase-grown bacteria, as these are most likely to resemble the meningococci present during invasive disease.

2. Materials

1. Heparin vacutainer (Becton Dickinson, Rutherford, NJ).
2. 96-well U-shaped microplates with sealing tape.
3. Dimethylsulfoxide (DMSO) (Sigma-Aldrich).
4. Dihydrorhodamine 123 (DHR) (Molecular Probe, Eugene, OR): 10 mg is dissolved in 1 mL DMSO, divided into small volumes and stored at −70°C.
5. Bovine serum albumin (BSA), without preservative.
6. Hanks' Balanced Salt Medium (HBSS) (Cat. no. 14025-043, Gibco BRL).
7. HBSS supplemented with 2 mg/mL BSA (HBSS-BSA).
8. Complement serum collected from a person without (or low) antibodies against meningococci, and stored to preserve the complement activity.

9. Erythrocyte-lysing solution, 10X concentrated: 8.29 g NH_4Cl, 1.0 g $KHCO_3$. 80.0 mg $EDTA-Na_2$, and distilled water to 100 mL.
10. Brain-heart infusion (BHI) agar plates.
11. Control sera: one serum with high and one with low RB activity.
12. Flow cytometer, e.g., EPICS XL (Coulter, Hialeah, FL).
13. Protein G-Sepharose (Amersham-Pharmacia biotech, Uppsala, Sweden).

3. Method

Extreme precaution must be taken when handling live meningococci. Follow the local guidelines for working with contagious, hazardous organisms. Always when possible, work in a safety hood, and use protective clothes, gloves, and mouth shields. The area around the flow cytometer must be carefully disinfected to avoid exposing other users at risk of contamination.

1. Grow the meningococci overnight on a BHI agar plate at 35°C in 5% CO_2. The next day, spread the meningococci on a new BHI agar plate and grow them for 4 h at 35°C in 5% CO_2.
2. Harvest the meningococci, wash by centrifugation ($2000g$ for 5 min.) twice with HBSS-BSA and adjust the concentration to approx 1×10^9/mL in HBSS-BSA (*see* **Notes 2–4**).
3. Inactivate the test sera and control sera by incubation at 56°C for 30 min (*see* **Note 5**).
4. Prepare a twofold dilution of the sera in HBSS-BSA on a microplate starting at 1:4 by adding 60 µL serum + 180 µL HBSS-BSA in the first well and 120 µL HBSS-BSA in wells 2–7. Use a multichannel-pipet to titrate by transferring 120 µL from one well to the other and mixing the solution by sucking 5 times up and down the pipet at each step.
5. Transfer 50 µL to two duplicate wells on a new microplate. If more than one microplate are needed, the control sera should be included at each microplate.
6. Controls: all sera should be tested at the highest concentration to check for the induction of RB in absence of meningococci (*see* **Note 6**). Also, a negative control must be included by substituting serum with HBSS-BSA.
7. Add 5 µL meningococci (1×10^9/mL in HBSS-BSA) to each well. Seal the microplate with tape and incubate for 30 min at 37°C by using a microplate shaker.
8. As complement source, add 5 µL of a serum without detectable antibodies against group B meningococci (*see* **Note 7**) and continue incubation for 10 min at 37°C by using a microplate shaker (*see* **Note 8**). (If it is difficult to obtain serum without antibodies against meningococci, such antibodies can be removed by passing the complement serum through a small column of Protein G-Sepharose at 4°C.)
9. The effector cells are prepared while the bacteria and serum are incubated. Collect 20 mL of heparin blood from a healthy volunteer by venesection. Prepare the

lysing solution by mixing 20 mL of the 10X concentrated lysing solution with 180 mL destilled water. Add the 20 mL heparinized blood to the 200 mL lysis solution and incubate at room temperature until the erythrocytes are lysed (3–5 min). Wash the cells two times with HBSS-BSA by centrifugation at 300g for 5 min. The cells are then counted in a Bürkerchamber and adjusted to 1×10^7/mL in HBSS-BSA (*see* **Notes 9, 10**).

10. About 3 min before the cells are to be used, add DHR to the effector cells (5 µL to 5 mL effector-cell suspension). Add 50 µL of the primed effector-cell suspension to each well and continue incubation by shaking for 10 min at 37°C (effector :target ratio ≈ 1:20) (*see* **Note 11**).

11. Place the plate on ice until ready for flow cytometric analysis (within 2 h) (*see* **Note 12**).

12. Prepare the samples for analysis by pipetting the sample from the microplate well into a sample tube containing 0.4 mL HBSS-BSA and pass it through the flow cytometer (*see* **Note 13**).

4. Notes

1. The method we describe here may easily be adjusted to analyze other samples than human sera. We have used it to study the opsonophagocytic activity of mouse monoclonal antibodies (MAbs), either as ascites fluid or as purified MAbs.

2. The concentration of the bacteria after harvesting can be coarsely determined by measuring the OD at 620 nm as you get a good estimate assuming that a concentration of 4×10^8 bacteria/mL gives an OD ≈ 1.

3. We prefer to measure the OP activity using viable meningococci as target cells as we have recently discovered that some antigens differ in surface expression between viable and dead bacteria. This is observed for the PorB (at least for the serotypes 4 and 15) (*6,11*), but also for the Rmp protein (*12*). These vaccine components elicit strong antibody responses, but these antibodies do not bind to viable bacteria. When comparing SBA activity and OP measured by flow cytometry, a discrepancy can occur on rare occasions if some epitopes are present in less than 50% of the meningococci. Antibodies against these epitopes will not give a significant SBA activity. In the OP assay, on the other hand, such antibodies will react with enough meningococci (there are 20 times more meningococci than PMNs during the test) to induce OP.

4. To minimize the hazard of working with potentially infectious organisms, the log-grown meningococci may be harvested in HBSS, pelletted by centrifugation (2000g for 5 min), and resuspended in 70% ethanol. After 1 h, the bacteria are centrifuged, washed in HBSS-BSA, and the concentration adjusted to 1×10^9/mL. These may be divided into samples and stored at –70°C.

5. We prefer to inactivate the sera and then add external complement to all samples. However, the amount of complement to be added will depend on the complement

source, and also on the meningococcal strain. Some strains spontaneously activate the complement system and may thus not be suitable as target for OP measurements as described here.

6. Other stimuli than antibody and complement may also trigger a RB. It is therefore necessary to test whether the sera alone (without meningococci) display any RB activity. For human sera this is seldom a problem if they have been properly collected and stored. However, repeated freezing and thawing, or prolonged storage at higher temperature may cause aggregation or microbial contamination that might induce RB.

7. The complement sera were divided into 200–500 µL volumes and stored at –70°C until use.

8. The various incubation periods may be slightly adjusted, but it is of great importance that all samples to be compared are analyzed under identical test conditions.

9. For a 96-well microplate 10 mL heparin blood is required.

10. There is some variation of FcγR expression on the PMNs among the effector-cell donors that may influence the results obtained. In particular, the allels of FcγRIIa have different affinity for different IgG subclasses *(8)*. One should therefore strive to use donors displaying identical FcγR allotypes throughout the experiment.

11. We have compared the RB activity with the internalization of FITC-labeled meningococci and we have always obtained virtually identical results (unpublished observations). As a probe for RB we use DHR, which is reported to be the most appropriate indicator for flowcytometric detection of RB in neutrophils *(10)*. One advantage of measuring RB is that we can use unmodified viable (or dead) target cells, thereby avoiding coupling fluorochrome to its membrane, which may disturb other membrane structures and possibly interfere with antibody binding.

12. The cell preparations obtained after the end of the phagocytic process can be fixed by adding paraformaldehyde to each well, giving a final concentration of 0.5%. By this means, the test samples can be stored over night before they are analyzed.

13. The configuration of the flow cytometer can be done in several ways. We prefer to use a two-parameter histogram showing the forward- and side-light scatter to discriminate the different leukocyte populations. Using this setup, an analytical gate can be drawn around the PMN population, excluding interference from monocytes or lymphocytes (**Fig. 1A**). The events within this gate are displayed in a single parameter histogram as log fluorescence on the x-axis. Running the negative sample, adjust the voltage on the fluorescence multiplier tube (FL1) so that the negative cells cover the first decade on the x-axis. An analytical region is drawn to exclude the negative population, thus covering the second, third, and fourth decade. Positive samples will cause the PMNs to emit fluorescence light within this region (**Fig. 1B**). The results can be presented as the percent positive

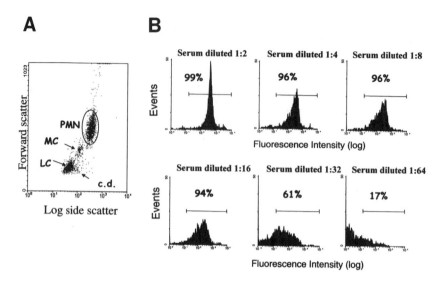

Fig. 1. **(A)** Light-scatter histogram showing the different cell populations of peripheral human blood after red cells have been removed by erythrolysis. (LC, lymphocytes; MC, monocytes; PMN, polymorphonuclear leukocytes; c.d., cell debris.) An analytical gate is set on the PMNs to analyze for fluorescence within this cell population. **(B)** The fluorescence from the PMNs after triggering a respiratory burst (RB) induced by a vaccinee serum. The activity of the serum with specific antibodies against meningococci was measured using serial twofold dilutions. The highest dilution giving a significant RB within the PMNs (e.g., >50%) may be recorded as the titer (=32 in this serum sample).

PMNs at each dilution tested. A titer can then be recorded as the highest dilution giving a positive response above a defined percentage. Alternatively, an analytical region can be set to cover the entire x-axis, and the results given as the median fluorescence intensity recorded at the different serum dilutions.

References

1. Goldscneider, I., Gotschlich, E. C., and Artenstein, M.S. (1969) Human immunity to the meningococcus. I. The role of humoral antibodies. *J. Exp. Med.* **129,** 1307–1326.
2. Halstensen, A., Haneberg, B., Frøholm, L. O., Lehmann, V., Frasch, C. E., and Solberg, C. O. (1984) Human opsonins to meningococci after vaccination. *Infect. Immun.* **46,** 673–676.
3. Ross, S., Rosenthal, P. J., Berberich, H. M., and Densen, P. (1987) Killing of *Neisseria meningitidis* by human neutrophils: implications for normal and complement deficient individuals. *J. Infect. Dis.* **155,** 1266–1275.

4. Aase, A., Bjune, G., Høiby, E. A., Rosenqvist, E., Pedersen, A. K., and Michaelsen, T. E. (1995) Comparison among opsonic activity, antimeningococcal immunoglobulin G response and serum bactericidal activity against meningococci in sera from vaccinees after immunization with a serogroup B outer membrane vesicle vaccine. *Infect. Immun.* **63,** 3531–3536.

5. Sjursen, H., Lehmann. V., Naess A., Hervig, T., Flo, R. W., Maehle, B., et al. (1992) Monocyte phagocytosis of opsonized Neisseria meningitidis serogroup B. *APMIS* **100,** 209–220.

6. Aase, A., Høiby, E. A., and Michaelsen, T. E. (1998) Opsonophagocytic and bactericidal activity mediated by purified IgG subclass antibodies after vaccination with the Norwegian group B menigococcal vaccine. *Scand. J. Immunol.* **47,** 388–396.

7. Lehmann, A. K., Halstensen, A., Aaberge, I. S., Holst, J., Michaelsen, T. E., Sørensen, S., et al. (1999) Human opsonins induced during meningococcal disease recognize PorA and PorB outer membrane proteins. *Infect. Immun.* **67,** 2552–2560.

8. Bredius, R. G., Fijen, C. A., De Haas, M., Kuijper, E. J., Weening, R. S., Van de Winkel, J. G., and Out, T. A. (1994) Role of neutrophil FcγRIIa (CD32) and FcγRIIIb (CD16) polymorphic forms in phagocytosis of human IgG1- and IgG3-opsonized bacteria and erythrocytes. *Immunology* **83,** 624–630.

9. Baggiolini, M. and Wymann, M. P. (1990) Turning on the respiratory burst. *TIBS.* **15,** 69–72.

10. Vowells, S. J., Sekhsaria, S., Malech, H. L., Shalit, M., and Fleisher, T. A. (1995) Flow cytometric analysis of the granulocyte respiratory burst: a comparison study of fluorescent probes. *J. Immunol. Methods* **178,** 89–97.

11. Michaelsen, T. E., Aase, A., Kolberg, J., Wedege, E., and Rosenqvist, E., (2001) PorB3 outer membrane protein on *Neisseria meningitidis* is poorly accessible for antibody binding on live bacteria. *Vaccine* **19,** 1526–1533.

12. Rosenqvist, E., Musacchio A., Aase, A., Høiby, E. A., Namork, E., Kolberg, J., et al. (1999) Functional activities and epitope specificity of human and murine antibodies against the class 4 (Rmp) outer membrane protein of *Neisseria meningitidis*. *Infect. Immun.* **67,** 1267–1276.

24

T-Cell Responses Against Meningococcal Antigens

Lisbeth Meyer Næss, Fredrik Oftung, Audun Aase, Terje E. Michaelsen, and Andrew J. Pollard

1. Introduction

1.1. Background

T-cells recognize protein antigens as short peptide fragments (8–20 amino acids) bound to major histocompatibility complex (MHC) molecules on the surface of antigen-presenting cells (APCs). A prerequisite for antigen-specific T-cell activation is antigen uptake, enzymatic degradation, and recycling of MHC-peptide complexes to the surface of APCs. Whereas CD8+ T cells recognize endogenously derived antigen (virus and other intracellular pathogens) bound to MHC class I molecules, CD4+ T cells recognize exogenously derived antigen in complex with MHC class II molecules. Hence, extracellular bacteria, such as meningococci during invasive disease, will be presented to CD4+ T cells in the context of MHC class II molecules, after uptake and processing by professional APCs like B cells, macrophages, or dendritic cells. Antigen-specific CD4+ T cells can be classified as Th1 or Th2 subpopulations on the basis of different cytokine production and effector functions (*1*). Intracellular microbes often induce Th1-dominated responses, whereas extracellular pathogens and parasites typically trigger Th2 responses. Th1 cells produce mainly interleukin (IL)-2, interferon (IFN)-γ, and tumor necrosis factor (TNF)-β, which represent important inducers of the cell-mediated immune responses. The principal Th1 cytokine IFN-γ activates macrophages by enhancing their ability to phagocytize and destroy microbes by intracellular bactericidal mechanisms. In contrast, Th2 cells produce IL-4, IL-5, IL-6, and IL-13, which are important factors for inducing and regulating B-cell responses (*1*).

From: *Methods in Molecular Medicine, vol. 66: Meningococcal Vaccines: Methods and Protocols*
Edited by: A. J. Pollard and M. C. J. Maiden © Humana Press Inc., Totowa, NJ

Although protective immunity against meningococci relies on antibody-mediated effector functions (bactericidal activity and opsonophagocytosis), Th2-cells play an important role in the regulation of the immune response, including stimulating B-cells to antibody production both at the systemic and mucosal level *(2)*. Cytokine mediated T-cell help is needed for the B cells to mature and differentiate and produce antibodies with high affinity of the relevant isotypes. IL-4 is involved in the induction of IgM, IgG, and IgE synthesis, whereas IL-5 and transforming growth factor (TGF)-β are involved in the differentiation of IgA producing B cells *(1)*. T cells are also necessary for the establishment of immunological memory and they promote activation of phagocytic cells, thereby facilitating the uptake and destruction of meningococci. The importance of T-cell activation is clearly demonstrated with vaccines solely based on polysaccharides: because carbohydrate antigens fail to induce T-cell help, polysaccharide vaccines against group A and C meningococci are poorly immunogenic in infants and do not induce long-term immunological memory *(3)*. To overcome this problem, conjugation of the polysaccharide to a protein carrier that contains T-cell epitopes has successfully been utilized in the recently developed meningococcal group C conjugate vaccines *(4,5)*.

Only a few studies of human T-cell responses induced by vaccination or meningococcal disease have been presented *(6–9)*. Until recently, such analyses have been time-consuming and logistically difficult to adapt to large-scale clinical studies. Both vaccination and meningococcal disease lead to activation and proliferation of antigen-specific CD4+ T-cells in peripheral blood. By using a thymidine incorporation assay based on the microtiter plate format in all steps, human CD4+ T-cell responses against meningococcal antigens can be measured as proliferation in vitro *(10)*. Furthermore, cytokine production by T-cells stimulated with antigen in vitro can be measured in the supernatant of proliferating cells by enzyme-linked immunosorbent assay (ELISA) *(11)*. We have used these techniques to map vaccine-induced T-cell responses against defined meningococcal antigens *(10,12)* (**Fig. 1**) as well as monitoring Th1 and Th2 cytokine production in children encountering meningococcal disease *(11)* (**Fig. 2**). Both systemic *(12)* and nasal vaccination *(10)* with outer-membrane vesicles (OMVs) from serogroup B meningococci-induced, antigen-specific T-cell proliferation against the PorA and PorB3 antigen, in addition to the vaccine antigen used. However, the T-cell response against the PorA antigen was considerably higher than measured against PorB3. In addition, the PorA-specific T-cell response correlated with mucosal IgA, serum IgG, and with bactericidal activity against meningococci *(10,12)*. These results indicate that PorA is more important than PorB3 with respect to T-cell help for production of protective antibodies, but a similar role for additional protein antigens (Opa

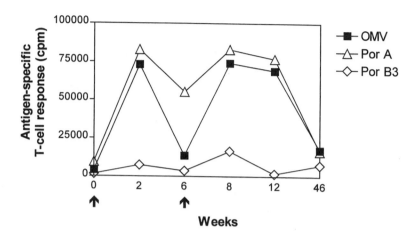

Fig. 1. Antigen-specific CD4+ T-cell proliferation to OMV, PorA, and PorB3 after intramuscular vaccination with the Norwegian meningococcal serogroup B vaccine. The vaccination schedule is defined by arrows, and the results are expressed as median cpm values of 10 vaccinees.

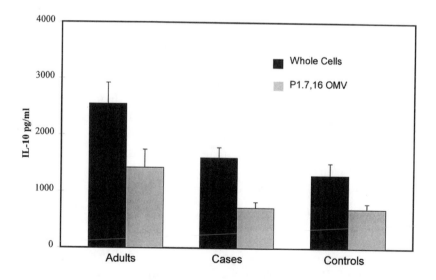

Fig. 2. Cytokine production (IL-10) by human PBMC from adults, cases (children after meningococcal infection) and control children following in vitro stimulation with heat-killed meningococci or OMV. Adapted from **ref. *11.***

and Opc) has also been suggested *(8)*. Cytokine responses after vaccination against meningococci have not been systematically analyzed. However, the observation that the cytokine pattern in young and older children convalescing from disease was skewed towards a Th1 and Th2 response, respectively *(11)*, suggests that inclusion of components favoring a Th2 response is especially important in vaccines designed to protect infants.

1.2. T-Cell Proliferation Assay

Peripheral blood mononuclear cells (PBMC) are isolated from freshly drawn whole blood and cultivated in vitro in the presence of meningococcal antigens (purified protein antigens, outer-membrane preparations, or whole inactivated bacteria). Recognition of meningococcal antigens presented, by APCs in the PBMC cultures will stimulate antigen-specific CD4+ T cells to proliferate. T-cell proliferation is measured by pulsing the cultures at day 6 with [^{3}H] thymidine, which is incorporated into the DNA of dividing cells. The amount of radioactivity present in DNA harvested from the cell cultures is detected in a scintillation counter and represents a measurement of antigen-specific CD4+ T-cell proliferation *(13)*. An overview of the assay is shown in **Fig. 3**. Although nonfractionated PBMC are used in the proliferation assay, the design of the assay allows detection of CD4+ T-cell responses against the antigens tested. Antigen-driven, polyclonal B-cell responses generally peak at day 2–3, whereas the detection of proliferation (thymidine pulsing) is performed at day 6, which generally corresponds to the peak in T-cell proliferation. We have confirmed that CD4+ T cells predominantly contribute to the proliferation observed by two different experimental approaches. By using flow cytometry, we have demonstrated that the blastoid and dividing cell population present at day 6 consisted of more than 90% CD4+ T cells (**Fig. 4**). The predominant contribution of CD4+ T cells was confirmed by showing that anti-MHC class II antibodies (anti-human leukocyte antigen [HLA]-DR) inhibited the proliferative responses to meningococcal antigens in a dose-dependent manner (**Fig. 5**). To exclude any potential mitogen or antigen-induced B-cell proliferation, this should ideally be confirmed for each antigen used in the assay.

1.3. Cytokine-Production Assay

Cytokines produced by T-cells in response to meningococcal antigens can be measured in the supernatants of antigen-stimulated PBMC cultures. Antigen stimulation of PBMC in vitro is undertaken as described in **Subheading 3.1., steps 1–10,** and cell-culture supernatants are aspirated at optimal timepoints and frozen for later analysis by cytokine-specific ELISA.

Isolate PBMC from whole blood by density
gradient centrifugation

⇩

Plate out PBMC in 96 wells microtiterplates and add
meningococcal antigens

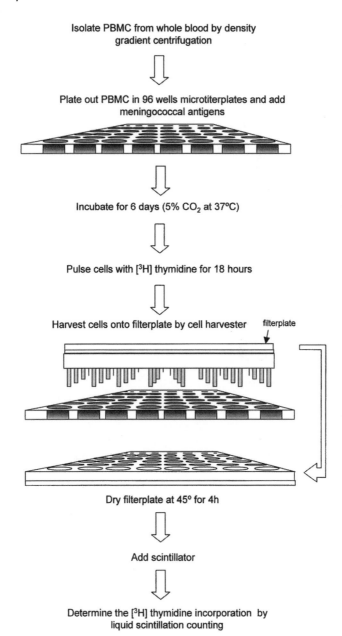

⇩

Incubate for 6 days (5% CO_2 at 37°C)

⇩

Pulse cells with [^{3}H] thymidine for 18 hours

⇩

Harvest cells onto filterplate by cell harvester   filterplate

Dry filterplate at 45° for 4h

⇩

Add scintillator

⇩

Determine the [^{3}H] thymidine incorporation by
liquid scintillation counting

Fig. 3. An overview of the T-cell proliferation assay.

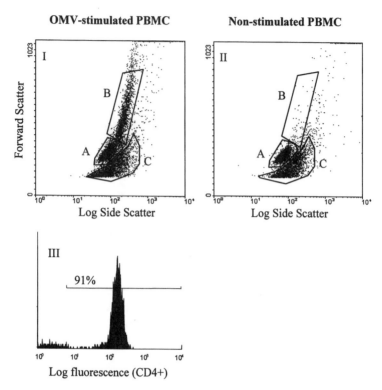

Fig. 4. The histograms I and II show the distribution of OMV-stimulated and nonstimulated PBMC, respectively. The cells in region A represent nonstimulated lymphocytes, in region B proliferating (activated) cells, and in C dead cells. Histogram III shows the distribution of CD4+ T-cells within region B in histogram I.

2. Materials

1. Heparin blood tubes (Becton Dickinson, Rutherford, NJ).
2. Physiological saline, NaCl, 9 mg/mL (Kabi, Pharmacia, Sweden).
3. Lymphoprep with density 1.077 g/mL (Nycomed Amersham, Oslo, Norway) or Histopaque-1077 (Sigma).
4. RPMI-1640 (Biowhittaker, Verviers, Belgium).
5. L-glutamine (Gibco).
6. Benzylpenicillin (Gibco).
7. Streptomycin (Gibco).
8. Phytohemagglutinin (PHA; Sigma).
9. Human serum, heat-inactivated (30 min at 56°C) from a serum pool (Sigma).
10. 96-well, flat-bottomed, microtiter cell-culture plates (Costar, Cambridge, MA).
11. Cell-counting chamber (Burker, Germany).
12. [³H] thymidine (Amersham, Little Chalfont, UK).

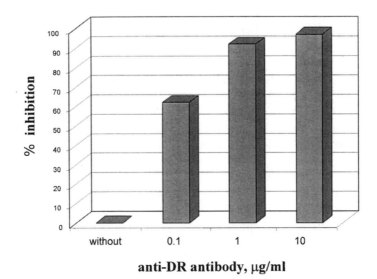

Fig. 5. Inhibition of OMV-induced PBMC proliferation by anti MHC class II antibodies (anti-HLA-DR: B8.11).

13. Cell harvester (FilterMate 196, Packard, Meriden, CT).
14. Filterplates (UniFilter GF/C, Packard) for scintillation counting or glassfiber filters (Packard) for direct β-counting.
15. Scintillation cocktail (Packard Microscint O) for scintillation counting.
16. Scintillation counter (Packard TopCount microplate scintillation counter) or a direct β-counter with gas-ionization detectors (Packard Matrix 96).
17. Cytokine ELISA kits (Pharmingen).

3. Methods
3.1. Proliferation Assay

1. Collect venous blood in blood tubes containing 10 U/mL of preservative-free heparin or ethylenediaminetetraacetic acid (EDTA) (*see* **Note 1**).
2. Dilute the blood with an equal volume of saline or RPMI 1640. Carefully layer the diluted blood (35 mL) onto the top of the Lymphoprep (or Histopaque) (15 mL) in 50-mL tubes and centrifuge at 580*g* for 20 min at 18–20°C (density gradient centrifugation modified after **ref. *14***).
3. Carefully aspirate PBMC from the interphase between the plasma and Lymphoprep (or Histopaque) with a Pasteur pipette and suspend the cells in RPMI 1640.
4. Wash the cells by centrifugation at 180*g* for 10 min. Pour off the supernatant and resuspend the cell pellet in RPMI 1640.

5. Repeat the washing of cells as described above twice and resuspend the PBMC pellet in 1 mL of RPMI 1640 medium supplemented with L-glutamine (2 mM), benzylpenicillin (100 IU/mL), and streptomycin (100 µg/mL) and containing 15% heat-inactivated human serum (*see* **Note 2**).

6. Count the isolated PBMC with a cell counting chamber and adjust the concentration of PBMC to 2×10^6 cells/mL in supplemented medium.

7. Plate out PBMC (50 µL per well) in flat-bottomed, 96-well microtiter plates (100,000 cells per well) (*see* **Note 3**). To increase the sensitivity of the assay, the cell concentration might be increased to 200,000 per well.

8. Add meningococcal antigens, control antigens (*see* **Note 4**) and PHA at optimal concentrations in triplicates (50 µL/well). Use medium without any antigen as a negative control in at least six wells (50 µL/well) to measure the background proliferation level. In addition, fill 3 wells with medium alone to allow early detection of bacterial or fungal contamination.
   The optimum stimulating concentration has to be determined for each antigen.
   We have used heat-killed whole meningococci at a final concentration of 5×10^7 bacteria/mL, OMVs from *N. meningitidis* strains at final protein concentrations between 0.1 and 5 µg/mL and purified PorA and PorB3 antigens at concentrations between 0.1 and 5 µg/mL. Final concentrations of PHA: 5 µg/mL.

9. Add RPMI 1640 supplemented medium (100 µL per well) to all wells, which gives a total volume of 200 µL per well.

10. Incubate cells for 6 d in a humidified atmosphere containing 5% CO_2 at 37°C.

11. Pulse cells with [³H] thymidine (1 µCi/well) for 18 h. A shorter time period could also be used but minimum 4 h (*see* **Note 5**). Follow the general guidelines for the use of [³H] thymidine.

12. Harvest cells onto filterplates or glassfiber filters by using a cell harvester with a 96-well microtiter format. Dry filterplates or filters overnight at room temperature or 4 h at 45°C.

13. Add scintillation cocktail to wells (25 µL per well) if a liquid-scintillation counter is used for the β-counting.

14. Determine the [³H] thymidine incorporation by liquid-scintillation counting or direct β-counting based on gas ionization detectors (*see* **Note 6**).

15. Express proliferative T-cell responses as counts per minute (cpm) or as stimulation index (SI). Cpm values (Δ cpm) are calculated by subtracting the mean of cpm values obtained without antigen (medium only) from the mean of triplicate cpm values obtained in the presence of antigen. SI is defined as the ratio of the mean of cpm triplicate values obtained in the presence of antigen to the mean cpm value obtained in the absence of antigen. SI values exceeding 3 or 5 are generally considered as positive responses.

3.2. Cytokine Production Assay

1. Carry out **steps 1–11** as described for the proliferation assay (*see* **Note 7**). Include wells for antigens of interest, control antigens and mitogens, medium alone, and nonstimulated PBMC (medium and PBMC).

2. At a specific time-point (or multiple time-points) during cell culture, aspirate supernatants from the wells and centrifuge at 4°C to pellet any cell debris.
3. Freeze the supernatants in aliquots at –70°C until use (*see* **Note 8**).
4. Thaw supernatants and measure cytokine concentrations using commercially available cytokine-specific ELISA kits.

4. Notes

1. ACD tubes are generally not recommended.
2. The least background proliferation is achieved by using human AB serum.
3. Proliferation assays can also be performed by combining a purified CD4+ T-cell fraction and nonfractionated irradiated PBMC as APCs. However, in a practical context with a large number of participants in clinical trials, this approach will be too time-consuming.
4. To ensure that the assay conditions are kept constant over time, which is important in longitudinal vaccination studies, a positive control antigen should be included. The positive control antigen has to be chosen on the basis of the immune status of donors participating in the study. *Mycobacterium bovis* Bacille Calmette Guerin (BCG) is a suitable control antigen that elicits strong proliferative T-cell responses in individuals previously vaccinated with BCG. In addition, the T-cell mitogen PHA should be used as a control for constant mitogenic activity.
5. The plates may be frozen after the thymidine incubation step and then thawed immediately before harvesting.
6. Direct counting of β-radiation based on gas ionization detectors are more convenient (faster) compared to scintillation counting, but the signal level (cpm values) obtained with a scintillation counter is considerably higher. High level cpm values are preferred in studies where individuals are followed over time, as the background level may vary and even small changes will affect the results expressed as SI. In comparative or longitudinal studies, we therefore recommend to use scintillation counting, which permits presentation of the results as cpm values.
7. Because the cell culture procedures of the proliferation and cytokine measurements are identical, the performance of these assays can be combined by using the same cell culture-plates. The optimum time-point for measuring each cytokine of interest must be determined for the cytokine and antigen(s) being studied. This is done by measuring the levels of cytokine released over time using daily time-points over the 6-d assay period. The supernatants should be maintained at 4°C until frozen.
8. In deciding the volume of each aliquot, consider the amount of supernatant that will be required for the quantitative ELISA (freeze and thaw only once).

References

1. Abbas, A. K., Murphy, K. M., and Sher, A. (1996) Functional diversity of helper T lymphocytes. *Nature* **383,** 787–793.
2. Ada, G. L. (1990) The immunological principles of vaccination. *Lancet* **335,** 523–526.

3. Frasch, C. E. (1995) Meningococcal vaccines, in *Meningococcal Disease* (Cartwright, K. A. V., ed.), John Wiley and Sons, NY, pp. 245–283.
4. MacDonald, N. E., Halperin, S. A., Law, B. J., Forrest, B., Danzig, L. E., and Granoff, D. M. (1998) Induction of immunologic memory by conjugated vs plain meningococcal C polysaccharide vaccine in toddlers. *JAMA* **280,** 1685–1689.
5. Richmond, P., Borrow, R., Miller, E., Clark, S., Sadler, F., Fox, A., et al. (1999) Meningococcal serogroup C conjugate vaccine is immunogenic in infancy and primes for memory. *J. Infect. Dis.* **179,** 1569–1572.
6. Greenwood, B. M., Oduloju, A. J., and Ade-Serrano, M. A. (1979) Cellular immunity in patients with meningococcal disease and in vaccinated subjects. *Clin. Exp. Immunol.* **38,** 9–15.
7. Wiertz, E. J., van Gaans-van den Brink, J. A., Schreuder, G. M., Termijtelen, A. A., Hoogerhout, P., and Poolman, J. T. (1991) T-cell recognition of *Neisseria meningitidis* class 1 outer membrane proteins. Identification of T-cell epitopes with selected synthetic peptides and determination of HLA restriction elements. *J. Immunol.* **147,** 2012–2018.
8. Wiertz, E. J. H. J, Delvig, A., Donders, E. M. L. M., Brugghe, H. F., van Unen, L. M. A., Timmermann, H. A. M., et al. (1996) T-cell responses to outer membrane proteins of *Neisseria meningitidis*: comparative study of Opa, Opc, and PorA proteins. *Infect. Immun.* **64,** 298–304.
9. Rouppe van der Voort, E. M., van Dijken, H., Kuipers, B., van der Biezen, J., van der Ley, P., Meylis, J., et al. (1997) Human B- and T-cell responses after immunization with a hexavalent PorA meningococcal outer membrane vesicle vaccine. *Infect. Immun.* **65,** 5184–5190.
10. Oftung, F., Næss, L. M., Wetzler, L. M., Korsvold, G. E., Aase, A., Høiby, E. A., et al. (1999) Antigen-specific T-cell responses in humans after intranasal immunization with a meningococcal serogroup B outer membrane vesicle vaccine. *Infect. Immun.* **67,** 921–927.
11. Pollard, A. J., Galassini, R., Rouppe van der Voort, E. M., Hibberd, M., Booy, R., Langford, P., et al. (1999) Cellular immune responses to *Neisseria meningitidis* in children. *Infect. Immun.* **67,** 2452–2463.
12. Næss, L. M., Oftung, F., Aase, A., Wetzler, L., Sandin, R., and Michaelsen, T. E. (1998) Human T-cell responses after vaccination with the Norwegian group B meningococcal outer membrane vesicle vaccine. *Infect. Immun.* **66,** 959–965.
13. Oppenheim, J. J. and Rosenstreich, D. L. (1976) Lymphocyte transformation: utilization of automatic harvesters, in *In Vitro Methods in Cell Mediated and Tumor Immunity* (Bloom, B. R. and David, J. R., eds.), Academic Press, NY, pp 573–585.
14. Bøyum, A. (1968) Separation of leukocytes from blood and bone marrow. *Scand. J. Clin. Lab. Invest.* **21(Suppl.),** 97.

25

CD4 T-Cell Epitope Mapping

Alexei A. Delvig and John H. Robinson

1. Introduction

The majority of T cells recognize peptide epitopes bound to major histocompatibility complex (MHC)-encoded glycoproteins on the surface of professional antigen-presenting cells (APC), principally dendritic cells, macrophages, and B cells *(1–3)*. Most T cells are specific for peptide epitopes in association with either classical MHC class Ia molecules (HLA-A, B, and C in humans and H2-K, D, and L in mice) in the case of CD8[+] T cells, or class II molecules (HLA-DR, DP, and DQ in humans and H2-A and E in mice) for CD4[+] T cells. However, a significant proportion of T cells recognize peptide antigens bound to nonclassical MHC class Ib molecules such as the human HLA-E (mouse analog Qa1) *(4)* and mouse H2-M3 *(5)*. In addition, some T cells recognize not peptides but lipid or glycolipid antigens bound to nonclassical MHC class Ib molecules such as CD1 in both humans and mice *(6)*.

In order for peptide epitopes to bind to MHC molecules, protein antigens require denaturation and enzymatic degradation, known as antigen processing, to different degrees within endosomal compartments of APC *(2,3,7)*. Most endogenous and some exogenous protein antigens can be degraded by cytosolic proteasomes, the products of which are delivered into the endoplasmic reticulum where short peptides bind to MHC class Ia molecules. MHC class Ia/peptide complexes are then exocytozed to the APC surface via the Golgi apparatus for subsequent recognition by specific T cells of the appropriate specificity leading to T-cell activation and differentiation. In contrast, most exogenous and some endogenous protein antigens can be denatured and degraded in early and late endosomal compartments, principally by lysosomal enzymes. Denatured or degraded polypeptides of variable length may then bind

From: *Methods in Molecular Medicine, vol. 66: Meningococcal Vaccines: Methods and Protocols*
Edited by: A. J. Pollard and M. C. J. Maiden © Humana Press Inc., Totowa, NJ

to MHC class II molecules newly synthesized in the endoplasmic reticulum and transported to endosomal compartments via the Golgi apparatus. Peptide epitopes may be subjected to further proteolytic exopeptidase activity referred to as trimming, before or after MHC class II/peptide complexes are exported to the APC surface. The structural properties of protein antigens dictate different requirements for denaturation and degradation, with examples ranging from a dependency on a series of cleavage steps to protein antigens requiring no enzymatic processing. Alternatively, existing surface MHC class I or class II molecules may be internalized into endosomal compartments, during which peptide exchange can occur, leading the presentation of new peptide epitopes upon recycling to the cell surface (8–10).

The size and structure of peptide epitopes that bind MHC class I and class II molecules have been confirmed by elution of naturally processed peptides from purified MHC class I or class II molecules and the structure of MHC class I and class II- peptide complexes have been determined by x-ray crystallography (1).

Mapping and characterization of T-cell epitopes of protein antigens implicated in allergic responses, tumor immunity, and protection against microbial pathogens such as *Neisseria meningitidis* has been a major goal of immunological research in the last decade. Knowledge of the localization of T-cell epitopes is of immense practical value as a pre-requisite for the design and evaluation of vaccines for development in animal models and eventual human trials (11). Several techniques have been described to localize T-cell epitopes to regions of protein antigens based either on protein fragmentation by chemical or enzyme treatment or achieved by employing molecular-genetic techniques (12). The latter include cDNA cloning followed by expression of the gene in cells with the appropriate MHC allotype using eukaryotic or viral expression systems and identification of positive clones by T-cell assay (13). Subsequently, localization of T-cell epitopes can be determined by studying truncation mutants of the original genes.

The seminal development of solid-phase peptide synthesis technology by Merrifield (14) broke away from solution-phase methods by using an insoluble resin support. This method allowed preparation of peptides much more rapidly at low cost. Subsequent developments in chemistry, resin supports, amino acid protecting groups, and coupling reagents led to the following variants of the solid-phase peptide synthesis: 1) the automated synthesis of up to 48 individual peptides in flow-through columns (15); 2) simultaneous multiple peptide synthesis of larger numbers of peptides (>100) on resin contained in polypropylene mesh bags using conventional *t*-boc chemistry ("tea bag" synthesis) (16); and 3) peptide synthesis on polypropylene pins performed in 96-well plates using fmoc chemistry (17). Using the latter method, more than a thousand peptides can be synthesized simultaneously, and then cleaved from the pins using trifluoroacetic acid (TFA) or formic acid if an aspartic acid-proline bond is used as a link to the pins *(18)*, or even at neutral pH into a physiologically compatible solution if a diketopiperazine linker is used.

The number of peptides that require synthesis can be reduced by attempting to predict the location of T-cell epitopes within the sequence of the test protein. Prediction is based on searching the protein sequence for motifs, which include a pattern of anchor amino acids known to be required for binding to a particular allele of individual MHC class I or class II molecules *(19)*. Interestingly, T-cell epitopes are often characterized by proline residues located close to both N- and C-termini, possibly reflecting stop signals for trimming MHC class II-associated protein fragments by exopeptidases and aminopeptidases *(20,21)*. The most comprehensive database for predicting MHC-binding peptides *(22)* is available for open internet access at: http://www.uni-tuebingen.de/uni/kxi/

Alternative approaches for identification of T-cell epitopes include sequencing of natural peptide epitopes eluted from purified MHC molecules *(23)* and the use of molecular libraries based on combinatorial peptide and nonpeptide chemistry *(24,25)*. In this chapter, we describe the synthetic peptide approach for mapping human and mouse MHC class II-restricted CD4$^+$ T-cell epitopes of meningococcal proteins.

2. Materials

2.1. Culture Media, Materials, and Equipment

2.1.1. Culture Media and Diluents

1. Culture medium used for mouse cell culture (MR10): RPMI 1640 medium (Sigma Chemical Co., supplied single strength in 500-mL bottles, #R0883) supplemented with 3.0 mM L-glutamine (Sigma, #G7513, supplied in 100-mL bottles), 0.05 mM 2-mercaptoethanol (2-ME, Sigma, #M7522, supplied in 100-mL bottles, 14.3 M stock) (*see* **Note 1**) and 10% fetal bovine serum (FBS) (v/v) (Sigma, #F7524, supplied in 500-mL bottles). MR2 is a variant medium containing 2% FBS for the preparation and assay of CTLL-2 cells used for synthetic peptide toxicity testing.
2. Culture medium used for human cell culture (HR10): RPMI 1640 supplemented with 3.0 mM L-glutamine, 25 mM HEPES buffer (Sigma, #H0887, stock 1.0 M, supplied in 100-mL bottles) and 10% autologous plasma from heparinized blood.
3. Phosphate-buffered saline (PBS) for dissolving soluble synthetic peptides (Dulbecco 'A', OXOID, #BR14a). Dissolve 1 tablet in 100 mL deionized water, autoclave at 115°C for 10 min.
4. Tris-HCl (0.2 M, Ultrol Grade, Calbiochem, #648311) plus 6 M Urea (Sigma, #U4128) adjusted to pH 7.0 for dissolving synthetic peptides with low solubility.

2.1.2. Materials

1. Gentamycin (Sigma, #G-1397, supplied in 10.0 mL vials of 50 mg/mL stock). Stored at 2–8°C.
2. Lymphoprep™ (Nycomed, #221395, density 1.077 g/mL) for separation of mononuclear cells by density centrifugation. Stored at 2–8°C.
3. Recombinant human IL-2 (Glaxo IMB, 100 µg). Stored at 4°C.
4. Titermax Gold Adjuvant (Sigma, #T2684, 1.0 mL) or TiterMax Classic Adjuvant (Sigma, #H4397, supplied in 0.5-mL vials) for immunizations of mice. Stored at 2–8°C (*see* **Note 2**).
5. Sterile round-bottomed 96-well microtiter plates with lids.
6. Tritiated thymidine (Amersham, #TRA310, 1 mCi/mL, specific activity 2.0 Ci/m*M*). A working stock of of 14.8 µCi/mL in RPMI 1640). Stored at 2–8°C.
7. Type A/E glass-fiber filters (Gelman Sciences, #p/n 61638, size 20.3 × 25.4 cm). Filter are cut to the size of a 96-well plate (8.0 × 12.5 cm).

2.1.3. Equipment

1. Cell harvester, such as Packard Micromate 196 (Packard, Canberra Packard, Berks, UK).
2. Beta counter, such as Packard Matrix 9600 direct beta-counter (Packard Instrument Company, Meridan, CT).

2.2. Synthetic Peptides and Antigens

2.2.1. Synthetic Peptides

The size of natural peptide epitopes eluted from MHC class II molecules is greater than 14 amino acids *(26)*, and synthetic peptides longer than 31 or shorter than 12 amino acids have been shown to be less effective for mapping T-cell epitopes *(27)*. There are also several other important parameters, which should be considered when designing and using synthetic peptides for mapping T-cell epitopes.

1. Design of peptide sets. At the initial screening of the entire sequence of the test protein peptides with their N-terminal residues offset along the sequence by 10 or more residues have been used. However, this design may result in missing some of the epitopes. In our mapping experiments, we used 18mer peptides overlapping either by 12 or 9 amino acids *(28,29)*.
2. Terminal amino acids. N-terminal glutamine residues should be avoided to prevent the formation of pyroglutamic acid. C-terminal proline residues can result in a decrease in the peptide synthesis efficiency and low yield. Peptides with either protected or unprotected termini can be used, although peptides with blocked termini are more effective. N-acetylation is recommended *(27)*.
3. Synthesis. If funds are available overlapping peptide sets can be synthesized on a 0.05-m*M* scale. Alternatively, several variants of small-scale MultiPin™ Synthe-

sis Kits are available from Chiron Technologies (*see* **Note 3**), which use the following linkers:

    a. Diketopiperazine. This linker gives rise to cyclic Lys-Pro dipeptide at the C terminus. This method has the advantage that peptides can be released into physiologically compatible medium, and therefore is recommended for mapping experiments.

    b. Glycine ester (GAP). Cleavage of peptides from this linker results in either acid or amide glycine C terminus depending on the cleavage methods used.

    c. Rink. This format results in forming C-terminal amide groups.

4. Yield. Conventional synthesis on a 0.05-mM scale yields 20 mg or more of each peptide as a lyophilized powder, which is a suitable quantity for repetitive in vitro screening as well as in vivo immunization. Using small-scale multiple peptide synthesis, up to 10 µmol of 20mer peptides can be obtained, sufficient for only very limited in vitro screening experiments. The purity of peptides is normally 70–90%, such that peptides can be used for mapping experiments without further purification.

5. Solubility and sterility of peptides. Concentrated stocks (4–5 mg/mL) of hydrophilic peptides are prepared either in PBS (*see* **Subheading 2.1.1., item 3.**) sometimes with application of gentle heat, whereas hydrophobic peptides are more of a problem and may require solubility in Tris-Urea buffer (*see* **Subheading 2.1.1., item 4.**). Unfiltered peptide solutions have been used successfully without contamination after in vitro culture in T-cell assays.

6. Concentration of peptides in the assay. Because the concentration of a particular peptide necessary to induce proliferation of T cells varies from 0.2 µM to more than 2.0 µM *(27)*, a range of concentrations of peptides should be used. We used synthetic peptides at 5.0 µM, 1.0 µM and 0.4 µM for mapping mouse T-cell epitopes on the PorB protein *(28)*, and at 6.0 µM for mapping T-cell epitopes on PorA, Opc, and Opa proteins *(29)*.

7. Pooling peptides for the initial screening. It is possible to test mixtures of 3 or more peptides to reduce number of wells in the assay and the positive pools can be re-tested using individual peptides. If many peptides are to be screened, larger pools of peptides can also be used and this approach is particularly important in the human studies because the amount of blood available may be limited for each experiment. However, with larger peptide pools, there is an increasing risk that epitopes will be missed owing to competition for MHC binding by peptides that do not stimulated a T-cell response.

8. Toxicity of peptides. Potential toxicity of peptides for T cells can be detected as reduction of proliferation of IL-2-dependent CTLL-2 cells (*see* **Subheading 3.1.**).

9. Storage. Lyophilized peptides should be stored desiccated at –20°C, and diluted peptide solutions are stored at –80°C.

2.2.2. Controls for T-Cell Assays

1. Concanavalin A (Con A) from *Canavalia ensiformis* type IV-S (ConA, Sigma, #C5275) is a lectin with mitogenic properties for all mouse T cells. High concen-

tration stock of ConA is prepared (1.0 mg/mL, sterile deionized water) and stored at −20°C.

2. Phytohemagglutinin (PHA-M. Calbiochem, #526511).

3. Lipopolysaccharide (LPS) (*Escherichia coli*, serotype 0111:B4, Sigma, #L4130) is potent B-cell mitogens in man and mouse. Stock solution of LPS is prepared (1.0 mg/ mL) and stored at −20°C.

4. An irrelevant control protein antigen such as Ovalbumin (OVA) (Albumin, Chicken Egg, grade VII, Sigma, #A7641) should be used to distinguish antigen-specific from antigen non-specific responses in activated T cells.

2.2.3. Test Proteins

A source of test protein antigen (recombinant of purified) is valuable, but not essential, as a specificity control for T-cell assays. However, purified (LPS-free!) test antigen is usually required to immunize mice to generate specific T cells for in vitro peptide-screening assays.

2.3. Sources of T Cells

2.3.1. Mouse T Cells

1. Cell suspensions from local lymph nodes are the preferred source of antigen specific T cells from immunized mice. Popliteal lymph nodes give yields of more than 10 million cells 7–14 d following footpad immunization with protein antigens in a suitable adjuvant. Alternatively, pooled inguinal and axillary lymph nodes yield a similar number of cells following subcutaneous immunization. Also, depending on the particular manner of natural immunization, cell suspensions from other relevant draining lymph nodes or the spleen provide a source of antigen-specific T cells.

2. It is important to consider which MHC haplotype or haplotypes of mice are chosen for T-cell epitope mapping. Most information is available for the common haplotypes H-2^b (e.g., C57BL/6 and C57BL/10 inbred strains), H-2^d (e.g., BALB/c inbred strain), and H-2^k (e.g., CBA and C3H inbred strains). Mouse strains expressing one or more of the remaining independent MHC haplotypes (H-2^f, H-2^p, H-2^q, H-2^r, H-2^s, H-2^u, and H-2^z), may be required to match a particular established animal model. The most useful source of information about MHC alleles is the Jackson Laboratory Mouse Genome Informatics website at: http://www.informatics.jax.org/

3. Intra–H2 recombinant strains of mice are available that allow determination of MHC class II locus, A or E, which restricts the response. For example, B10.GD (A^{d}E^b) or B10.A(4R) (A^{k}E^b).

4. Epitopes can be mapped for several MHC haplotypes to determine regions of the molecule, that include several overlapping epitopes. These regions have potential as universal immunogens in the development of peptide vaccines. It is an

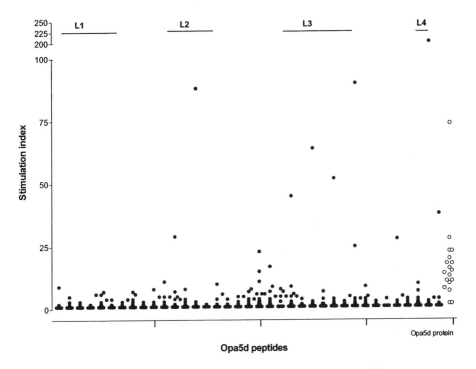

Fig. 1. Proliferative responses of PBMCs from 17 normal donors to 37 synthetic peptides corresponding to Opa5d protein *(29)*. Closed circles indicate individual responses to the particular peptides. Open circles show responses to Opa5d protein. L1–4 show portion of loops in the Opa5d protein.

advantage to consider the use of congenic strains of mice expressing different MHC haplotypes but shared background non-MHC genes, such as the C57BL/10 congenic strains B10.D2 (H-2^d) and B10.BR (H-2^k). Note also that several H2 haplotypes fail to express E molecules owing to defective Eα and/or Eβ genes *(30,31)*. These haplotypes include H-2^b, H-2^f, H-2^s, and H2^q.

2.3.2. Human T Cells

1. Peripheral blood from naturally immunized or vaccinated individuals is normally used for mapping human T-cell epitopes. Cord blood or peripheral blood from nonvaccinated individuals can be used as negative controls.
2. HLA haplotype is a major consideration in choosing individuals for study, as different MHC class II alleles binds largely different peptide epitopes. This point is illustrated in **Fig. 1**, which shows the proliferation responses of 17 normal donors to overlapping synthetic peptides corresponding to the complete sequence of Opa5α protein *(29)*.

3. Methods

The procedure described in **Subheading 3.1.** is essential for establishing whether or not particular peptides are toxic for T lymphocytes. The lack of toxicity is established if lymphocyte proliferation to the control mitogen or antigen is not inhibited by the test peptide used at the same concentration range as used in the mapping experiments. The procedure described in **Subheading 3.2.** uses mouse lymphoid cells for mapping T-cell epitopes following immunization with the test protein or peptide antigen. The frequency of specific T cells is enhanced by immunization with test protein or peptide in adjuvant or following infection. This method allows also evaluation of the relative immunodominance of T-cell epitopes. Peptide immunization allows confirmation of the specificity of T-cell responses in peptide-immunized mice as well as evaluation of whether peptide immunization recalls proliferative responses to the test protein, which has important implications for immunodominance of T-cell epitopes and the development of peptide vaccines.

Human studies described in **Subheading 3.3.** use peripheral blood as a source of T lymphocytes. Those studies rely on therapeutic or natural exposure to immunogens, such that the frequency of peptide-specific T cells can be very low.

3.1. Testing for Toxicity of Peptides

1. Grow CTLL-2 cells in MR10 supplemented with 2.0 ng/mL IL-2 in 24-well plates.
2. One day before required, collect CTLL-2 cells, count, wash twice in MR2 and incubate overnight. The following day, resuspend cells in MR2 supplemented with 50 µg/mL gentamycin and 2.0 ng/mL IL-2. Add CTLL-2 cells (2×10^4/well) in 100 µL volumes to the triplicate wells of flat-bottomed, 96-well plates.
3. Distribute synthetic peptides in 100 µL volumes into the wells of flat-bottomed 96-well plates at the same concentrations as for mapping T cell epitopes. Dissolve peptides in MR10 supplemented with 50 µg/mL gentamycin and 2.0 ng/mL IL-2. Incubate the cultures for 6 h at 37°C in a humidified CO_2 incubator.
4. Pulse the cultures with 0.3 µCi of ^{3}H-thymidine (20 µL of concentrated stock 15.0 µCi/mL). 16–18 h later, and harvest the plates on Type A/E Glass fiber filters using a cell harvester. Measure the amount of radioactivity in each well using a beta counter, and express results as mean cpm plus standard deviation.
5. Use the following controls:
   a. Proliferation of CTLL-2 cells in MR10 without IL-2 or peptides.
   b. Proliferation of CTLL-2 cells in MR10 supplemented IL-2 in the absence of peptides.

3.2. Proliferation Assay Using Popliteal Lymph Node Cells from Protein-Immunized Mice

1. Immunize mice in foot pads with 20 µg test antigen or 30 µg ovalbumin emulsified in TiterMax adjuvant according to the manufacturer's instructions (*see* **Note 2**). Seven

to fourteen d later, remove popliteal lymph nodes and tease lymph nodes to a single cell suspension. Resuspend the cells in MR10 and distribute them (2×10^5/well) in 100 μL volumes in triplicate wells of round-bottomed, 96-well microtiter plates.

2. Add synthetic peptides or pools of several peptides in 100 μL volumes at 20, 4, and 0.8 μg/mL and the test protein at 10–0.01 μg/mL. Incubate the cultures for 72 h at 37°C in a humidified CO_2 incubator.

3. Add tritiated thymidine (0.3 μCi) to the wells, incubate overnight, and harvest on glass-fiber membranes. Measure the radioactivity incorporated as described in **Subheading 3.1., step 4**. Use popliteal lymph-node cells from 3 mice or more to compare peptide responses.

4. Use the following controls:
   a. Proliferation of popliteal lymph-node cells from the test protein-immunized mice to the control antigen OVA (a 10-fold dilution series starting from 100.0 μg/mL).
   b. Proliferation of popliteal lymph-node cells from OVA-immunized mice to the test protein and synthetic peptides.
   c. Proliferation to ConA (5.0 μg/mL).

5. Use the same method for mice that were footpad immunized with 30 μg of one or more synthetic peptides. The proliferation mixture consists of popliteal lymph node cells and synthetic peptides covering the immunodominant region.

3.3. Proliferation Assay Using Peripheral Blood Mononuclear Cells (PBMCs) from Humans

1. Use HR10 culture medium as in **Subheading 2.1.1., item 2**. The frequency of T cells specific for the particular peptide epitope is likely to be very low, therefore test each peptide in at least 6 wells to allow an estimate of the frequency of peptide-specific T cells to be performed (*see* **Note 3**).

2. Add synthetic peptides (2.0 μg/well) in 100 μL volumes to the wells of U-bottomed 96-well plates.

3. Obtain venous blood and dilute it 1:1 with RPMI 1640. Separate human PBMCs by density-gradient centrifugation (using Lymphoprep™. The approximate number of PBMC in 10 mL blood is 10×10^6, which can help to estimate the amount of blood needed for each experiment.

4. Resuspend PBMC in HR10 and add them to the wells (10^5/well) containing peptides. Adjust the total volume to 200 μL.

5. After 5 d of incubation at 37°C in humidified 5% CO_2/air, pulse the cultures with 0.3 μCi of ^{3}H-thymidine, harvest, and quantitate the amount of radioactivity in each well, as described in **Subheading 3.1., step 4**.

6. Use the following controls:
   a. Proliferation of PBMC in HR10 alone.
   b. Proliferation to PHA (50 μg/mL) and LPS (10 μg/mL).
   c. Proliferation of PBMC isolated from cord blood in the presence of test antigen or synthetic peptides.

4. Notes

1. Mouse T cells require 2-mercaptoethanol for proliferation in vitro, whereas human T cells do not *(32)*.
2. TiterMax Classic and Titermax Gold Adjuvant are equally effective in our experience.
3. Chiron Technologies supply MultiPin Synthesis Kits. Chiron Technologies have also developed software that assists with the design of the T-cell mapping assays, as well as with data analysis. In addition, the program calculates a precursor frequency of peptide-specific T cells *(33)*.

Acknowledgments

We thank E. J. H. J. Wiertz and J. T. Poolman for useful comments on mapping human T-cell epitopes on meningococcal outer membrane proteins. This project was supported by The Wellcome Trust.

References

1. Germain, R. N. (1999) Antigen processing and presentation, in *Fundamental Immunology*, 4th ed. (Paul, W. E., ed.), Lippincott-Raven, Philadelphia, 287–340.
2. Harding, C. V. (1997) MHC Molecules and Antigen Processing. Springer-Verlag, Heidelberg.
3. Watts, C. (1997) Capture and processing of exogenous antigens for presentation on MHC molecules. *Annu. Rev. Immunol.* **15,** 821–850.
4. Seaman, M. S., Perarnau, B., Lindahl, K. F., Lemonnier, F. A., and Forman, J. (1999) Response to *Listeria monocytogenes* in mice lacking MHC class Ia molecules. *J. Immunol.* **162,** 5429–5436.
5. Fischer-Lindahl, K., Byers, D. E., and Dabni, V. B. (1997) H2-M3, a full-service class Ib histocompatibility antigen. *Annu. Rev. Immunol.* **15,** 851–879.
6. Moody, D. B., Besra, G. S., Wilson, I. A., and Porcelli, S. A. (1999) The molecular basis of CD1-mediated presentation of lipid antigens. *Immunol. Rev.* **172,** 285–296.
7. Parham, P. E. (1999) Pathways of antigen processing and presentation. *Immunol. Rev.* **172,** 1–343.
8. Pinet, V. and Long, E. O. (1998) Peptide loading onto recycling HLA-DR molecules occurs in early endosomes. *Eur. J. Immunol.* **28,** 799–804.
9. Delvig, A. A. and Robinson, J. H. (1998) Two T cell epitopes from the M5 protein of viable Streptococcus pyogenes engage different pathways of bacterial antigen processing. *J. Immunol.* **160,** 5267–5272.
10. Zhong, G., Romagnoli, P., and Germain, R. N. (1997) Related leucine-based cytoplasmic targeting signals in invariant chain and Major Histocompatibility Complex class II molecules control endocytic presentation of distinct determinants in a single protein. *J. Exp. Med.* **185,** 429–438.
11. Ben-Yedidia, T. and Arnon, R. (1997) Design of peptide and polypeptide vaccines. *Curr. Opin. Biotechnol.* **8,** 442–448.

12. Benjamin, D. C., Berzofsky, J. A., and East, I. J. (1987) The antigenic structure of proteins: a reappraisal. *Annu. Rev. Immunol.* **2,** 67–101.
13. Walden, P. (1996) T-cell epitope determination. *Curr. Opin. Immunol.* **8,** 68–74.
14. Merrifield, R. B. (1963) Solid phase synthesis: I The synthesis of a tetrapeptide. *J. Am. Chem. Soc.* **85,** 2149–2154.
15. Merrifield, R. B., Stewart, J. M., and Jernberg, N. (1966) Instrument for automated synthesis of peptides. *Anal. Chem.* **38,** 1905–1914.
16. Houghten, R. A. (1985) General method for the rapid solid-phase synthesis of large numbers of peptides: specificity of antigen-antibody interaction at the level of individual amino acids. *Proc. Natl. Acad. Sci. USA* **82,** 5131–5135.
17. Geysen, H. M., Meloen, R. H., and Barteling, S. J. (1984) Use of peptide synthesis to probe viral antigens for epitopes to a resolution of a single amino acid. *Proc. Natl. Acad. Sci. USA* **81,** 3998–4002.
18. Van der Zee, R., Van Eden, W., Meloen, R. H., Noordzij, A., and Van Embden, E. J. (1989) Efficient mapping and characterization of a T cell epitope by the simultaneous synthesis of multiple peptides. *Eur. J. Immunol.* **19,** 43–47.
19. Hammer, J. (1995) New methods to predict MHC-binding sequences within protein antigens. *Curr. Opin. Immunol.* **7,** 263–269.
20. Rotzschke, O. and Falk, K. (1994) Origin, structure and motifs of naturally processed MHC class II ligands. *Curr. Opin. Immunol.* **6,** 45–51.
21. Ansorge, S., Scho, E., and Kunz, D. (1991) Membrane-bound peptidases of lymphocytes: functional implications. *Biochim. Biophys. Acta.* **50,** 799–807.
22. Rammensee, H. G., Bachmann, J., Emmerich, N., Bachor, O. A., and Stevanovic, S. (1999) SYFPEITHI: database for MHC ligands and peptide motifs. *Immunogenetics* **50,** 213–219.
23. Hunt, D. F., Henderson, R. A., Shabanowitz, J., Sakaguchi, K., Michel, H., Sevilir, N., et al. (1992) Characterization of peptides bound to the class I MHC molecule HLA-A2.1 by mass spectrometry. *Science* **255,** 1261–1263.
24. Sparbier, K. and Walden, P. (1999) T cell receptor specificity and mimotopes. *Curr. Opin. Immunol.* **11,** 214–218.
25. Pinilla, C., Martin, R., Gran, B., Appel J. R., Boggiano, C., Wilson, D. B., and R. A. Houghten. (1999) Exploring immunological specificity using synthetic peptide combinatorial libraries. *Curr. Opin. Immunol.* **11,** 193–202.
26. Chicz, R. M., Urban, R. G., Gorga, J. C., Vignali, D., Lane, W. S., and Strominger, J. L. (1993) Specificity and promiscuity among naturally processed peptides bound to HLA-DR alleles. *J. Exp. Med.* **178,** 27–47.
27. Reece, J. C., McGregor, D. L., Geysen, H. M., and Rodda, S. J. (1994) Scanning for T helper epitopes with PBMC using pools of short synthetic peptides. *J. Immunol. Meth.* **172,** 241–254.
28. Delvig, A. A., Rosenqvist, E., Oftung, F., and Robinson, J. H. (1997) T-cell epitope mapping the PorB protein of serogroup B Neisseria meningitidis in B10 congenic strains of mice. *Clin. Immunol. Immunopathol.* **85,** 134–142.
29. Wiertz, E., Delvig, A. A., Donders, E., Brugghe, H. F., van Unen, L. M. A., Timmermans, H. A. M., et al. (1996) T cell response to outer membrane proteins

of *Neisseria meningitidis*: comparative study of the Opa, Opc and PorA proteins. *Infect. Immun.* **64,** 298–304.

30. Mathis, D. J., Benoist, C., Williams, V. E., Kanter, M., and McDevitt, H. O. (1983) Several mechanisms can account for defective Eα gene expression in different mouse haplotypes. *Proc. Natl. Acad. Sci. USA* **80,** 273–277.

31. Sant, A. J., Braunstein, N. S., and Germain, R. N. (1987) Predominant role of amino-terminal sequences in dictating efficiency of class II major histocompatibility complex αβ dimer expression. *Proc. Natl. Acad. Sci. USA* **84,** 8065–8069.

32. Knight, S. C. (1987) Lymphocyte proliferation assays, in *Lymphocytes: A Practical Approach* (Klaus, G. G. B., ed.), IRL Press, Washington, 189–207.

33. Deane, R. (1993) T cell epitope mapping with PIN peptides. *Pinpoints Mimotopes Peptide Technol.* **6,** 1–8.

26

Epitope Mapping

John E. Heckels and Myron Christodoulides

1. Introduction

An epitope is defined as the site on an antigen at which an antibody binds. In the case of proteins the epitopes can be classified as continuous (or sequential) and discontinuous according to whether or not the amino acids recognized are close together in the primary sequence or are well-separated but brought together by the folding of the protein. The methods described have permitted the localization or "mapping" of continuous epitopes on meningococcal outer-membrane proteins (OMPs), which are recognized by both monoclonal and polyclonal antibodies (MAbs/PAbs).

The differentiation of meningococci into serotypes and subtypes results from antigenic differences in the PorB and PorA OMPs, respectively. Following the initial cloning and sequencing of the *porA* gene from *Neisseria meningitidis* isolate MC50 *(1)*, the inferred amino acid sequences of several meningococci of different subtypes became available *(6,8,13)*. The identity of the antigenic determinants recognized by the MAbs used in subtype classification was of particular interest not only for understanding the molecular basis of subtype specificity, but also because in vitro studies had revealed that the antibodies were more effective than those directed against other surface antigens, in protection against meningococcal infection. Despite the antigenic diversity of the PorA proteins, sequencing studies revealed that they showed considerable homology with structural differences largely confined to two discrete variable regions designated VR1 and VR2. These regions therefore appeared to be responsible for the antigenic specificity of the protein either singly as continuous epitopes or by combining to form a discontinuous epitope. Epitope-mapping experiments have confirmed this conclusion and have also demonstrated that

From: *Methods in Molecular Medicine, vol. 66: Meningococcal Vaccines: Methods and Protocols*
Edited by: A. J. Pollard and M. C. J. Maiden © Humana Press Inc., Totowa, NJ

variations within a subtype, which presumably arise as a result of point mutations, may have a profound effect on recognition by the standard subtyping MAbs *(7,8)*.

The technique for defining continuous epitopes on a protein involves the synthesis of a large number of small peptides that span the amino acid sequence of the protein. This requires not only knowledge of the protein sequences, which are usually available from gene cloning and sequencing, but also a method that permits the synthesis of large numbers of peptides. Traditional methods of peptide synthesis, which produced milligram amounts of pure peptides, were not suitable for large-scale epitope mapping methods because of the high costs involved. Detailed epitope mapping became practical with the development by Geysen and colleagues of the "pin" technology in which microgram amounts of a large number of peptides could be economically synthesized bound to polystyrene pins in the format of a 96-well microtiter plate *(4)*. This system is available as a commercial kit (Mimotopes) in which the polyethylene pins are derivatized with a spacer arm with a Nα-9-flourenylmethoxycarbonyl (Fmoc) protected β-alanine residue. This provides a free amino group onto which the peptide can be synthesized using conventional peptide chemistry with pentafluorophenyl (pfp)-activated esters of Fmoc-L-amino acids. After an experiment in which antibodies have been bound to the pins, the antibody can be dissociated and the pins reused up to 50 times. A modification of the system allows the synthesis of peptides that can be cleaved from the polystyrene support to produce soluble peptides for mapping of epitopes recognized by T-cells *(5)*.

These methods have been used to define the epitopes recognized by protective subtype-specific MAbs on the meningococcal PorA protein and to analyze the immune response to immunization with candidate vaccines *(2)*. They have also been used for mapping epitopes on Rmp (class 4) *(14)*, pilin *(15)*, and Opc proteins *(9)*, either from meningococci or the equivalent proteins in the closely related gonococci. They have not been successful in defining the epitopes responsible for type specificity on the PorB protein as these appear to be largely discontinuous in nature *(11,16)*.

2. Materials

2.1. Synthesis of Peptides on Polyethylene Pins

1. Multipin peptide synthesis kit: The methods described are based on the use of the Multipin™ Non-Cleavable Peptide Synthesis Kit (Mimotopes, Heswell, UK). This contains a block of derivatized pins and 96-well reaction trays. In addition, a computer program is provided that prints a daily synthesis schedule based on the amino acid sequence of the peptides to be synthesized.

2. Activated amino acid esters: For most amino acids, the synthesis uses pfp-active esters of Fmoc-L-amino acids with t-butyl side-chain protecting groups. The

exceptions to this are arginine in which the side chain is protected by the methoxytrimethylphenylsulphenyl group and serine and threonine in which oxobenzatriazine, rather than pfp, active esters are used. All active amino acid esters are purchased from Novabiochem (Beaston, Nottingham) and are stored at −20°C over desiccant.

3. 1-hydroxybenzatriozole (HOBt) from Novobiochem, stored at −20°C over dessicant.

4. Piperidene (analytical grade, Merk BDH).

5. Dimethylformamide DNA grade (DMF) from Romil Chemicals Ltd (Cambridge, UK). This is stored in airtight bottles flushed with nitrogen over molecular sieve (type 4A, Merk BDH; previously activated by heating to 200°C) in order to remove contaminating amines that would react with the Fmoc-amino acid active esters. Before use the DMF is assayed for amine content *(12)*; samples of DMF are mixed with an equal volume of fluorodinitrobenzene (FDNB) solution (1 mg/mL^{-1} in 95% (v/v) ethanol). After standing in the dark for 30 min, the A_{381} is measured against a FDNB blank (0.5 mg/mL^{-1}). Only batches of DMF with A_{381} less than 0.15 are used.

6. Solvents and reagents: Methanol, dichloromethane (DCM), acetic anhydride and trifluoroacetic acid (TFA) are from Romil Chemicals Ltd. Diisopropylethylamine and 1,2 ethanedithiol are from Aldrich Chemical Company Ltd. (Poole, UK). All reagents are of analytical grade.

   Warning: many of the solvents and reagents used are flammable, toxic, corrosive, and/or have an offensive odor. The toxicological properties of some of the reagents have not been fully determined. All manipulations should be carried out in a fume cupboard with adequate personal protection (*see* **Notes 2–4**).

7. Wash baths: domestic polypropylene "sandwich" boxes (155 × 100 × 55mm) with lids. A larger box (240 × 170 × 100mm) for holding blocks and reaction trays during overnight coupling of amino acids.

2.2. Assay of the Immunological Reactivity of Antibodies Reacting with Synthetic Peptides

1. Disruption buffer: 0.1 *M* phosphate buffer, pH 7.2, containing 0.1% (w/v) sodium dodecyl sulphate (SDS), and 0.1% (v/v) mercaptoethanol.

2. Phosphate-buffered saline (PBS): 0.01 *M* phosphate buffer containing 0.8% (w/v) NaCl

3. Antibody diluent: PBS containing 1% (w/v) ovalbumin (Sigma; grade II), 1% (w/v) bovine serum albumin (BSA) (Sigma; fraction V) and 0.1% (v/v) Tween 20 (Merck BDH). The solution is centrifuged at 850 g for 30 min to remove any insoluble material before use. For long-term storage the solution can be frozen at −20°C and thawed as required.

4. Enzyme-linked immunosorbent assay (ELISA) wash: 0.05% (w/v) Tween 20, 0.15 *M* NaCl in phosphate buffer containing 0.0025 *M* NaH$_2$PO$_4$ and 0.006 *M* Na$_2$HPO$_4$ adjusted to pH 7.2 with phosphoric acid.

5. Substrate buffer solution: 0.1 M Na$_2$HPO$_4$, 0.08 M citric acid, stored at 4°C.
6. ABTS substrate solution: dissolve 0.5 mg/ml of 2,'-azino-bis[3-thylbenxthiazoline-6-sulphonate] in substrate buffer, which has been equilibrated to room temperature, then add hydrogen peroxide to a final concentration of 0.01% (w/v). The substrate solution should be prepared immediately before use; 15 mL are required for each plate tested.
7. ELISA plates: flat-bottomed polystyrene ELISA plates from Sterilin.

3. Methods
3.1. Synthesis of Peptides on Polyethylene Pins

The basic strategy involved in identifying continuous epitopes is twofold; in the first phase, the area of the sequence containing the epitopes is located and in the second phase the epitope is defined to the resolution of a single amino acid. In the first phase we have synthesized a series of dodecameric peptides in which adjacent peptides in the series have an overlap of six common residues and in which the starting amino acids differ by six positions (offset = 6). This represents an economical method of ensuring that that all possible six amino acid sequences have been synthesized. When the area in which the epitope is located has been identified, a further series of peptides are synthesized comprising all possible octamers encompassing the region (i.e., offset = 1, overlap = 7).

The peptides to be synthesized are determined using the known amino acid sequence of the protein and the strategy for epitope scanning described in the previous paragraph. The sequences of the peptides to be synthesized can be generated by the software if the strategy is based on a standard peptide length, offset, and overlap; alternatively, the peptides can be determined manually and then fed into the program in the form a series of sequences in an ASCII file. The program will then generate a series of daily synthesis schedules that will give the volumes of the HOBt and each of the activated amino acid ester solutions required for each day. The overall scheme for the synthesis of peptides is shown in **Fig. 1**.

1. Weigh out the activated amino acid esters into small glass bottles, according to the requirements of the daily synthesis schedule. Similarly, weigh out the HOBt required into a glass flask.
2. Removal of the Fmoc Protecting group. The Fmoc protecting group is base-labile and is removed by treatment with piperidine in DMF. On the first day of the schedule, the Fmoc is removed from the β-alanine on the pins, and on subsequent days the Fmoc is removed from the N-terminus of the amino acid, that was added on the previous day. All reactions are carried out in polypropylene sandwich boxes with gentle shaking on an orbital shaker (approx 50 rpm; there should be

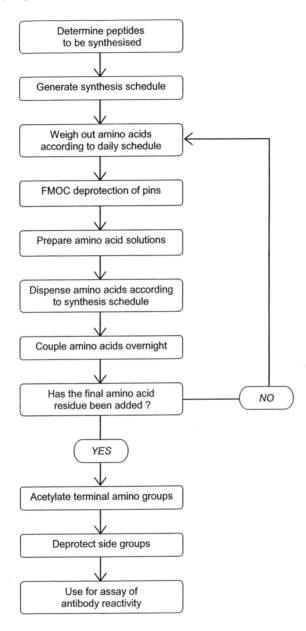

Fig. 1. The procedures for synthesis of solid-phase peptides to be used in epitope mapping.

sufficient liquid to cover the pins to half their height. All steps should be carried out in a fume cupboard.

   a. Place the blocks of pins in a bath containing 20% (v/v) piperidene in DMF (100 mL) and incubate for 30 min at room temperature.
   b. Remove the blocks from the bath and shake off excess liquid. Wash the pins in DMF (100 mL) for 5 min.
   c. Shake off excess DMF and wash the pins in a bath of methanol (100 mL) for 2 min. Repeat the methanol wash a further three times.
   d. Remove the blocks and allow the pins to air-dry for a minimum of 30 min.
   e. Wash the blocks in a fresh DMF bath for 5 min. The pins are now ready to be transferred to the solutions of the activated amino acid esters.

3. Coupling of the Fmoc-amino acid active esters.

   a. Dissolve the HOBt in the volume of DMF determined by the daily synthesis schedule to produce a 120 mM solution.
   b. Dissolve each of the activated amino acid esters in the volume of HOBt solution specified by the daily synthesis schedule. Each solution should be prepared immediately prior to dispensing and should not be left to stand at room temperature. This is particularly important with the arginine ester, which is the most labile and should be dispensed last.
   c. Dispense the individual solutions of the activated amino acids into the appropriate wells of a 96-well reaction tray as directed by the daily synthesis schedule (100 µL per well).
   d. Carefully lower the blocks of washed and deprotected pins into the wells of the reaction plate taking great care to ensure correct orientation of pins and tray. Place the blocks into a container that can be sealed (e.g., a large plastic sandwich box) and incubate at room temperature overnight.
   e. After overnight incubation, remove the blocks of pins from the reaction tray and wash in a DMF (100 mL) bath for 10 min.
   f. Shake off excess DMF and wash in methanol (100 mL) for 10 min. Repeat the methanol wash for three further periods of 2 min.
   g. Finally, wash the blocks in DMF (100 mL) for 2 min.

4. Repeated addition of amino acid residues: If further amino acids are to be added, repeat the deprotection (**Step 4**) and coupling steps (**Step 5**) each day until the final residue has been added. If peptides of differing lengths are to be synthesized, then only the pins for the longest peptides are present in the block on day 1, the remaining pins are added on subsequent days so that the amino-terminal residue of each peptide is on the final day of the synthesis schedule.

5. Acetylation of the terminal amino groups: After the final coupling reaction, wash the pins as usual and then place the blocks in a reaction tray in which the wells each contain 150 µL of acetylation mixture (DMF:acetic anhydride:diisopropylamine 50:5:1) and allow to react at room temperature for 90 min. Then wash the pins, once in DMF (100 mL) for 2 min, four times in methanol for 2 min each, then air-dry for a minimum of 15 min. The pins are then ready for side-chain deprotection.

6. Side-chain deprotection: The groups used to protect the amino acid side chains during the coupling process must be removed before use of the peptides. Place the blocks in a reaction tray in which the wells each contain 150 μL of cleavage mixture, TFA:phenol:ethanedithiol (190:5:5; v:w:v), and allow to react at room temperature for 4 h. Then wash the pins, twice in DCM (100 mL) for 2 min, twice in DCM containing 5% (v/v) diisopropylethylamine (100 mL) for 5 min each, and once in DCM for 5 min before air-drying for 15 min. Then wash the pins in water for 2 min, then for 18 h in methanol. Finally dry *in vacuo* over silica gel for 18 h. The pins and are then ready for assay of antibody reactivity.

3.2. Assay of the Immunological Reactivity of Antibodies Reacting with Synthetic Peptides

1. Disruption: Before use, place the blocks with the pins downwards in an ultra-sonic bath containing disruption buffer that has previously been heated to 60°C. Subject the pins to sonication at 35KHz for 30 min and then wash thoroughly by complete immersion and shaking in distilled water, three times at 60°C. Then place the blocks in a glass tray containing sufficient boiling methanol to cover the reactive end of the pins, and leave for 3 min. Allow the blocks to air-dry; they are then ready for reaction with antibodies (or can be stored in sealed polythene bags at 4°C with silica gel as a desiccant).

2. Immunological reactivity of antibodies with the peptides immobilized on the polythene pins is determined by ELISA using ABTS as the color reagent.
   a. First "block" the pins by placing in antibody diluent in a 96-well, flat-bottomed microtiter tray (125 μL per well) and incubating at room temperature for 1 h.
   b. Dilute the antibodies of interest into antibody diluent at an appropriate concentration (1:10–1:1000 for MAbs or hyperimmune polyclonal serum) and dispense the solution into a 96-well flat-bottomed microtitre tray (125 μL per well). Carefully lower the blocks containing pins into the trays and then place in a sealed plastic container and incubate at 4°C overnight.
   c. Remove the pins from the primary antibody and wash four times, with shaking, in a bath of ELISA wash (100 mL).
   d. Dilute an appropriate second antibody, conjugated with horseradish peroxidase (HRP) (e.g., HRP conjugated goat anti-mouse IgG (Biorad) for MAbs), into antibody diluent (approx 1:2000). Incubate the pins in a flat-bottomed microtiter tray with the second antibody (125 μL per well), at room temperature for 1 h and then wash four times in ELISA wash.
   e. Dispense freshly prepared ABTS substrate into a 96-well, flat-bottomed microtiter tray (125 μL per well), and react the pins with the substrate, in the dark, until color develops (10–30 min). Then remove the pins and determine the A_{405} of each well in an ELISA plate reader.
   f. Determine the specificity of the antibody reaction by comparing the positions of the positive wells with the amino acid sequence of the corresponding peptide, identified from the synthesis schedule.

g. Remove the bound antibody from the pins by disruption as in **Subheading 3.2.1.**. Either reuse the pins with a different antibody or store in sealed polythene bags at 4°C with silica gel as a desiccant.

4. Notes

1. It is essential that all equipment is kept scrupulously clean to avoid interference with the chemical reactions of the synthesis.
2. Many of the reagents used in the peptide synthesis are potentially hazardous. It is essential that all reactions are carried out in a fume cupboard and it is strongly advised that gloves and safety glasses should be worn at all times. All coupling reagents should be regarded as toxic; many of the solvents are toxic and flammable.
3. The thiol-containing solutions used for side chain protection have an offensive odor. It is recommended that the baths used for these reagents and the subsequent washes should be reserved for this purpose.
4. Under no circumstances should TFA solutions be mixed with any of the coupling, deprotection, or wash solutions containing DMF. TFA and DMF undergo a highly exothermic reaction on mixing.
5. Dispensing of the amino acid derivatives into the correct wells of the reaction plates is simplified by the availability of a PinAID™ (Chiron Mimotopes), which lights up the wells that require a particular activated amino acid to be added during the coupling step, eliminating the possibility of filling a well with the wrong solution. However, this device is by no means essential.
6. The activity of HRP is destroyed by sodium azide. Do not add azide as a preservative to any of the solutions used for immunological detection.
7. The general technique described above is used to identify continuous epitopes recognized by MAbs or polyclonal serum. In some cases the separate regions of discontinuous epitopes recognized by MAbs can be identified by the same methods that reveal reactivity in two discrete regions of the protein *(6)*.
8. The same basic technique can be used to produce soluble peptides for investigation of epitopes recognized by T-cells. The peptides are synthesized as described above on polythene pins via a labile linkage. After synthesis and deprotection, the peptides are cleaved from the pins for use in T-cell stimulation experiments *(3,10)*.
9. The activated ester of the Fmoc protected amino acids and HOBt are available from a number of suppliers including Novabiochem (Beaston, UK), PE Biosystems (Warrington, UK) and Bachem (Torrence, CA).

References

1. Barlow, A. K., Heckels, J. E., and Clarke, I. N. (1989) The class 1 outer membrane protein of *Neisseria meningitidis*: gene sequence and structural and immunological similarities to gonococcal porins. *Mol. Microbiol.* **3,** 131–139.

2. Christodoulides, M. and Heckels, J. E. (1994) Immunisation with multiple anti-gen peptides containing B- and T- cell epitopes: production of bactericidal antibodies towards *Neisseria meningitidis*. *Microbiology* **140,** 2951–2960.
3. Fahrer, A. M., Geysen, H. M., White, D. O., Jackson, D. C., and Brown, L. E. (1995) Analysis of the requirements for class II-restricted t-cell recognition of a single determinant reveals considerable diversity in the T-cell response and degeneracy of peptide binding to I-E(D1). *J. Immunol.* **155,** 2849–2857.
4. Geysen, H. M., Rodda, S. J., Mason, T. J., Tribbick, G., and Schoofs, P. G. (1987) Strategies for epitope analysis using peptide synthesis. *J. Immunolog. Methods* **102,** 259–274.
5. Maeji, N. J., Bray, A. M., and Geysen, H. M. (1990) Multi-pin peptide-synthesis strategy for T-cell determinant analysis. *J. Immunolog. Methods* **134,** 23–33.
6. McGuinness, B. T., Barlow, A. K., Clarke, I. N., Farley, J. E., Anilionis, A., Poolman, J. T., and Heckels, J. E. (1990) Deduced amino acid sequences of class 1 protein (porA) from 3 strains of *Neisseria meningitidis*: synthetic peptides define the epitopes responsible for serosubtype specificity. *J. Exp. Med.* **171,** 1871–1882.
7. McGuinness, B. T., Clarke, I. N., Lambden, P. R., Barlow, A. K., Poolman, J. T., Jones, D. M., and Heckels, J. E. (1991) Point mutation in meningococcal porA gene associated with increased endemic disease. *Lancet* **337,** 514–517.
8. McGuinness, B. T., Lambden, P. R., and Heckels, J. E. (1993) Class 1 outer membrane protein of *Neisseria meningitidis*: epitope analysis of the antigenic diversity between strains, implications for subtype definition and molecular epidemiology. *Mol. Microbiol.* **7,** 505–514.
9. Merker, P., Tommassen, J., Kusecek, B., Virji, M., Sesardic, D., and Achtman, M. (1997) Two-dimensional structure of the Opc invasin from *Neisseria meningitidis*. *Mol. Microbiol.* **23,** 281–293.
10. Nanda, N. K., Arzoo, K. K., Geysen, H. M., Sette, A., and Sercarz, E. E. (1995) Recognition of multiple peptide cores by a single T-cell receptor. *J. Exp. Med.* **182,** 531–539.
11. Sacchi, C. T., Lemos, A. P., Whitney, A. M., Solari, C. A., Brandt, M. E., Melles, C. E., et al. (1998) Correlation between serological and sequencing analyses of the PorB outer membrane protein in the Neisseria meningitidis serotyping system. *Clin. Diagn. Lab. Immunol.* **5,** 348–354.
12. Stewart, J. M. and Young, J. D. (1984) *Solid Phase Peptide Synthesis*, Pierce Chemical Company, Rockford, IL.
13. Suker, J., Feavers, I. M., Achtman, M., Morelli, G., Wang, J. F., and Maiden, M. C. J. (1994) The porA gene in serogroup A meningococci: evolutionary stability and mechanism of genetic variation. *Mol. Microbiol.* **12,** 253–265.
14. Virji, M. and Heckels, J. E. (1989) Location of a blocking epitope on outer membrane protein III of *Neisseria gonorrhoeae* by synthetic peptide analysis. *J. Gen. Microbiol.* **135,** 1895–1899.

15. Virji, M., Heckels, J. E., Potts, W. J., Hart, C. A., and Saunders, J. R. (1989) Identification of epitopes recognized by monoclonal antibodies SM1 and SM2 which react with all pili of *Neisseria gonorrhoeae* but which differentiate between 2 structural classes of pili expressed by *Neisseria meningitidis* and the distribution of their encoding sequences in the genomes of *Neisseria* spp. *J. Gen. Microbiol.* **135,** 3239–3251.

16. Zapata, G. A., Vann, W. F., Rubinstein, Y., and Frasch, C. E. (1992) Identification of variable region differences in *Neisseria meningitidis* class 3 protein sequences among five group B serotypes. *Mol. Microbiol.* **6,** 3493–3499.

27

Meningococcal Vaccine Trials

Paddy Farrington and Elizabeth Miller

1. Introduction

The evaluation of meningococcal vaccines in humans is a challenging task. Issues of safety, and benefit to the individual patient and to the community may raise difficult ethical problems. The inherent variability of human responses, the rarity of clinical disease, age-dependence in the immune response, and the role of carriers complicates the evaluation process.

Carrying out a meningococcal vaccine trial is a collaborative undertaking requiring laboratory, epidemiological, clinical, statistical, data processing, and management skills. The experimenter can now draw upon a vast body of experience and knowledge about the conduct of clinical trials, much of it of direct relevance to the conduct of meningococcal vaccine trials. In particular, the basic statistical framework for the design, analysis, and interpretation of clinical trials is covered in most texts on the subject (1,2). The topic is too broad for detailed description within a single chapter. Instead, rather than attempt to describe in detail the planning and conduct of vaccine trials, we will review the broad principles and stages involved, concentrating on the issues that arise specifically in the context of meningococcal vaccines. Finally, it is important to bear in mind that vaccine evaluation is a rapidly advancing topic. Although several generations of meningococcal vaccines have been tested in the field (3), many aspects of the transmission and epidemiology of meningococcal disease remain mysterious, and there is still relatively little experience with full efficacy trials. The evaluation of meningococcal vaccines and vaccination programs thus remains an active research area.

From: *Methods in Molecular Medicine, vol. 66: Meningococcal Vaccines: Methods and Protocols*
Edited by: A. J. Pollard and M. C. J. Maiden © Humana Press Inc., Totowa, NJ

Table 1
The Evaluation Process

Stage	Rationale	Main characteristics		
		Primary outcome	Subjects	Design
Phase I	First trials in humans	Safety and immunogenicity	Adult volunteers Typical study size: 10–100	Controlled or uncontrolled
Phase II	Initial evaluation in target population	Safety and immunogenicity	Target population Typical study size: 50–500	Randomized, double-blind, controlled trial
Phase III	Full evaluation in target population	Protective efficacy	Target population Typical study size: 10,000–150,000	Randomized, double-blind, controlled trial
Phase IV	Post-licensure surveillance	Safety, effectiveness and population effects	Vaccinees or total population Variable study size	Epidemiological studies

2. The Vaccine Evaluation Process

Vaccines are evaluated in a sequence of clinical trials that provide increasingly stringent tests of the vaccine's safety, immunogenicity, and protective efficacy. Successful completion of the first three experimental stages (phase I, II, and III trials) is normally required for licensure, after which further observational studies are undertaken to monitor the performance of the vaccine in the field. The main features of these various phases are compared in **Table 1**. These categorizations are not rigid: for example, phase III field evaluations can be difficult to undertake, and are usefully complemented by experience obtained through use of the vaccine in outbreaks. For vaccines or diseases for which there is already an established serological correlate of protection, phase III efficacy trials may not be required for licensure as, for example, with the meningococcal C conjugate vaccines, which were recently licensed in the UK. Under these circumstances, a comprehensive phase IV evaluation strategy is essential to assess safety and efficacy in the target population (*see* for example, http://www.phls.co.uk/advice/mensurvw.pdf

Clinical trials are undertaken in accordance with a protocol that sets out the rationale for the study and the detailed plan of the investigation. **Table 2** shows typical headings for a vaccine trial protocol, which may be expanded in suitable appendices to include model letters and forms, laboratory protocols, and

Table 2
Main Protocol Headings

Protocol Headings	
1. Introduction	Background and rationale
2. Aims and objectives	Primary and secondary objectives
3. Study design	Outcome measures, hypotheses, plan of study, trial size, and duration
4. Study population	Inclusion and exclusion criteria
5. Methods and Procedures	Recruitment, vaccine handling and allocation, vaccine delivery, follow-up, laboratory methods, statistical analysis
6. Trial monitoring	Data monitoring, quality assurance of data, and laboratory methods
7. Timetable	Start and end of recruitment, end of follow-up, date of report
8. Ethical approval and indemnity	

details of other procedures. The protocol forms the basis of the submission to an institutional review board (IRB) or independent ethics committees (IEC) and hence must demonstrate that the study meets both the necessary ethical and scientific requirements. These requirements have been made explicit in the International Committee for Harmonisation (ICH) Guideline for Good Clinical Practice (GCP) (CPMP/ICH/135/95, Jan 97) and are based on the principles articulated in the Declaration of Helsinki, first adopted by the World Medical Assembly in 1964 *(4)*. The ICH GCP guideline was developed to provide a unified standard for the European Union, Japan, and the United States and hence to facilitate the mutual acceptance of clinical-trial data by the regulatory authorities in these different jurisdictions. The guideline covers all aspects of the conduct of clinical trials and is now accepted as the industry standard. A more detailed discussion of some of the ethical issues involved in clinical trial design and implementation may be found in *(5)*.

The regulatory framework that governs the conduct of clinical trials is country-specific. In the United Kingdom, the relevant legislation is the Medicines Act (1976); in the United States, it is the Federal Food, Drug and Cosmetic Act. Under this legislation, suitable trial certificates or exemptions are required before the trial can begin. Information on the method of manufacture, the results of toxicity and immunogenicity testing in animals, and evidence of protection in an animal model are considered before approval is given. For phase II and phase III trials, the clinical experience already available for the vaccine is also reviewed as part of the regulatory submission.

2.1 Phase I Trials

These are the first trials in which the vaccine is used in humans. Phase I trials are usually conducted in adult volunteers, and tend to be small, increasing in size as experience with the vaccine grows. The primary aim of such trials is to obtain initial data on the tolerability and immunogenicity of the vaccine prior to conducting larger phase II studies. The safety data available from phase I trials is necessarily limited to documenting the more common reactions and identifying serious or unusual adverse reactions.

In some cases, prior exposure to the meningococcus or other vaccine component may be problematic. For example, in a trial of a diphtheria conjugate meningococcal A and C vaccine, 80 adult volunteers were recruited, but only 8 had sufficiently low diphtheria antibody titers to allow them to receive the vaccine, a further 8 being given a placebo *(6)*. Another problem, particularly with polysaccharide vaccines, is that the immune response is age-dependent *(7)*, and hence immunogenicity results obtained in a phase I trial in adults may be of limited relevance to predicting their performance in a pediatric population. Where possible, phase I trials should be used to investigate underlying immunological mechanisms, such as immunological memory, as well as measuring the immediate post-vaccination antibody levels. For example, a trial of a serogroup C tetanus toxoid conjugate vaccine found a rapid drop in serum bactericidal antibodies 6 mo post-vaccination, while avidity of meningococcal C antibodies increased *(8)*. This trial also illustrates a further role of phase I studies, namely to gain experience with assays under controlled experimental conditions; in this case, correlating serum bactericidal antibodies with IgG antibodies to C-meningococcal polysaccharide.

Phase I studies may *(6)* or may not *(8)* be controlled. In small, early phase I experimental studies there may be little point in including a control group because comparisons may be biased and certainly lack power. For example, in one phase I study *(6)* 6/8 vaccinees and 2/7 placebo recipients experienced local pain after the second dose. The difference of 46% in reaction rates is not significant ($p = 0.13$) but the power to detect such a difference, if genuine, is only 40% with this sample size. On the other hand the use of a control group, preferably randomized, in later phase I studies may be valuable in generating hypotheses to be tested in subsequent trials.

2.2. Phase II Trials

Following successful completion of phase I studies, the next stage is to evaluate the vaccine in those individuals for whom it is intended for use after licensure.

2.2.1. Rationale for Phase II Studies

Phase II trials may be regarded as preliminary investigations, laying the groundwork for phase III protective efficacy trials if required. Of particular importance is the optimization of the immunization schedule for the efficacy trial based on the results of the phase II immunogenicity data. If efficacy trials are not required, then phase II trials may be designed to underpin policy decisions about how the vaccines should be used in the target population. This was the rationale for the co-ordinated series of phase II trials that preceded the implementation of the national meningococcal C conjugate vaccination programme in the UK *(9)*. Because a correlate of protection based on the serum bactericidal assay (*see* **Chapter 20**) already existed for C polysaccharide vaccines *(10)*, formal efficacy trials of the C conjugate vaccines were not considered necessary for licensure by the UK Medicines Control Agency. However, a number of key policy-related questions needed to be answered in phase II trials before a national campaign with these vaccines could be planned in the target high-risk population (namely all individuals under 18 years of age). These were as follows: What is the minimum number of doses required for immunization of children aged 1 year and above? Are there any interactions between the diphtheria and tetanus proteins used in the conjugates vaccines and other DT-containing vaccines given to the target population? What is the safety profile of the vaccine in a school age population? What is the response in children who have already received the unconjugated meningococcal C vaccine? An integrated series of phase II trials, funded by the Department of Health, was therefore designed to answer these questions and to provide comparative immunogenicity and safety data on different manufacturers' vaccines *(9)*. The DH-funded trials were carried out in parallel with the manufacturer-sponsored trials designed to provide the immunogenicity and safety data needed to support a licence application.

Whatever the rationale of a phase II trial, its aim should be to extract as much information as possible about the vaccine. Typically several hypotheses will be tested, concerning dose, vaccination schedule, vaccine composition, immunogenicity to homologous and heterologous meningococcal strains, age-specific responses, shape, and duration of the immune response, and local and systemic reactions. In this respect, phase II studies differ radically from phase III studies, in which the emphasis is on the primary criterion of protective efficacy.

The need to obtain maximum information about the vaccine must nevertheless be weighed against the problem of multiple significance testing. As the number of independent significance tests increases, the probability that one test comes up significant purely by chance increases; after 14 tests, there is over 50% chance that one will come up significant at the 5% significance level. The comparisons to be made should be specified a priori in the trial protocol to avoid any suspicion of data-dredging, and the interpretation of trial results should not depend unduly on one particular p-value. Note that more stringent criteria are required in phase III trials, in particular the specification of a primary hypothesis.

2.2.2. Target and Study Populations, Recruitment

The primary objective of a phase II trial is to evaluate the safety and immunogenicity of one or several meningococcal vaccine preparations in their target populations. These may include one or several age groups. For example, a trial of 2 serogroup B OMP meningococcal vaccines in Chile recruited participants in three age groups: infants <1 yr, children aged 2–4 yr, and adults aged 17–30 yr *(11)*. The term 'target population' refers to the collection of individuals to whom the vaccine may be administered after licensure. This is distinct from the study population, which comprises those invited to participate in the trial.

Individuals in the study population are recruited to the trial on the basis of selection criteria. Inclusion criteria define, in broad terms, the age and other characteristics required of the participants. Exclusion criteria, on the other hand, comprise a detailed list of the operational and medical factors precluding enrolment into the study. These may include a stated intention to move out of the study area before the end of the trial, a previous history of meningococcal disease or vaccination, or specific contra-indications to vaccination.

The individuals recruited to the trial cannot usually be described as a random sample of the population. However, selection criteria should be objective and should not be so stringent as to make the trial cohort completely unrepresentative of the target population. Finally, a realistic assessment of the likely recruitment rate is required at an early stage in planning the trial, because this will influence the overall duration of the trial (recruitment plus follow up) and whether or not it is designed as a single or multi-center trial. These issues may have a substantial bearing on the cost of the trial.

2.2.3. Design

Phase II trials are usually comparative, involving one or more vaccine groups and a control group. The control group may receive a control vaccine or a placebo. Phase II studies should be individually randomized to treatment; the rationale for this is covered in greater detail in the section on phase III trials. The trial should also be double-blind; that is, group membership should be known neither to the participant nor to the staff undertaking the clinical evaluation, for example, study nurses. Ideally, group membership should also be concealed to the laboratory staff undertaking the serological testing.

The sample sizes should be sufficient to identify clinically important differences in reaction rates and immune responses, a requirement that seldom necessitates more than a few hundred participants. The precise details of sample size calculations may be found in standard references *(12)*; tables of sample sizes are available for a wide variety of clinical-trial designs *(13)*.

2.2.4. Logistics and Quality Control

In view of their appreciable size, phase II trials require careful attention to logistical issues. Forms and data-handling procedures should be tested. Clear procedures are required for handling vaccines, including labeling, storage, and transport. The condition of the vaccines should be monitored, for instance using temperature-sensitive devices to identify any that may have been exposed to temperatures outside the recommended range during storage or distribution. Careful attention to practical details of this kind (down to the quality of the adhesives to fix the labels on the vaccine ampoules!) is required to reduce protocol violations to a minimum. Under GCP guidelines, Standard Operating Procedures (SOPs) must be drawn up to describe in detail how each of these processes should be carried out and their execution by the trial staff must be independently audited. The accuracy of the data recorded on the case-report forms, particularly compliance with the inclusion and exclusion criteria, and the prompt notification to the vaccine manufacturer of any severe or serious adverse events is also independently validated by a trial monitor.

2.3. Phase III Trials

The primary purpose of a phase III trial is to assess the protective efficacy of the vaccine in the target population. Vaccine efficacy is usually defined as the percentage reduction in the incidence rate of disease in vaccinated compared to unvaccinated individuals. Thus,

$$VE = 100 \times \frac{IRU - IRV}{IRU}$$

where *IRU* denotes the incidence rate in unvaccinated and *IRV* the incidence rate in vaccinated individuals. The incidence rates IRU and IRV are usually calculated as numbers of events per total person-time of follow-up, thus allowing for different observation times between individuals. Note that the definition of vaccine efficacy given here refers to protection against meningococcal disease.

The material on target and study populations, recruitment, logistics, and quality control covered under phase II studies also applies to phase III trials. It is worth emphasizing that these are large trials, which may last for several years, and hence the logistics need very careful preparation. Pilot studies may be needed. In trials involving several centers or many staff in the field, it is particularly important to ensure that the protocol is applied consistently. This might require special training programs for trial staff.

In trials of long duration, it is particularly important to maintain a high level of enthusiasm and commitment for all participants. This is necessary to maintain the standard of the trial, but also to minimize drop-out rates and to respond rapidly to any problems that may arise.

2.3.1. Primary Aim and Trial Hypothesis

A phase III trial must be designed with a clear and explicit primary goal. This is necessary to avoid lack of focus in the trial organization and problems of interpretation arising from the use of multiple end-points and data-dependent inferences.

In the context of meningococcal-vaccine trials, the emphasis will normally be on demonstrating evidence of protective efficacy against meningococcal disease. The choice of null hypothesis should depend primarily on the purpose of the trial and on the policy options available. The minimum requirement is usually to demonstrate that the vaccine affords some protection, and to this end the trial would be designed to reject the null hypothesis that VE = 0% with high power (say 90%). In some circumstances it will also be required to obtain a precise estimate of the vaccine efficacy. This may be required, for instance, if the vaccine will only realistically be introduced into the vaccination schedule if its efficacy is greater than some value. For instance, if a new group B meningococcal vaccine will not be introduced into the routine vaccination schedule unless its efficacy is, say, more than about 25% in children aged 1–3 yr, then the trial should be sufficiently large that the lower 95% confidence limit on vaccine efficacy is above 25%. This, of course, assumes that the true efficacy of the vaccine is indeed greater than 25%. Such considerations played a role in the Norwegian trial of group B meningococcal vaccine; the estimated efficacy was deemed too low to warrant inclusion of the vaccine in the routine immunization program (14). Professional statistical advice on design issues including formulating hypotheses should be sought at an early stage in the planning of a clinical trial.

2.3.2. Case Definitions and Case Ascertainment

As with all phase III trials, it is essential that the case definitions for the trial endpoints are clearly defined at the outset. The precise case definition chosen will depend on whether the protection from the vaccine is expected to be serogroup-specific (as with vaccines based on capsular polysaccharides), serosubtype-specific (as with vaccines based on Por A OMPs) or generic against any meningococcus (as may be the case with a live attenuated type vaccine). Even if protection is expected to be serogroup- or serosubtype-specific, secondary analyses using any confirmed meningococcal infection as the case definition may be undertaken to assess the proportion of the overall burden of morbidity from meningococcal disease, that the vaccine can be expected to prevent. This measure is important both in public-health terms and also under circumstances where the vaccine might possibly allow expansion of nonvaccine serogroups/serosubtypes into the niche provided by removal of the vaccine strains as suggested by Gotschlich et al. *(15)* or more recently by Maiden and Spratt *(16)*.

Whatever the case definition, laboratory confirmation is essential and can be achieved by culture or antigen detection with phenotypic characterization of serogroup/serosubtypes, or by PCR with appropriate sequencing to identify serogroup and serosubtype (*see 16a*). Serology may also be employed to confirm cases, as in the Norwegian trial of an outer membrane vesicle vaccine *(14)* providing a specific antigen is available which allows differentiation of serogroup or serosubtype if required. (*see 16a*). Usually, clinical criteria would be added to the laboratory criteria to ensure that the trial endpoint reflects meningococcal disease rather than infection.

Use of additional endpoints based on purely clinical case definitions may be considered for secondary analyses in phase III trials, particularly if the sensitivity of the laboratory methods for case confirmation is low or there is reason to suspect differential sensitivity of the method between vaccinated and unvaccinated groups. This may be the case with serological methods for which prior exposure to the test antigen in vaccinated individuals may mitigate against the demonstration of a fourfold rise in titer to that antigen following natural infection. This bias could result in falsely high efficacy estimates. On the other hand, use of a clinical case definition with low specificity will inevitably result in an underestimate of the true vaccine efficacy by the inclusion in both vaccinated and control groups of cases that are not attributable to meningococcal infection. Providing such potential sources of bias are recognized at the outset, the use of an additional clinical case definition in an efficacy trial may usefully contribute to the information generated by a potentially restrictive laboratory case definition.

The case definition employed for the main analysis will necessarily determine the case-ascertainment methods employed in the trial. For example, use of serological methods that depend on the demonstration of a fourfold rise in titer between acute and convalescent sera will require case-ascertainment methods that ensure the collection of early serum samples from all suspected cases.

In any event, it is desirable to have an agreed-upon protocol to define which specimens should be collected, when, and from whom. For this, a suspected case definition is needed that triggers the appropriate investigations for patients presenting with symptoms that meet this definition. In the case of meningococcal infection, such symptoms would include the presence of a purpuric rash or neck stiffness. Standardization between laboratories in the methods used to culture swabs or detect meningococci by polymerase chain reaction (PCR) is also essential. These issues are generic to phase III trials and are nicely illustrated in the technical reports on the recent series of efficacy trials of acellular pertussis vaccines conducted in Sweden (17,18).

2.3.4. Trial Design

Efficacy trials of meningococcal vaccines are usually large, because the disease is comparatively rare. For example, in the Norwegian group B meningococcal vaccine trial in Norway, a total 171,800 participants were recruited, and only 36 cases of group B meningitis were ascertained (14). In an even more striking example, only 8 cases occurred in a trial cohort of 124,349 children recruited into a group A meningococcal polysaccharide vaccine trial in Egypt (19). These examples illustrate the central conundrum of phase III meningococcal vaccine trials: the organizational and management problems of conducting a large-scale trial are compounded by the power limitations and potential biases stemming from low incidence rates. Furthermore, the protective efficacy of meningococcal vaccines may not be high, at least in some age groups; in the Norwegian trial mentioned earlier, the estimated efficacy was 57%. The lower the efficacy, the larger the sample size required to detect a significant difference between vaccinees and controls. Thus great care is required in the design of meningococcal vaccine trials to maximize efficiency and eliminate bias. Such difficulties did not arise to any comparable extent in the early trials of vaccines against the common infections of childhood, in which the vaccine effects were generally sufficiently large that the trials were robust-to-moderate biases (1).

The target populations for phase III trials are usually selected in age groups with higher attack rates, most frequently children and teenagers. Many vaccine trials have also been organized in army or marine recruits. Trials in adults present the additional problem that individuals may have acquired protection from prior exposure. For example, in a trial in army recruits in Finland, it was found that 71% of participants had bactericidal antibodies to group A meningococci (20).

In some cases, smaller sample sizes can be achieved by focusing on other outcomes than clinical disease. Thus a trial involving 3018 Marines successfully demonstrated reduced rates of carriage of group C meningococcus in vaccinated recruits using a Group C polysaccharide vaccine *(21)*.

2.3.5. Double-Blind, Individually Randomised Controlled Trials

The gold-standard design for a phase III evaluation is the double-blind, individually randomized controlled trial. In such a trial, participants are recruited and, after informed consent has been obtained, randomly allocated to vaccine or placebo using unique identifiers. Which individuals receive the vaccine and which the placebo is known neither to the participants nor to the organizers; the code matching identifiers with treatment allocation is kept securely and is normally only broken at then end of the trial.

The purpose of double-blinding is to ensure that there can be no bias in case ascertainment or reporting of adverse events owing to knowledge of vaccination status. For classical meningococcal meningitis or septicemia, differential case ascertainment between vaccinated and placebo groups is unlikely as the clinical presentation necessitates hospital admission. However, the ascertainment of milder cases for which initiation of appropriate investigations may not be automatic, could be affected by knowledge of vaccination status. The purpose of randomization is to remove any subjective bias in the allocation of participants to vaccine groups, and to provide a formal statistical basis for significance tests. Randomization does not in itself guarantee that the groups have identical characteristics, although in large trials they should be roughly balanced. If important potential confounders are known prior to the trial, it is best to achieve balance by block randomization within such categories. For instance, meningococcal disease may cluster in geographical localities: it is therefore advisable that each locality should have a mix of vaccine and placebo recipients. This might be achieved by ensuring that blocks of study numbers are assigned to each locality and that vaccine and placebo are randomized within blocks.

Individually randomized trials require careful planning. Most meningitis vaccines are administered in several doses, requiring meticulous record-keeping to ensure that the right ampoules are matched to the right individuals. Ideally each set of ampoules comprising one immunization course should be labeled with a unique study number and the participant who is randomized to that number should receive these appropriately numbered ampoules for each dose. This is logistically complex, and usually means that the trial cannot easily be incorporated within the existing vaccine-delivery infrastructure, but requires dedicated staff and separate management. It is, however, the best way of ensuring that double-blinding is maintained. An alternative is to label the vaccine vials as A and the placebo as B, which simplifies allocation in the clinic but runs the risk of unblinding owing to obvious differences between the groups in post-vaccination symptoms or disease incidence. Splitting the vaccine group into, for example, A, C, E subgroups and the placebo into B, D, and F and using different subgroups at different clinics may help to preserve blinding without unduly complicating trial management. Alternative approaches to simplifying trial design and reducing costs are described in **Subheading 2.3.6.**

2.3.6. Cluster-Randomised Double-Blind Controlled Trials

One way to simplify trial design is to use cluster randomization. Under this scheme, groups of individuals are randomized to the vaccine or control group. Such designs are normally used when treatments are applied to communities rather than individuals, for instance, water fluoridation or STD treatment policy. Vaccination programs may sometimes be thought of as applying to communities rather than individuals, the aim of the trial being to measure both direct protection conferred by vaccination individuals and indirect protection of unvaccinated individuals through herd immunity *(22)*. The Norwegian and Cuban trials of group B meningococcal vaccine were a cluster randomized trial, the unit of randomization being schools *(14,23)*. There is plenty of scope for varying the randomization unit according to context; Devine et al., for example, randomized military platoons *(21)*.

The arguments for and against cluster randomization in the case of meningococcal vaccines may be finely balanced and need careful consideration. First, the evidence for herd immunity is often indirect and remains controversial *(3)*. Furthermore, most trials target specific age groups and so are unlikely to generate substantial herd immunity, though this depends on the details of the transmission dynamics of the infection that are poorly understood. Thus any benefit of cluster randomization is likely to come through simplification of trial procedures rather than increased power owing to herd immunity. This is partially offset by the fact that the total sample size required in cluster randomized trials is larger than in individually randomized trials, at least when the cluster sizes are themselves large, to compensate for the extra between-cluster variability.

The main problem with cluster randomization is the possibility of bias. Bias may arise through confounding, the risk of meningococcal disease in some units being related to variables such as the socio-economic status of the locality or its geographical location. Such bias may be controlled by matching units on known confounding variables and allocating the vaccine randomly within matched pairs. Bias may also arise owing to chance, for instance, if cases of meningococcal disease are themselves clustered, as within schools or localities. This can only be controlled by increasing the number of randomization units, which may of course negate any cost or organizational advantages of cluster randomization. Careful power and sample-size calculations are necessary to evaluate the relative advantages of different designs.

2.3.7. Other Designs

A wide range of variations on these basic trial designs have been used in the evaluation of meningococcal vaccines. Several authors describe nonrandomized, unblinded trials with no placebo in army recruits *(20,24,25)*. Peltola et al. describe a large double-blind trial with Hib vaccine control, in which randomized allocation has been replaced by systematic alternate allocation of vaccine and control *(26)*. Wahdan et al. describes a cluster trial with systematic allocation of vaccines to classes within schools *(19)*. It should be noted, however, that abandoning randomization or blinding constitutes substantial departures from the ideal trial design, and may produce biased or contested results.

The 'stepped wedge' design has been suggested as a way of evaluating meningococcal vaccine efficacy *(27)*. In this design, the vaccine is gradually introduced into the study population over a period of time; randomization units such as health districts would be randomly assigned to times of introduction *(28)*. This is a variant on the cluster design, but combines comparison of incidence rates before and after introduction of the vaccine with comparisons between randomization units.

2.3.8. Power and Sample Size

Power and sample-size calculations are a key element of phase III clinical-trial design. Suitable references for individually randomized trials have already been mentioned; for cluster randomised trials, see *(29)*. The calculation of trial size and duration should be based on the primary outcome of interest, additional calculations perhaps illustrating the power available for secondary outcomes. The sample size depends on the power and significance level required and on the vaccine effect that the trial is to be designed to detect. A value is also required for the rate (per person-years of follow-up) of cases of meningococcal disease in unvaccinated individuals. This should be calculated on the basis of the case definition to be used in the trial, preferably on the basis of real data. The duration of the trial depends on the required total sample size and recruitment rate. Other factors, such as a requirement to obtain information on duration of immunity, might also affect the planned duration of the trial. Finally, sample sizes should be adjusted for individuals dropping out of the trial.

For example, if an individually randomized, placebo-controlled phase III trial were to be conducted in England and Wales with a meningococcal B vaccine that had a true efficacy of 80% against all laboratory-confirmed invasive meningococcal B (from 1 mo after the third dose given at 4 mo of age), then a 3-yr study with 1 yr recruitment and 2 yr follow-up would require 12% of the birth cohort (*n* = 78,000) to show efficacy is greater than zero and 68% of the birth cohort (*n* = 442,000) to show efficacy is greater than 50%. This calculation is based on a study with 80% power at a 5% significance level and uses the average age-specific incidence of laboratory-confirmed serogroup B disease in England and Wales during 1995-1999. No allowance has been made in these estimates for post-randomization losses, which could increase sample sizes by up to a further 10%. If a serosubtype specific Por A OMP vaccine was evaluated then the trial size would need to be increased further to reflect the proportion of the prevalent strains that would be covered by the vaccine. Because the UK has a relatively high incidence of group B disease compared with other countries and given the size of the trial population needed, it is clear that the opportunities for conducting efficacy trials of meningococcal B vaccines in infants is limited.

The sensitivity of the power calculations to assumptions about disease incidence and vaccine efficacy should be investigated. For cluster-randomized trials, an estimate of the coefficient of variation of the rates between clusters (schools, localities, general practitioner (GP) practices) is also required. This is often difficult to obtain and in this case a range of likely values can be used; Hayes and Bennett describe how such values might be obtained *(29)*.

It is also worth bearing in mind that all sample-size formulae are based on asymptotic statistical theory, which might not be appropriate for rare diseases like meningococcal disease. In this case, the theoretical formulae provide guidelines to be checked by computer simulation. Simulations can also help in getting a feel for the impact of localized outbreaks on the power of a cluster-randomized trial.

2.3.9. Safety and Data Monitoring

Whatever the trial design, an essential requirement of any phase III trial is active monitoring of vaccine safety. The incidence of common, mild reactions will already be known through phase II studies, so the main concern is more serious events potentially related to vaccination. For these, background rates should ideally have been documented prior to the trial, because in large trials some deaths or other serious events are likely to occur by chance. The task of reviewing the safety data as the trial progresses is usually undertaken by an independent Data Monitoring Committee, with the power to stop the trial if the evidence supports a causal link with the vaccine. The Data Monitoring Committee may also undertake interim efficacy analyses, ideally according to the pre-planned specifications set out in the trial protocol. The decision whether or not to stop a trial early and to offer vaccine to all participants once protective efficacy has been established often poses difficult dilemmas. Continuing the trial yields better estimates of efficacy and more information on safety, but might result in preventable deaths. Clarity is also required on what procedure to follow should an outbreak of meningococcal disease affect the trial area, a problem that could generate acute public concern, particularly for cluster-randomized trials. A discussion of the issues confronting Data Monitoring Committees may be found in **ref. 5**.

2.3.10. SECONDARY OBJECTIVES

In addition to the primary aim of assessing protective efficacy and essential safety monitoring, a phase III vaccine trial provides an opportunity to investigate other aspects of vaccine efficacy relevant to future vaccination policy. We consider three such aspects: laboratory correlates of protection, age effects, and duration of vaccine protection. The effect of the vaccine on other features relevant to the control of meningococcal disease, such as carriage, infectiousness, and ecological effects, are discussed later.

Phase III trials provide a unique opportunity of establishing laboratory correlates of protection. These are required in order to verify the potency of future batches of a vaccine that has been shown to be effective in a phase III trial, and to enable similar vaccines to be licensed without direct evidence of protective efficacy.

For some meningococcal vaccines, efficacy against clinical disease varies considerably with age. For example a trial in Brazil of a group C meningitis polysaccharide vaccine found that the vaccine had no effect on attack rates in children aged <24 mo, but reduced them by half in children aged 24–36 mo *(30)*. If the target population of the trial spans a suitably broad age range, it is important to calculate age-specific vaccine efficacy estimates. Age-specific efficacy at age a is usually defined as:

$$VE_a = 100 \times \frac{IRU_a - IRV_a}{IRU_a}$$

where IRU_a and IRV_a are, respectively, the incidence rates in unvaccinated and vaccinated individuals of age a without natural immunity. However the prevalence of natural immunity, which increases with age *(31)*, may be difficult to measure. A simple alternative is to base age-specific efficacies on attack rates in all vaccinated and unvaccinated individuals. The interpretation of these various measures of age-specific efficacy can be complex in older individuals, and depends on the mechanism of vaccine-induced immunity *(32)*.

A further issue of considerable importance for the long-term impact of meningococcal vaccination programs is the duration of protection. Most phase

III clinical trials are too short (3–5 yr) to offer substantial evidence of sustained or waning efficacy. In a large trial, plans should be made to follow up individuals in an open study after the end of the trial.

2.3.11. ANALYSIS OF TRIAL DATA

The statistical analysis of individually randomized trials is relatively simple provided the trial has been well-designed and well-conducted. The key analysis is the comparison of disease incidence in the two trial groups, or within centers if the trial is multi-center. This comparison may be done directly or, particularly for trials of long duration, using survival techniques. The standard analysis of comparative trials follows the intention to treat principle; groups are compared according to the original allocation, irrespective of subsequent interventions or departures from the protocol. Such interventions may arise, for instance, if a serious outbreak occurs in the study population and standard control measures are introduced.

The analysis of cluster-randomized trials should take account of the design; analysis of cluster designs using methods suitable for individually randomized trials has been described as an exercise in self-delusion *(33)*. In particular, it is essential to take into account variation between the randomization units. Note, however, that with rare diseases such as meningococcal disease, it may be difficult to interpret the results of a cluster-randomized trial. For instance, the Norwegian trial involved 1335 schools randomized to vaccine or placebo *(14)*. Twelve of the 36 cases in trial participants occurred in vaccinees. However of the 24 cases in nonparticipants, 16 occurred in pupils attending schools allocated to vaccine *(34)*. This suggests that exposure to infection was greater by chance in schools allocated to vaccine than in schools allocated to placebo; in this case a trial individually randomized within schools may have produced a rather higher estimate of efficacy.

2.4. Phase IV Post-Licensure Evaluation

Phase IV studies are undertaken after a vaccine has been licensed, to monitor its performance under field conditions. Such observational studies differ fundamentally from randomized controlled clinical trials, in that a randomized control group is not available. In consequence, such studies may be subject to bias and their results can be difficult to interpret. On the other hand, they provide a unique opportunity to study population-level aspects of the vaccine, which cannot usually be evaluated in clinical trials; some of these are touched upon in the next section. However the main reason for undertaking phase IV studies is to monitor vaccine effectiveness and document the less-frequent adverse reactions.

2.4.1. Vaccine Effectiveness: Estimation Methods

Many of the methods used are standard epidemiological designs such as case-control and cohort studies, and will not be described in detail here *(35–37)*. One non-standard method that is particularly suitable when dealing with surveillance data is the screening method. All or a random sample of meningitis cases are collected, and the proportion of cases vaccinated (PCV) is calculated. Given knowledge of the proportion of the population vaccinated (PPV), the vaccine efficacy is then estimated as:

$$VE = 100 \times \frac{PPV - PCV}{PPV(1 - PCV)}$$

Blanket application of this formula can yield misleading results owing to confounding by age or location, either of which is likely to be associated with both vaccine-coverage and disease incidence. However both vaccine coverage statistics and case information are usually available by age and location. Simple methods have been developed to stratify the analysis by such potential confounders *(39)*.

2.4.2. Studies in Outbreaks

Meningococcal vaccines are frequently used for control of disease in hyperendemic situations or outbreaks. These offer important opportunities for evaluating effectiveness, though in some instances no controls may be available, in which case no convincing demonstration of efficacy is possible *(39)*. Comparisons of rates before and after a vaccination campaign are necessarily confounded with temporal effects *(40)*. Vaccination campaigns targeted at some localities, with others used as controls, can offer some evidence of vaccine effect *(41)*. Cohort or case-control methods are generally the best methods for demonstrating efficacy in an outbreak. A mass vaccination campaign in Quebec analyzed using cohort methods enabled the authors to estimate efficacy, investigate age dependencies in efficacy, and demonstrate a herd immunity effect *(42)*; a similar approach has also been used in Spain *(43)*. Case control studies of a Cuban group B meningococcal vaccine in Brazil using community *(44)* and hospital *(45)* controls have also been used to investigate age-specific vaccine efficacy.

2.4.3. Adverse Events

Phase IV studies in populations in which the vaccine has been given to large numbers of individuals provide important information on the incidence of rare adverse events. Rare reactions cannot be investigated with any substantial power in any but the very largest phase III meningococcal vaccine trials. On the other hand, passive reports of possible vaccine reactions inevitably under-estimate the true risk. Moreover, for nonspecific events, passive reports poten-tially attributable to vaccine cannot be used to estimate relative risks, because some temporally associated events may occur by chance. Methods for investi-gating possible associations include cohort and case-control designs *(37,46)*. Recently, simple but powerful case-series methods, which eliminate bias by indication by using individuals as their own controls, have been developed *(47,48)*. These are particularly suitable for use with linked databases of clinical events and vaccination records *(49)*.

3. Population Effects

The primary aim of phase III clinical trials of meningococcal vaccines is to evaluate the vaccine's protection against meningococcal disease, with a view to incorporating such vaccines in routine immunization programs. Clinical trials, even when large, primarily provide information on the direct individual effects of vacci-nation, namely the extent to which vaccinated individuals are protected from men-ingococcal disease. However, vaccination programs can have indirect population effects *(22)* stemming both from herd immunity *(51)* and from complex individual effects that cannot easily be estimated in vaccine trials.

3.1. Herd Immunity

There has been considerable speculation about the extent to which menin-gococcal vaccines induce herd immunity. The evidence for such an effect is generally indirect. It has been suggested that herd immunity might influence the results of some cluster-randomized trials; *see*, for example, the discussion following the Norwegian trial *(34,51)*. Makela and Kayhty *(20)* report that group A meningococcal disease rates in army recruits were reduced to zero after 36% had been vaccinated with a polysaccharide vaccine, despite an ongo-ing epidemic in the general population; the authors ascribed this effect to herd immunity. Similarly, in another trial of a polysaccharide group A meningitis vaccine, Peltola et al. *(26)* found that the disease rates in nonparticipants were lower than expected, and suggested that this was owing to herd immunity gen-erated by the vaccination of 38% of the target age group (children aged 3 mo to 5 yr). Sbyrakis and Galanakis *(52)* also report reduced meningococcal morbid-ity after introduction of a group C meningococcal polysaccharide vaccine in Crete. Long-term surveillance of partially vaccinated populations is required to resolve the issue.

3.2. Vaccine Effect on Carriage

In some trials, attempts have been made to measure directly the effect of vaccination on carriage rates. This is often impossible owing to low carriage rates for the relevant strains; for example, Makela and Kayhty *(20)* found total meningococcal carriage rates of 54% in their group A vaccine trial participants, but only 3.2% of group A strains. In the Norwegian trial of group B vaccine, carriage was not investigated as rates for the dominant virulent strain were less than 0.5% in the general population *(34)*. Nevertheless some trials of group C meningococcal vaccines in army and marine recruits have demonstrated directly that vaccination reduces carriage *(21,25)*.

3.3. Reduction in Infectiousness

Even if vaccination with a meningococcal vaccine does not protect against carriage acquisition, it may reduce carriage duration or reduce infectiousness to others. Such effects are not measured by standard vaccine-trial designs that focus on protective efficacy; that is, efficacy against susceptibility. To measure the vaccine effect on infectiousness would require a meningococcal carriage trial supplemented by a randomized secondary attack-rate study. Such designs are discussed in Datta et al. *(54)*, but appear impractical for meningococcal vaccines owing to low carriage rates.

Nevertheless, the population effect of vaccine-induced reduction in infectiousness is substantial *(54)*. For example, suppose that a meningococcal vaccine offers no protection against acquisition of carriage, but vaccinated carriers are some amount $p < 1$ times as infectious as unvaccinated carriers. Carriage may then be eliminated from the population by vaccinating the proportion $(1-1/R_0)/(1-p)$ where R_0 is the reproduction number of the infection, namely the average number of individuals infected by a single carrier in a wholly susceptible population. For instance if $R_0 = 2$ and $p = 0.25$, then carriage would be eliminated by vaccinating two-thirds of the population, even if vaccination had no impact on susceptibility to becoming a carrier.

3.4. Ecological Effects

The ecological effects of large-scale vaccination are discussed in **refs. 16** and **24**; these authors conclude that mass vaccination with a monovalent vaccine may result in the emergence of other serogroups as causes of disease. Specifically, Maiden and Spratt *(16)* have postulated that if serogroup C carriage is largely eradicated under the pressure of vaccination with C conjugate vaccines, there is a possibility of expansion of serogroup B strains in the niche provided. The majority of serogroup C disease in the UK at the time of introduction of C conjugate vaccines in November 1999 was associated with hypervirulent strains belonging to the ET-37 complex. With the possibility of capsular switching, the emergence of hypervirulent clones of the ET-37 complex bearing a serogroup B capsule is a possibility. Meningococcal carriage rates among the groups targeted by the conjugate vaccination program are highest in 15–17-yr-olds and emergence of serogroup B disease associated with the ET-37 hypervirulent clones may therefore first become apparent in this age groups. A further possibility is the emergence of hypervirulent clones of other serogroups by strain replacement such as the ET501/508 Y clones as in the US. In the UK, extensive carriage studies in adolescents were therefore carried out at the time of vaccination and will be repeated in the same cohorts in successive years. The phenotypic and genotypic characteristics of the meningococcal strains will be analyzed and mathematical models developed to explore the impact of the vaccination program on the population biology of the organism.

References

1. Farrington, P. and Miller, E. (1996) Clinical Trials, in *Methods in Molecular Medicine: Vaccine Protocols* (Robinson, A., Farrar, G., and Wiblin, C., eds.), Humana Press, Totowa, NJ, pp. 251–268.
2. Pocock, S. J. (1983). *Clinical Trials: A Practical Approach.* Wiley, Chichester, UK.
3. Riedo, F. X., Plikaytis, B. D., and Broome, C. V. (1995) Epidemiology and prevention of meningococcal disease. *Pediatr. Infect. Dis. J.* **14,** 643–657.
4. Anon (1997) World Medical Association Declaration of Helsinki. *JAMA* **277,** 925–926.
5. Pocock, S. J. (1993) Statistical and ethical issues in monitoring clinical trials. *Stat. Med.* **12,** 1459–1469.
6. Costantino, P., Viti, S., Audino, P., Velmonte, M. A., Nencioni, L., and Rappuoli, R. (1992) Development and phase I clinical testing of a conjugate vaccine against meningococcus A and C. *Vaccine* **10,** 691–698.
7. Gold, R., Leplow, M. L., Goldchneider, I., Draper, T. F., and Gotschlich, E. (1979) Kinetics of antibody production to group A and C meningococcal polysaccharide vaccines administered during the first six years of life: prospects for routine immunization of infants and children. *J. Infect. Dis.* **140,** 690–697.
8. Richmond, P., Goldblatt, D., Fusco, P. C., et al. (2000) Safety and immunogenicity of a new *Neisseria meningitidis* serogroup C tetanus toxoid conjugate vaccine in healthy adults. *Vaccine* **18,** 641–646.
9. Miller, E., Richmond, P., Borrow, R., Kaczmarski, E., Cartwright, K., Morris, R., et al. (1998) UK strategy for the introduction of meningococcal C conjugate vaccines. Eleventh International Pathogenic *Neisseria* Conference, Paris (abstract), p. 57.
10. Goldschneider, I., Gotschlich, E. C., and Artenstein, M. S. (1969) Human immunity to the meningococcus. I. The role of humoral antibodies. *J. Exp. Med.* **129,** 1307–1326.
11. Tappero, J. W., Lagos, R., Ballesteros, A. M., et al. (1999) Immunogenicity of 2 serogroup B outer membrane protein meningococcal vaccines. *JAMA* **281,** 1520–1527.
12. Lachin, J. M. (1981) Introduction to sample size determination and power analysis for clinical trials. *Controlled Clin. Trials* **2,** 93–113.

13. Machin, D. and Campbell, M. J. (1987) *Statistical Tables for the Design of Clinical Trials*. Blackwell Scientific, Oxford, UK.

14. Bjune, G., Holby, E. A., Gronesby, J. K., et al. (1991) Effect of outer membrane vesicle vaccine against group B meningococcal disease in Norway. *Lancet* **338,** 1093–1096.

15. Gotschlich, E. C., Goldschneider, I., and Artenstein, M. S. (1969) Human immunity to the meningococcus V. The effect of immunization with meningococcal group C polysaccharide on the carrier state. *J. Exp. Med.* **129,** 1385–1395.

16. Maiden, M. C. J. and Spratt, B. G. (1999) Meningococcal conjugate vaccines: new opportunities and new challenges. *Lancet* **354,** 615–616.

16a. Pollard, A. J. and Maiden, M. C. J., eds. *Meningococcal Disease* (2001) Humana Press, Totowa, NJ, in press.

17. Gustafsson, L., Hallander, H., Olin, P., Reizenstein, E., and Storsaeter, J. (1995) Efficacy trial of acellular pertussis vaccines. Swedish Institute for Infectious Disease Control. Technical report Trial I.

18. Olin, P., Gustafsson Rasmussen, F., Hallander, H., Heijbel, H., and Gottfarb, P. (1997) Efficacy trial of acellular pertussis vaccines. Swedish Institute for Infectious Disease Control. Technical report Trial II.

19. Wahdan, M. H., Rizk, F., El-Akkad, A. M., et al. (1973) A controlled field trial of a serogroup A meningococcal polysaccharide vaccine. *WHO Bull.* **48,** 667–673.

20. Makela, P. H. and Kayhty, H. (1975) Effect of group A meningococcal vaccine in army recruits in Finland. *Lancet* **ii,** 883–886.

21. Devine, L. F., Pierce, W. E., Floyd, T. M., et al. (1970) Evaluation of group C meningococcal polysaccharide vaccine in marine recruits, San Diego, California. *Am. J. Epidemiol.* **92,** 25–32.

22. Halloran, M. E., Haber, M., Longini, I. M., and Struchiner, C. J. (1991) Direct and indirect effects in vaccine efficacy and effectiveness. *Am. J. Epidemiol.* **133,** 323–331.

23. Sierra, G. V. G., Campa, H. C., Varcael, N. M., et al. (1991) Vaccine against group B *Neisseria meningitidis*: protection trial and mass vaccination results in Cuba. *NIPH Ann.* **14,** 187–192.

24. Gold, R. and Artenstein, M. S. (1971) Meningococcal Infections 2: Field trial of group C meningococcal polysaccharide vaccine in 1969-70. *Bull. WHO* **45,** 279–282.

25. Artenstein, M. S., Gold, R., Zimmerly, J. G., Wyle, F. A., Schneider, H., and Harkins, C. (1970) Prevention of meningococcal disease by group C polysaccharide vaccine. *N. Engl. J. Med.* **282,** 417–420.

26. Peltola, H., Makela, P. H., Kayhty, H., et al. (1977) Clinical efficacy of meningococcus group A capsular polysaccharide vaccine in children three months to five years of age. *N. Engl. J. Med.* **297,** 686–691.

27. Fairley, C. K., White, J. M., and Begg, N. T. (1994) Fast-tracking meningococcal vaccination. *Lancet* **344,** 1164–1165.

28. Gambian Hepatitis Study Group (1987) The Gambia hepatitis intervention study. *Cancer Res.* **47,** 5782–5787.

29. Hayes, R. J. and Bennett, S. (1999) Simple sample size calculation for cluster-randomized trials. *Intl. J. Epidemiol.* **28,** 319–326.

30. Taunay, A. E., Feldman, R. A., Bastos, C. O., Galvao, P. A. A., Morais, J. S., and Castro, I. O. (1978) Avaliacao do efeito protetor de vacina polissacaridica antimeningogocica do grupo C, em criancas de 6 a 36 meses. *Revista Instit. Adolfo Luz* **38,** 77–82.

31. Goldschneider, I., Gotschlich, E. C., and Artenstein, M. S. (1969) Human immunity to the meningococcus II. Development of natural immunity. *J. Exp. Med.* **129,** 1327–1348.

32. Farrington, C. P. (1992) The measurement and interpretation of age-specific vaccine efficacy. *Intl. J. Epidemiol.* **21,** 1014–1020.

33. Cornfield, J. (1978) Randomization by group: a formal analysis. *Am. J. Epidemiol.* **108,** 100–102.

34. Bjune, G. (1992) Herd immunity and the meningococcal vaccine trial in Norway. *Lancet* **340,** 315.

35. Begg, N. and Miller, E. (1990) Role of epidemiology in vaccine policy. *Vaccine* **8,** 180–189.

36. Orenstein, W. A., Bernier, R. H., Dondero, T. J., et al. (1985) Field evaluation of vaccine efficacy. *WHO Bull.* **63,** 1055–1068.

37. Rodrigues, L. C. and Smith, P. G. (1999) Use of the case-control approach in vaccine evaluation: efficacy and adverse effects. *Epidemiolog. Rev.* **21,** 56–72.

38. Farrington, C. P. (1993) Estimation of vaccine effectiveness using the screening method. *Intl. J. Epidemiol.* **22,** 742–746.

39. Masterton, R. G., Youngs, E. R., Wardle, J. C. R., Croft, K. F., and Jones, D. M. (1988) Control of an outbreak of group C meningococcal meningitis with a polysaccharide vaccine. *J. Infect.* **17,** 177–182.

40. Mimouni, D., Gdalevich, M., Mandel, Y., et al. (1998) Meningococcal polysaccharide vaccination of military recruits in Israel: Preliminary assessment of vaccine effect. *Scand. J. Infect. Dis.* **30,** 263–264.

41. Kriz, P., Vlckova, J., and Bobak, M. (1995) Targeted vaccination with meningococcal polysaccharide vaccine in one district of the Czech Republic. *Epidemiol. Infect.* **115,** 411–418.

42. De Wals, P., Dionne, M., Douville-Fradet, M., Boulianne, N., Drapeau, J., and De Serres, G. (1996) Impact of a mass immunization campaign against serogroup C meningococcus in the Province of Quebec, Canada. *WHO Bull.* **74,** 407–411.

43. Pintos, A. M. (1998) Evaluacion de la campana de vacunacion de la enfermedad meningococica en Galicia. Metodologia empleada, ventajas e inconvenientes. Estudio de portadores. *Rev. Esp. Salud Publica* **72,** 393–400.

44. Moraes, J. C., Perkins, B. A., Camargo, M. C., et al. (1992) Protective efficacy of a serogroup B meningococcal vaccine in Sao Paulo, Brazil. *Lancet* **340,** 1074–1078.

45. Noronha, C. P., Struchiner, C. J., and Halloran, M. E. (1995) Assessment of the direct effectiveness of BC meningococcal vaccine in Rio de Janeiro, Brazil: a case control study. *Intl. J. Epidemiol.* **24,** 1050–1057.

46. Fine, P. E. M. and Chen, R. T. (1992) Confounding in studies of adverse reactions to vaccines. *Am. J. Epidemiol.* **136,** 121–135.

47. Farrington, C. P. (1995) Relative incidence estimation from case series for vaccine safety evaluation. *Biometrics 51, 228–235.*

48. Farrington, C. P., Nash, J., and Miller, E. (1996) Case series analysis of adverse reactions to vaccines: a comparative evaluation. *Am. J. Epidemiol.* **143,** 1165–1173.

49. Miller, E., Waight, P., and Farrington, P. (1998) Safety assessment post-licensure. *Dev. Biol. Standard.* **95,** 235–243.

50. Fine, P. E. M. (1993) Herd immunity: History, theory, practice. *Epidemiol. Rev.* **15,** 265–302.

51. Fine, P. E. M. (1991) Meningococcal vaccine trial in Norway. *Lancet* **338,** 1456–1457.

52. Sbyrakis, S. and Galanakis, E. (1999) Meningococcal vaccine and herd immunity. *Lancet* **354,** 1733.

53. Datta, S., Halloran, M. E., and Longini, I. M. (1999) Efficiency of estimating vaccine efficacy for susceptibility and infectiousness: randomization by individual versus household. *Biometrics* **55,** 792–798.

54. Longini, I. R., Sagatelian, K., Rida, W. N., and Halloran, M. E. (1998) Optimal vaccine trial design when estimating vaccine efficacy for susceptibility and infectiousness from multiple populations. *Stat. Med.* **17,** 1121–1136.

28

The Introduction of Group C Conjugate Meningococcal Vaccine into the UK

David M. Salisbury

1. Introduction

Throughout the 1990s, the incidence of meningococcal disease was higher in England and Wales than in most other European countries *(1)*. In addition to the high incidence, the pattern of disease changed, with shifts to more cases caused by serogroup C strains, and more cases occurring in older teenagers, among whom the case fatality rate is higher than in any other age group *(2,3)*. Not surprisingly, market research undertaken by the UK Health Education Authority consistently showed that meningococcal disease is the most feared disease by parents of young children (unpublished reports based on British Market Research Bureau surveys). By 1999, serogroup C accounted for 41% of laboratory confirmed cases; 49% were serogroup B *(3)*.

Based on the numbers of confirmed cases through culture or polymerase chain reaction (PCR), and the increasing availability of PCR, estimates have been made by the Public Health Laboratory Service of the likely burden of group C meningococcal disease. This took account of confirmed cases annually as well as those clinically diagnosed without laboratory evidence, or where the organism was not typable. When the case fatality rate by age from confirmed cases was applied to these estimates, then the probable numbers of deaths by age group could be calculated *(4)*.

Figures 1 and **2** show the estimated numbers of cases and deaths respectively, by age, for England and Wales. PCR confirmation became increasingly available from 1997. Based on these analyses, estimates for the burden of Group C meningococcal disease in 1998–1999 were for 1,530 cases and 130 deaths in England and Wales *(4)*.

From: *Methods in Molecular Medicine, vol. 66: Meningococcal Vaccines: Methods and Protocols*
Edited by: A. J. Pollard and M. C. J. Maiden © Humana Press Inc., Totowa, NJ

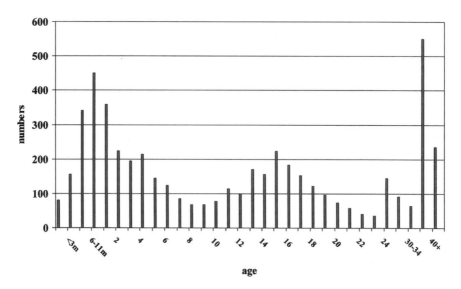

Fig. 1. Estimated total number of cases of Group C meningococcal disease, England and Wales 1993–1998, by age group (PHLS data).

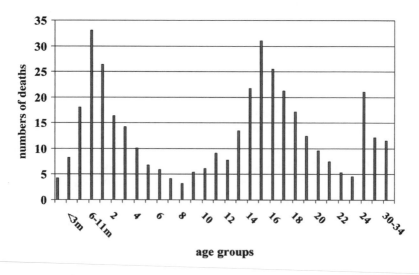

Fig. 2. Estimated total numbers of deaths from Group C meningococcal disease, England and Wales, 1993–1998, by age group (PHLS data).

2. Development of the Research Program

Since the early 1990s, the Department of Health, London, has been funding a vaccine evaluation program. The purpose of the program has been to identify new vaccines that may be needed for the UK program and to evaluate these vaccines, using the standard UK schedule, in order to generate data in UK children that will be valuable in the development of subsequent national immunization policy. The key collaborators in this consortium have been the Communicable Disease Surveillance Centre (of the Public Health Laboratory Service), the National Institute for Biological Standards and Control, the Centre for Applied Microbiology Research, and the Institute for Child Health, University of London. The early priorities of the consortium were to evaluate combination vaccines that had acellular pertussis vaccine as one component. In 1994, two factors were influential in the decision to change the direction of the consortium's work. Firstly, there was awareness of the increase of Group C cases in Canada (and subsequently Spain), and secondly the dramatic impact of the introduction of Hib vaccine in the UK showed how effective conjugated polysaccharide vaccines could be *(5)*.

Discussions then started with all major vaccine manufacturers that could possibly be able to develop conjugated Group C meningococcal vaccines. In the event, three manufacturers (Wyeth Lederle, Chiron Biocine, North American Vaccines) indicated an interest in a collaboration to accelerate vaccine development through a structured clinical-trials program in partnership with the UK Vaccine Evaluation Consortium. The first two vaccines to be evaluated were based on meningococcal polysaccharide conjugated to CRM197 diphtheria toxoid; the third vaccine is conjugated to tetanus toxoid. Throughout the development program, there was close collaboration between the manufacturers and lead individuals from the Department of Health and the consortium. Manufacturers committed themselves to the development program with no guarantes that, even after completion of the studies, there would be a national campaign.

3. Research Studies

Studies were identified to investigate immunogenicity and reactogenicity, across a broad range of ages of target groups, when vaccines would be given according to the UK schedule. Thus studies were under taken when meningococcal C conjugate vaccine was given at the same time as:

- DTP/Hib/OPV at 2, 3, and 4 mo of age.
- MMR at 13 mo of age.
- MMR/DT/OPV at 3.5 yr of age (pre-school boosters).
- Td/OPV at 14 yr of age (school leaving boosters).

In the latter case, studies were undertaken when meningococcal C conjugate vaccine was given either 1 mo before the school-leaving boosters, simultaneously, or 1 mo after the boosters. The purpose of these studies was to ensure that there would be no untoward effect from the prior or subsequent administration of diphtheria- or tetanus-containing vaccines because the meningococcal vaccines were conjugated to either diphtheria (CRM197) or tetanus toxoids; the pre-school and school-leaving boosters contain both diphtheria and tetanus toxoid. Immunization sessions were also carried out in schools when large numbers of children or young people were immunized simultaneously in order to gain experience in operational issues, and for any common adverse events to be identified. The results of the studies confirmed that the vaccines, given according to the UK schedule, were highly immunogenic. In all ages, putative protective levels of antibodies were achieved in very high proportions of individuals. In infants, the vaccines were well tolerated with fewer local reactions than the concurrent DTP/Hib immunization and there was no increase in systemic reactions, compared with historical controls receiving DTP/Hib alone *(6,7)*. Toddlers were given a single dose that was shown to be immunogenic, well tolerated, and primed for immunological memory *(8,9)*. In teenagers, local reactions such as pain, swelling, and redness occurred as frequently as seen with Td vaccines; there was a small increase in the number of those reporting headaches.

4. Implementation Phase

In the course of the vaccine-evaluation program, it was anticipated that the studies that were essential to support the development of new national policy would be completed in late 1999 and early 2000. Allowing for a lead-in time for granting of product licenses and manufacturing, and rollout of a new national campaign, a target date was chosen for starting the new program in the autumn of 2000. However, recruitment to the studies was excellent and results, which were all supportive, became available earlier than anticipated. Furthermore, the previously noted changes in epidemiology were becoming even more evident, with increasing numbers of outbreaks affecting school pupils over the winter of 1998–1999. Manufacturers were therefore asked to accelerate their plans, and the program was brought forward by one year to start in the autumn of 1999.

This acceleration significantly curtailed the time available for resource mobilization, implementation planning at national and local level, vaccine manufacturing, and other elements essential for the successful launch. Nevertheless, it was recognized that the gains from preventing one year's worth of cases would outweigh disadvantages from a campaign being implemented without the opportunities for development that a further year would allow.

The campaign was announced in mid-July 1999 with a target start date for the autumn. Because the three vaccine manufacturers were at different stages in their pre-license studies, it was clear that the introduction would be dictated by vaccine availability. Therefore, the selection of groups to be targeted for immunization, and the time when they could be called for immunization, was a rationalization of the epidemiological priorities and the manufacturers' projections of when vaccine would be available. The campaign started with school health services providing immunization for the whole of the 15–17-yr-old group over a 6-wk period. Shortly after the start of this phase, immunization started in primary care with children receiving meningococcal C conjugate vaccine concurrently with their DTP/Hib/OPV immunizations, or with MMR at 13 mo. A catch-up program then was undertaken in primary care, first for the remaining children less than 2 yr old, then for children under 5 yr. This program was scheduled to be completed by the summer 2000.

Based on the results of the research studies, children were recommended to have three doses of meningococcal C conjugate vaccine at the same time as their primary immunizations, two doses if over the age of 4 mo but less than 1 yr. All children over 1 yr have one dose; no boosters are given.

All children were invited for immunization by computer-generated scheduling, and not through opportunistic immunization, in order to preserve supplies for priority groups. School health services are working towards completion of all of the child population aged 5 up to 18 yr by the autumn of 2000. This campaign, aiming to immunize 15 million children and young people in less than a year, is on course.

5. Impact of the Campaign

The enhanced surveillance of meningococcal disease *(2)*, which became nationwide in January 1999, provides weekly data on numbers of confirmed cases of Group C disease, by age and by locality, and by immunization status. In addition to overall trends, the staggered introduction of the vaccine allows nonvaccinated age groups to serve as controls to evaluate the vaccine impact. Historic data by age band, in conjunction with current data in immunized and unimmunized groups, allows projections to be made of the expected numbers of cases in the immunized groups. Similar analyses can be made for the numbers of deaths.

As immunization has been completed for each age band, so a clear impact has been seen. In nonimmunized age bands, levels of Group C (and Group B) meningococcal disease were higher in the winter of 1999–2000 than in previous years, making the early introduction of the vaccine all the more important.

Figures 3 and **4** show the cumulative numbers of confirmed cases of Group C meningococcal disease in the first two groups to be offered vaccine: young people aged 15–17 yr inclusive, and children less than 1 yr. In each group, the impact has been considerable. When compared with expected numbers of cases

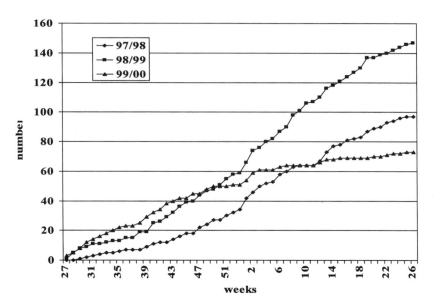

Fig. 3. Cumulative numbers of confirmed meningococcal C cases in ages 15–17 yr, by epidemiological week, England and Wales; 1997–2000. (PHLS data.) Vaccine introduced wk 43 of 1999.

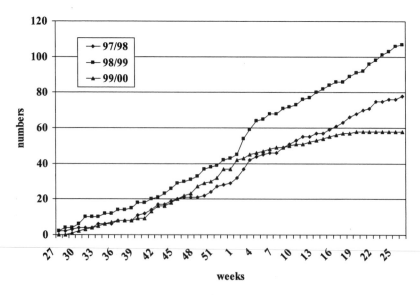

Fig. 4. Cumulative numbers of confirmed meningococcal C cases in children under 1 yr, by epidemiological week, England and Wales; 1997–2000. (PHLS data.) Vaccine introduced wk 46 of 1999.

in these age groups, based on previous years' data and the increases in cases in non-immunized age groups, the reductions against expected numbers are of the order of 75%. It is of note that in the under 1 yr group, the numbers of confirmed cases started to fall when many children could only have received a single dose of vaccine. At that time, vaccine had only been offered to older teenagers so it is unlikely that this was an indirect effect of the wider immunization program reducing the exposure to carriage from older siblings.

6. Adverse Events

Considerable data was available on adverse events before the start of the campaign as a result of UK studies (approx 8,000 immunized children), and from US and other studies on pneumococcal conjugate vaccine, for which meningococcal C conjugate vaccine had been used for the control (approx 20,000 immunized children).

In children under 2 yr, local reactions occurred in 2–4%; generalized symptoms of irritability were highest among infants <12 mo (50%) falling to 19% in children 12–17 mo. These rates were similar to those seen in studies on reactions after DTP/Hib vaccination. Higher rates of local reactions were observed in school aged children (26–29% according to age group); fever was uncommon (1–2.5%) but headaches were reported relatively often (10–14%).

Post-licensure follow-up has been implemented through the routine UK Yellow Card system used for reporting adverse events. For the first time, yellow cards submitted by nurses have been accepted for entry into the database. From the outset of the campaign, reports have been monitored regularly for occurrence of previously unreported serious reactions, clusters of reports, or any deaths after immunization. By early June 2000, close to 14 million doses of vaccine had been distrubuted, all having been supplied by either Wyeth Lederle or Chiron Biocine: both vaccines are CRM197 conjugates. The rates and types of reports have been similar between the two products. A total of 4764 reports of patients experiencing adverse events had been submitted, a rate of 1 in 2875 distributed doses. The reactions were similar to those identified in the pre-license studies. The reactions reported most frequently included dizziness, pyrexia, headache, nausea, vomiting, and fainting (449). Myalgia (42), arthralgia (45), lymphadenopathy, and allergic reactions were also reported. Anaphylaxis appeared to be very rare with only one report for each 500,000 distributed doses. Seizures (133) were reported at a rate of approx 1 for each 100,000 doses distributed. Some of the reported seizures may have been faints, febrile convulsions, or were coincidental. Late-onset seizures were thought to be unlikely to be caused by the vaccine.

7. Conclusions

- Group C conjugate meningococcal vaccines were introduced into the UK 1 yr ahead of schedule, after a unique collaboration between industry and government agencies.
- The UK is the first country in the world to use these vaccines.
- The program aims to immunize all 15 million children and young people under 18 yr of age within 1 yr, and is on course to achieve that objective.
- The impact is already apparent, with cases falling by up to 75% in groups where the immunization has been completed.
- The vaccines appear to have excellent safety profiles.

References

1. Connolly, M. and Noah, N. (1999) Is Group C meningococcal disease increasing in Europe? A report of surveillance of meningococcal infection in Europe 1993–6. European Meningitis Surveillance Group. *Epidemiol. Infect.* **122,** 41–49.
2. Anonymous (1999) Enhanced surveillance of meningococcal disease. *Commun. Dis. Rep.* **9(30),** 263–264.
3. Ramsay, M., Kaczmarski, E., Rush, M., Mallard, R., Farrington, P., and White, J. (1997) Changing patterns of case ascertainment and trends in meningococcal disease in England and Wales. *Commun. Dis. Rep. Rev.* **7,** R49–R54.
4. Anonymous (1999) Vaccination program for group C meningococcal infection is launched. *Commun. Dis. Rep.* **9(30),** 261, 264.
5. Slack, M. P., Azzopardi, H. J., Hargreaves, R. M., and Ramsay, M. E. (1998) Enhanced surveillance of invasive Haemophilus influenzae disease in England, 1990 to 1996; impact of conjugate vaccines. *Pediatr. Infect. Dis. J.* **7,** S204–S207.
6. Richmond, P., Borrow, R., Miller, E., Clark, S., Sadler, F., Fox, A., et al. (1999) Meningococcal Serogroup C Conjugate Vaccine is immunogenic in Infancy and primes for memory. *JID* **179,** 1569–1572.
7. Richmond, P., Borrow, R., Fox, A., Clark, S., Sadler, F., Morris, R., et al. (1999) Evaluation of meningococcal C conjugate vaccines in UK infants. Proceedings of the Royal College of Paediatrics and Child Health, Spring Meeting. *Arch. Dis. Child.* **(Suppl.1),** pA71.
8. Richmond, P., Cartwright, K., Borrow, R., Morris, R., Clark, S., Burrage, M., et al. (1998) An investigation of the immunogenicity and reactogenicity of three meningococcal serogroup C conjugate vaccines administered as a single dose in UK toddlers. Eleventh International Pathogenic *Neisseria* Conference. Paris, p. 156.
9. Richmond, P., Borrow, R., Clark, S., Findlow, J., Morris, R., Kaczmarski, E., et al. (1999) A single dose of meningococcal C conjugate vaccine is immunogenic and primes for memory in toddlers. Proceedings of the Royal College of Paediatrics and Child Health, Spring Meeting. *Arch. Dis. Child.* **80(Suppl.1),** p. A73.

Index